Benvenutus Grassus' On the well-proven art of the eye

Practica oculorum &
De probatissima arte oculorum

Late Middle English Texts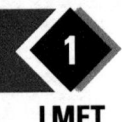

LMET

Antonio Miranda-García
Santiago González Fernández-Corugedo

Benvenutus Grassus' On the well-proven art of the eye
Practica oculorum &
De probatissima arte oculorum
Synoptic Edition and Philological Studies

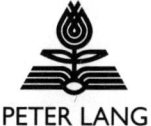

PETER LANG

Bern · Berlin · Bruxelles · Frankfurt am Main · New York · Oxford · Wien

Bibliographic information published by die Deutsche Nationalbibliothek
Die Deutsche Nationalbibliothek lists this publication in the Deutsche National-
bibliografie; detailed bibliographic data is available on the Internet
at ‹http://dnb.d-nb.de›.

British Library Cataloguing-in-Publication Data: A catalogue record for this book is
available from The British Library, Great Britain

Library of Congress Cataloging-in-Publication Data

Grapheus, Benvenutus.
 [De probatissima arte oculorum. Polyglot]
 Benvenutus Grassus' On the well-proven art of the eye = Practica oculorum & de
probatissima arte oculorum : synoptic edition and philological studies / Antonio
Miranda-García, Santiago González Fernández-Corugedo.
 p. cm. – (Late Middle English texts, ISSN 2235-0136 v. 1)
 Gathers together Benvenutus Grassus' work as it was presented in six different
manuscripts: the Latin text (Bibliothèques-Médiatèques de Metz, Ms. 176), the Provençal
version (Ötentliche Bibliothek der Universität, Basel, Ms. D.II.11) and the four Middle
English versions identified so far (Glasgow University Library, Hunter Ms. 503;
Glasgow University Library Hunter Ms. 513; British Library, Sloane Ms. 661; and
Bodleian Library, Ashmole Ms. 1468) and includes analysis by Santiago González and several
others. Includes bibliographical references.
 ISBN 978-3-0343-0698-0
 1. Grapheus, Benvenutus. De probatissima arte oculorum. 2. Eye–Diseases–Early
works to 1800. 3. Medicine, Medieval–Sources. I. Miranda García, Antonio. II. Fernández-Corugedo, S. G. (Santiago González) III. Title. IV. Title: On the well-proven art of the
eye. V. Title: Practica oculorum & de probatissima arte oculorum.
 RE48.G68512 2011
 617.7'1–dc23
                                    2011042358

Facsimile on page 5: © The University of Glasgow Library, Special Collections Department.

ISBN 978-3-0343-0698-0
ISSN 2235-0136

© Peter Lang AG, International Academic Publishers, Bern 2011
Hochfeldstrasse 32, CH-3012 Bern, Switzerland
info@peterlang.com, www.peterlang.com

All rights reserved.
All parts of this publication are protected by copyright.
Any utilisation outside the strict limits of the copyright law, without the permission
of the publisher, is forbidden and liable to prosecution.
This applies in particular to reproductions, translations, microfilming, and storage
and processing in electronic retrieval systems.

Printed in Switzerland

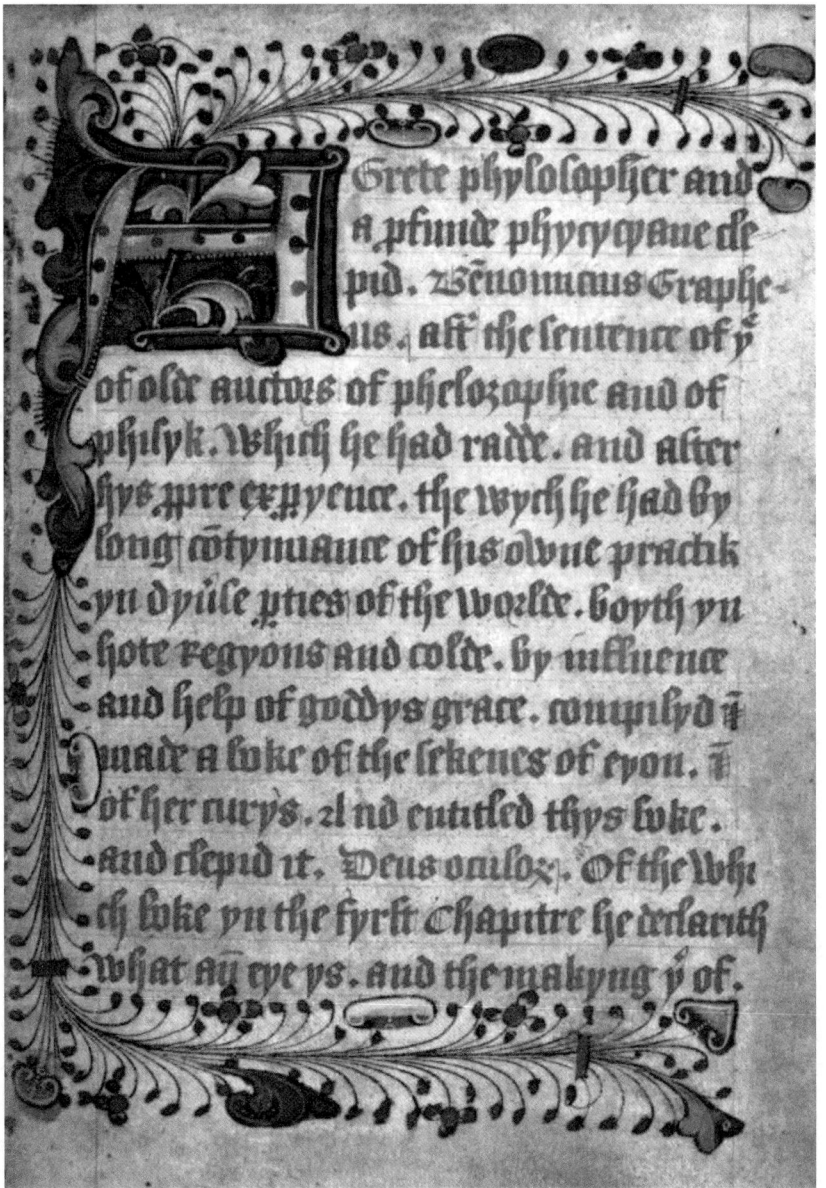

A Grete phylosopher and a pfunde physycyane clepid, Zenonicus Graphaeus, aft the sentence of ye of olde auctors of phelozophie and of phisyk. Which he had radde. and after hys pre experience. the wych he had by long cotynuance of his owne prachk yn dyuise pties of the worlde. boyth yn hote regyons and colde. by influence and help of goddys grace. compylyd & made a boke of the sekenes of eyon. & of her curys. and entitled thys boke. and clepid it. Deus oculoꝝ. Of the whiche boke yn the fyrst chapitre he declarith what an eye ys. and the makyng y of.

Glasgow, Glasgow University Library, Hunter MS 503 (V.8.6), p. 1

Contents

Acknowledgements 9

SANTIAGO GONZÁLEZ
Prologue 11

LAURENCE M. ELDREDGE
The Latin Manuscripts of Benvenutus Grassus' Treatise
on Diseases and Injuries to the Eye 19

JAVIER CALLE MARTÍN
Through the Looking Glass: The Palaeography
of Benvenutus Grassus' English Vernacular Tradition 35

TERESA MARQUÉS AGUADO
Depunctuating the Middle English Benvenutus Grassus:
The Cases of GUL, MSS Hunter 503 and 513 55

LAURA ESTEBAN-SEGURA
Syntactic Aspects of MSS Hunter 503 and 513:
Relatives and Negation 75

ALEJANDRO ALCARAZ SINTES
A Textual Analysis of MSS Hunter 503 and 513 89

ANTONIO MIRANDA GARCÍA
Setting MSS Hunter 503 and 513 apart:
A Quantitative Analysis 143

DAVID MORENO OLALLA
Foreword to the Synoptic Edition 167

LAURENCE M. ELDREDGE, DAVID MORENO OLALLA
AND TERESA MARQUÉS AGUADO
Benvenutus Grassus' *De probatissima
arte oculorum*: A Synoptic Edition 182

References 507

Notes on Contributors 523

Aknowledgements

We would like to acknowledge the funding of the Ministry of Science and Innovation (Dirección General de Investigación) of Spain for granting research project FFI2008-02336/FILO, and to the Council of Economy, Innovation and Science of the Andalusian Autonomous Government (Dirección General de Universidades) for awarding publication grant Res. 2/2008.

We would also like to thank the permission granted by the University of Glasgow Library, Special Collections Department, and the Bibliothèques-Médiathèques de Metz / Département Patrimoine to use their images.

We are particularly grateful to Dr David Moreno for his formatting of the manuscript, Dr José Angel Narváez, Vice-chancellor of Research at the University of Malaga for his support, Mr David Weston, Keeper of the Hunterian Collection, for his valuable cooperation, and Mr Joaquín Garrido, our computer wizard, for his willingness to help at all times.

Santiago González

Prologue

The inaugural book in this series, *Benvenutus Grassus' On the well-proven art of the eye (*Practica oculorum & De probatissima arte oculorum*)*, is a comprehensive study and edition of a Late Middle English medical treatise on Ophthalmology whose Latin or Provençal origins are attributed to Benvenutus Grassus (a "composite author" who may be placed in the late 13th century), and whose catalogue titles have a certain variation (Marqués/Miranda/González 2008).

That is why we have decided, after long discussions (not necessarily fruitful most of the times), to settle with a comprehensive (and long) title such as *On the well-proven art of the eye*, rendering the Latin *Practica oculorum* and *De probatissima arte oculorum* into the modern English vernacular. The importance of the Late Middle English Grassus's works for the history of medicine is well known, as it was one of the most widely used scientific texts in the period between the 14th and the 16th centuries. It is also a significant group of texts for the study of Late Middle English scientific prose (Taavitsainen/Pahta 2004).

We have indeed chosen the Hunterian collection manuscripts numbered 503 and 513 (as David Moreno explains in his Foreword to the synoptic edition) because Laurence Eldredge has documented in his thorough review and study of the Grassus MSS sources, together with the University of Glasgow's accesibility to its library collections and remarkable digitizing facilities, which already resulted in the previous edition of MS Hunter 513 (Marqués/Miranda/González 2008). We truly acknowledge the spirit of the University of Glasgow's staff and curators as, in quite a different mood and mode from other rather narrow-minded Anglo-Saxon examples, but much in line with the opinion of other Scottish institutions, wish to preserve the legacy of their cultural artifacts by facilitating access to their singular collections without overcharge and with a free spirit.

The reasons why we have centred on these Late Middle English versions of Grassus's treatises are justified and expounded in the Foreword, and then by the very nature of the specific studies on the palaeography of both manuscripts by Javier Calle and punctuation by Teresa Marqués, Antonio Miranda's quantitative scrutiny of the morphology and lexicon, Alejandro Alcaraz's textual analyses, and then further by Laura Esteban's panorama of the MSS's relatives and negation.

The book as a whole is a tentative answer to a still ongoing problem posed (among others) by A. Houseman back in 1921:

> There is no science in which it is more necessary to take precautions against error arising from internal causes. Those who follow the physical sciences enjoy the great advantage that they can constantly bring their opinions to the test of fact, and verify or falsify their theories by experiment. Our conclusions regarding the truth or falsehood of a manuscript reading can never be confirmed or corrected by an equally decisive test, for the only equally decisive test would be the production of the author's autograph. It is therefore a matter of common prudence and common decency that we should neglect no safeguard lying within our reach; that we should look sharp after ourselves; that we should narrowly scrutinise our own proceedings and rigorously analyse our springs of action.

Since the advenement of the personal computer in the 1980's, the possibility of accessing networks via hypertextual interfaces in the 1990's and the extensive and almost universal access to the Internet in the first decade of the 21st century – all in less than 30 years – the changes in Textual Criticism, Textual Analysis, Ecdotics and what one is still tempted to call Philology, have also been revolutionary inasmuch as technological approaches are concerned. But I dare say not that much in what Houseman called "common prudence and common decency". What we have acquired is the possibility of reproducing (virtually) with extreme accuracy, comfort, and economy all the artifacts of times past, because, among other machines, digital photography today is only hindered (in the case of manuscripts and similar items) by their curators' zeal and the protectionist (even mercantile) regulations of many traditionally-minded repositories, libraries, archives and other seats of learning. The expensive and elitist late 19th century facsimiles, either photographic or otherwise, have been completely superseded by today's electronic editions in their various filing formats, although their former price is comparatively similar to fees charged today by different institutions, which also turn access to such items a comparatively expensive luxury for the select minority of acquisition officers of University and Reseach Institutions Libraries.

As to the nature and contents of digital and electronic editions in 2010, one wonders what the Modern Languages Association Committee for Scholarly editions would say today of the previous Committee's recommendations of 1976:

> Whatever additional materials are included, however, the CSE considers the following essential for a scholarly edition:
> 1. A textual essay, which sets forth the history of the text and its physical forms, describes or reports the authoritative or significant texts, explains how the text of the edition has been constructed or represented, gives the rationale for all decisions affecting its construction or representation, and discusses the verbal composition of the text as well as its punctuation, capitalization, and spelling.
> 2. An appropriate textual apparatus or notes or both, which (1) records alterations and emendations in the basic text(s), (2) discusses problematical readings (if not treated in the textual essay), (3) reports variant substantive readings from all versions of the text that might carry authority, and (4) indicates how the new edition treats ambiguously divided compounds (if any) in the basic text as well as which end-of-line hyphens in the new edition should be retained in quoting from the text. These four kinds of information need not be presented in any specific arrangement, and not all obtain in every situation, but the CSE requires that, when applicable, they should be either in each volume bearing the "Approved Edition" emblem or otherwise available at the time of publication.
> 3. A proofreading plan that provides for meticulous proofreading at every stage of production so that the accuracy of the text, the textual essay, arid the textual apparatus is not compromised.[1]

Because several remarkable authors such as for instance Richard Finneran were already adapted to the changing paradigm twenty years later (1996):

---

1 <http://www.iupui.edu/~peirce/writings/cse.htm>.

> The development of digital technology and its widespread availability on the personal computer are bringing about a fundamental paradigm shift in the ways that literary texts are created, preserved, disseminated, and studied – a revolution that many scholars have argued is as profound as that created by Gutenberg's invention of movable type. At the same time, a major shift in textual theory – away from the notion of a "Definitive Edition" and toward a recognition of the integrity of discrete versions – has highlighted the fundamental limitations of the printed book. The Literary Text in the Digital Age addresses these developments from a wide range of perspectives. The essays discuss topics from the history of electronic editions to problems in encoding to the relationship between contemporary literary theory and the capabilities of digital technology... Individually and together the contributions show how these projects will go beyond the "electronic book" and exploit the full potential of the new medium.

Futher developments in the concept of the new types of electronic editions have taken place since Peter Robinson, one of the first scholars who revolutionised the core concepts of the apparatus of textual studies with his 1990 thesis on Icelandic texts by writing *Collate*, said in 2005:

> § 30 Throughout this article, I have expressed what I think should be our aim: that some time quite soon scholars wishing to make scholarly editions will naturally choose the electronic form. It follows then that all major series of scholarly editions, including those now published by the major academic presses, also will become digital. There will be exceptions: there always will be a place for a printed "reader's edition" or similar. But we should expect that for most of the purposes for which we now use editions, the editions we use will be electronic. We should do this not just to keep up with the rest of the world, but because indeed electronic editions make possible kinds of reading and research never before available and offer valuable insights into and approaches to the texts they cover.
> § 31 But this will not happen simply because we will it, or because this conclusion is obvious. We need some things we do not yet have: software that does not exist and established online publication systems that have yet to be created. Let us not wait too long.

Martin Foys, in a quite interesting summary of the evolution of computing and technologies applied to the Humanities and in our case, to Textual Criticism, while emphasizing the uneven changes in the concepts of progress, referring to the seminal concept of Robinson's general extension of the electronic edition, told us in 2008:

§5. Until very recently, this technological illiteracy has been excusable: humanities researchers and students, quite properly, concerned themselves primarily with their disciplinary work. The early Humanities Computing experts were working on topics, such as statistical analysis, the production of concordances, and building the back-ends for dictionaries, that were of no real interest to those who intended simply to access the final results of this work. Even after the personal computer replaced the typewriter, there was no real need for humanities scholars to understand technical details beyond such basics as turning a computer on and off and starting up their word-processor. The principal format for exchange and storage of scholarly information remained paper and the few areas where paper was superseded – such as in the use of email to replace the memo – the technology involved was so widely used, so robust, and above all so useful and so well supported that there was no need to learn anything about it: if your email and word-processor weren't set up at the store when you bought a computer, you could expect this work to be done for you by the technicians at your place of employment or over the phone by the Help Desk at your Internet Service Provider: nothing about humanities scholars' use of the technology required special treatment or distinguished them from the University President, a lawyer in a one-person law office... or their grandparents.

§6. In the last half-decade, this situation has changed dramatically. The principal exchange format for humanities research is no longer paper but the digital byte – albeit admittedly as represented in PDF and word-processor formats (which are intended ultimately for printing or uses similar to that for which we print documents). State agencies are beginning to require open digital access to publicly-funded research. At humanities conferences, an increasing number of sessions focus on digital project reports and the application. And as Peter Robinson has recently argued, it is rare to discover a new major humanities project that does not include a significant digital component as part of its plans (Robinson 2005). Indeed some of the most interesting and exciting work in many fields is taking advantage of technology such as GIS, digit.[2]

One may not fully agree with all the nuances that Robinson and Foys mention (although my presentation is biased and partial by the very nature of what a scholarly edition should be, and by my basic adscription to what they state), but there are sound reasons for that. When, back in 1990, and after several years of the typical training in the use of

---

[2] Stuart D. Lee was one of the pioneers of the PDF format for scholarly editions. His 1999 online edition of *Ælfric's Homilies on Judith, Esther, and the Maccabees* was among the very first to help establish a trend that has become extended only 10 years later.

xerocopies, facsimilar editions (of different kinds and nature), microfilms and photographs, apart from the traditional printed editions and texts, the only feasible way of consulting the manuscript and most incunabula sources that researchers and academics in the fields of textual studies needed for their work had, was to physically travel to the library or other sort of repository where the actual volumes or codices were kept, obtain (preferably well in advance to avoid expensive disappointments) the adequate permissions, eventually pay the establised fees, and at long last sit down usually on a wooden chair or bench (not rarely if not as old as the manuscripts themselves, at least well soiled by decades – or a couple of centuries, sometimes – of previous scholar's bottoms sitting on them, carrying a convenient amount of notebooks and pencils to scribble one's notes, having an eraser at hand, to read. And read, and read and handwrite very much under the same conditions (one may count electricity as one of the true amenities of the modern times for light and heating) of the scribes who had produced the copies of the texts that the 1990's textual editor was interested in.

Since the times of the Egyptian scribes (inkhorn and stylus in hand), and for almost four thousand years very little (apart from the technical implements such as computers, digital cameras and the like) had changed substantially. In 1990 for most people 'books' were still 'printed books' and very much similar to those first handwritten texts that were bound in the fourth or fifth centuries in a codex format, once the parchment rolls were superseeded by the codices in most of Europe. As for printed texts, since the late 15th century, nothing substantial had changed. Ten years later *all* was changing fast. It basically begun in 1984 when the first really desktop personal computers were massively sold, but it took another decade at least to catch, and another decade more to become really pervasive. It might not completely out of place here to remind the reader that most word-processing programs' interface still work today under the papyrus/parchment paradigm, while some of the fanciest and fashionable electronic book reading devices (in 2010) seem to prefer the "turning pages" mode (the bookish paradigm), unless we deal with the PDF page-under-page/unfolding method. In any case, there are not technical computing reasons to prefer one form to the other.

As usual, most things tend to follow what has been long established in the eye of the beholder (the mind of the reader this time) as customary, and changing one paradigm for another seems to have similar problems in most fields of science. It is certainly difficult to do so in the field of Litterae Humaniores, for instance.

To mention one of my favourite examples, one may refer to the fact that George Hickes, the Jacobite supporter and finally suffragan bishop of Thetford, some years after his return to England in 1694, published the texts in his *Linguarum vetterum septentrionalium thesaurus grammatico-criticus et archæologicus* (1705) in a format that we can label as "printed palaeographical edition", which, by the way, were much more accurate than most of the so-called "great philological editions" of the English 19th century scholars. Hickes' printers reproduced – after Hickes' instructions – all the Old and Middle English graphemes that were blended into thorn and eth (or modernised to ⟨th⟩), or used the yogh and the several Old English types of yogh and ⟨g⟩, just to mention a more "archaeological" systematicity than the one we may have found in, say, the Early English Society's editions, Henry Sweet's Primers and Readers, or even in later 20th century early electronic corpora strongly influenced by the textual reductionist tradition. In that sense, electronic editions that digitally reproduce the original are more than welcome. And that is why this book is really a complement and an expansion to the online digital electronic edition of manuscripts *Hunter 503* and *513*,[3] a collaborative project started at the Universities of Málaga, Glasgow and Oviedo, to which colleagues from Murcia, Jaén and Oxford have been added for this publication.

Although the time of the individual scholar has not ended completely (yet?), as much sound and worth-reading scholarship is produced in that form, electronic editions are likely to become a much more collaborative job than they had been twenty years ago. Again, the mid 1990's saw the first attractive and truly replicable electronic projects. In the field of English texts, the best early example that comes to my memory dates from 1994: the Windows-3 based 3.5" disks of *The Dream of the Rood* produced by Ann Squires and Nicola Timbrell.

---

3 <http://hunter.uma.es>.

It may be too soon to write (or compile) a history of the origins and development of electronic and digital editions, but it may be worth trying before many of the early cases slip into oblivion. Also, the term "digital humanist" may be too recent for an evaluation of its nature and true meaning.[4] However, online editions and their derived work are here to stay and to supersede the traditional printed ones because they are much more attractive to the specialist and allow us a range of critical approaches that the physical book does not. But I must emphasize the point again: they are for the specialist. For the apprentice and for those who still need help with either the former stages of a language or with languages no longer having an extensive community of speakers, for those who need training in the letterform and handwriting of other ages, and for those who wish to pursue their search of an elitist and arcane group of disciplines and who have still a way (or wish) to read, something in between the pure printed text and the handwritten witnesses of older times is what we offer, both here and in the virtual interface of the online readership.

---

[4] Martin Foys (2008) summarises the dilemma of such scholars in this way: "§15. Not all humanists need to become Digital Humanists. Indeed, in attending conferences in the last few years and observing the increasingly diverging interests and research questions pursued by those who identify themselves as "Digital Humanists" and those who define themselves primarily as traditional domain specialists, I am beginning to wonder if we are not seeing the beginnings of a split between "experimentalists" and "theorists" similar to that which exists today in some of the natural sciences. But just as theoretical and experimental scientists need to maintain some awareness of what each branch of their common larger discipline is doing if the field as a whole is to progress, so too must there remain an interaction between the traditional humanistic and digital humanistic domains if our larger fields are also going to continue to make the best use of the new tools and technologies available to us. As humanists, we are, unavoidably, making increasing use of digital media in our research and dissemination. If this work is to take the best advantage of these new tools and rhetorics – and not inadvertently harm our work by naively adopting techniques that are already known to represent poor practice – we need to start treating a basic knowledge of relevant digital technology and rhetorics as a core research skill in much the same way we currently treat bibliography and research methods."

LAURENCE M. ELDREDGE

The Latin Manuscripts of Benvenutus Grassus' Treatise on Diseases and Injuries to the Eye

1. Introduction

In the following essay I should like to do three things: first, give a brief description of the contents of Benvenutus' *De Probatissima Arte Oculorum*; second, discuss the Latin manuscripts of the work and their relation to one another; and third present a brief description of Benvenutus' implied theory of vision and his pharmacology. The reference numbers used in the essay are those numbering the paragraphs of the text of Bibliothèques-Médiathèques de Metz/Département Patrimoine, MS 176, ff. 1r–16r, edited in this same volume.

2. Contents

The text begins with what seems more like a mountebank's spiel[1] than the introduction to a serious medical document (§§1, 2), addressed as it is not to prospective medical students but rather to a group of bystanders. There are, as with all mountebanks, certain constants: the author names himself, boasts of both his knowledge of ancient philosophers and his own experience, boasts of his observations in several countries, and warns his listeners against quacks and mountebanks. But Benve-

---

1 See Pormann (2005), Porter (2001), Katritzki (2006) and Nicoud (2004). See also Alcock/Wilmot ([1687] 1961).

nutus also notes, contrary to most mountebanks, that he has written it all down, has given it a title, and claims that it fills a gap in medical knowledge. From there he moves easily to a presentation of the anatomy of the eye (§§3–14) and, within limits, the function of some of the anatomical parts. At this point the intended audience shifts from the bystanders to a group of prospective ophthalmologists, whom he treats with respect, addressing them as "karissimi," throughout the rest of the text. The anatomy begins with a description of the tunics and humours of the eye (these humours are not the same as the four Galenic humours described below), the colours of the eye and their relation to vision, and the composition of the eye in the head.

Benvenutus next describes the seven cataracts (§§15–25), four curable (§§15–23) and three incurable (§§24, 25), and he describes the operation necessary to cure the curable ones. This is essentially the same operation as that in use up to the introduction of lens implants. During the Middle Ages, it was called *acuare*, that is "needling," but more recently it was known less descriptively as "couching." In brief, the procedure requires the physician to insert a needle into the eye and push the cataract out of place into the lower part of the eye. Benvenutus' description of the incurable cataracts would help his students to recognise diseases that were beyond their abilities.

Apart from cataracts the treatise takes up some 19 other eye diseases, and these are grouped according to the humour that Benvenutus assigns to each. These humours are the sanguine, related to blood; the phlegmatic, related to phlegm in the stomach; the choleric, related to yellow bile; and the melancholic, related to black bile. Where a physician like Galen might diagnose a disease and find several humour-related causes for it, each requiring a different treatment, Benvenutus uses the humours as a simple cataloguing device and treats each ailment according to its symptoms. The six diseases attributed to the sanguine humour, most of which seem to be characterised by a mark on the outer surface of the eye, are dealt with in §§26–38. The four attributed to the phlegmatic humour, with tears as the consistent symptom, in §§39–46. The two attributed to choler (§§47–49) are characterised by a clouded vision, and the melancholic in §§50–55, a sort of catch-all for the seven remaining diseases that Benvenutus has identified.

At §56 there is an admonition to all prospective ophthalmologists always to have a supply of an ointment that Benvenutus called *Unguentum Alabastrum*, for, in his opinion, it bolsters whatever medicines have already been applied. This admonition marks the end of the shorter recension of the text, of which more is said below in the section on the manuscripts.

The longer version of the treatise continues at §57 with the addition of two more melancholic diseases, which Benvenutus describes from §57 to §60. Paragraphs 61–71 deal with typical injuries that may happen to the eyes, from various blows that damage the eye, bits and pieces that can become lodged in the eye, and the bites in the eye of various insects. At §72 the text moves away from injuries and back to diseases, and from §72 through §79 offers remedies for a condition called a *Nebula*. And from §80 to §82, the final paragraph of the treatise, Benvenutus discusses diseases that may afflict the eyelid. Paragraphs 72 to the end may seem like additions made by someone else, after Benvenutus has finished discussing injuries. But the manuscripts consistently reproduce these paragraphs, and I conclude that the author himself added them.

3. Manuscripts

The twenty five Latin manuscripts, along with one incunable edition, of Benvenutus' treatise divide into two recensions, a longer and a shorter.[2] The longer contains all the parts of the shorter, that is §§1–56, plus an addtional section dealing with injuries to the eye and remedies for

---

[2] Eighteen of the manuscripts are described in Lindberg (1975: 102–105). Eldredge (1993) lists these eighteen plus six more; Eldredge (2004) adds a manuscript from Ansbach; and Beaujouan (1972: 177) describes a manuscript from the Biblioteca Nacional in Madrid. Eldredge (1993) discusses fully the relation of the manuscripts to each other. The printed editions listed are quite difficult to find, but see Eldredge (2007).

a *Nebula*, in §§57–82. The title, *De Probatissima Arte Oculorum*, is supplied by Benvenutus in the opening section of the treatise and is repeated frequently throughout. Many manuscripts give it a different title in the heading to the text or on the title page,[3] but Benvenutus' own title is consistently reported throughout the majority of the manuscripts.

The shorter recension of the treatise is found in the following twelve manuscripts, with their abbreviations listed to the left:

Be   Besançon, Bibliothèque Municipale, MS. 475, ff. 59r–76r. Fifteenth century. Described in Castan (1897: 271–272). Printed in Laurans (1903).

Ber2   Bergamo, Biblioteca Civica Angelo Mai, MS. inc. h. 301/6 (olim sala I, P. 1. 25), ff. 361–399. Fifteenth century. Described in Agrimi (1976: 44). The scribe, Giorgio de Richi of Florence, dates his work between 1469 and 1476 and notes that it is copied from the printed edition of Ferrara 1474. Unpublished.

C   Caen, Bibliothèque Municipale, MS. 93, ff. 40r–62v. Fourteenth century. Described in Couderc/Lavalley/Albanès (1890: 236–237). Unpublished.

Clm1   Munich, Bayerische Staatsbibliothek, MS. CLM 259, ff. 105r–112v. Fifteenth century. Described in Halm et al. (1873–1894: I.1, 66). Printed in Berger/Auracher (1884–1886).

Clm2   Munich, Bayerische Staatsbibliothek, MS. CLM 331, ff. 49r (100r)–51v (102v). Fifteenth century. Described in Halm et al. (1873–1894: I.1, 84). Incomplete, but printed *sparsim* as variants to Clm1 in Berger/Auracher (1884–1886).

Clm3   Munich, Bayerische Staatsbibliothek, MS. CLM 23907, ff. 1r–6r. Dated 1490 on f. 6r. Described in Halm et al. (1873–1894: II.4, 108). Condensed, but used by Berger/Auracher (1884–1886).

---

3   Lindberg (1975: 102) lists these titles.

G	Wolfenbüttel, Herzog August Bibliothek, MS. Guelf 51.1. Aug. fol. (= 2584), ff. 60r–69r. Fourteenth century. Described in von Heinemann (1898: 288–290). Unpublished.
Mad	Madrid, Biblioteca Nacional, MS. 3066, ff. 15v–21v. Fifteenth century. Described in Biblioteca Nacional de España (1953–2002: X, 11). Unpublished.
N	Naples, Biblioteca Nazionale, MS. VIII. G. 100, ff. 48r (51r)–67v (70v). Fifteenth century. Described in Albertotti (1902: 1–2); printed in Albertotti (1902), in parallel columns with VV, Al, and VR.
Ric	Florence, Biblioteca Riccardiana, MS. 2150, ff. 286r–292r. Dated on f. 293v 1453 and 1455. Described in Albertotti (1896: 27–101), and printed in Albertotti (1898: 10–57) in parallel columns with the Paris manuscript of the French translation.
Sl	London, British Library, MS. Sloane 284 (*olim* Bernard 3650), ff. 77r (79r)–81v (83v). Fifteenth century. Described in British Museum ([1837–1840]: 44). Incomplete.
VV	Vatican, Biblioteca Apostolica, MS. Vat. Lat. 5373, ff. 166v–181v. Dated 1475 on f. 181v. Described in Albertotti (1902: 2–6). Printed in Albertotti (1902: 10–140) in parallel columns with Al, N, and VR.

The fifteen manuscripts of the longer recension, adding descriptions and treatments of injuries to the eye, are the following, again with their abbreviations to the left:

Al	G. Albertotti (*olim* Boncompagni 330), ff. 108r–128v. Fifteenth century. Described in Albertotti (1902: 6–8). Printed in Albertotti (1902: 11–139), in parallel columns with N, VV, and VR. Purchased in February 1898 by Albertotti from the estate of Prince Baldassare Boncompagni, present location unknown.

Am	Erfurt, Universitäts Bibliothek, MS. Dep. Erf. CA. 4° 193 (*olim* Wissenschaftliche Bibliothek, MS. Amplonianische Q. 193), ff. 102r-117v. Late thirteenth to mid-fourteenth century. Described in Schum (1887: 451–454). Printed in Finzi (1900: 25–52).
Ans	Ansbach, Staatliche Bibliothek, MS. 120, ff. 230v–242r. Fifteenth century. Described in Keller/Schmolinski (1994–2001: II, pp. 85–98). Unpublished.
Ash	Florence, Biblioteca Medicea Laurenziana, MS. Ashburnham 225, ff. 1–21. Fifteenth century. Described in Paoli/Rostagno/Lodi (1887: 245). Printed in Albertotti (1898: 58–81).
Berl	Bergamo Biblioteca Civica Angelo Mai, MS. MA 294 (*olim* Ψ viii. 19), ff. 48v–51v. Fifteenth century. Described in Agrimi (1976: 7–8). Unpublished.
Bo	Oxford, Bodleian Library, MS. Bodley 484, ff. 56r–102v. Fifteenth century. Described in Madan et al. (1895–1953: II.1, 191–192). Complete, despite catalogue description. Unpublished.
F	Ferrara, incunable edition of 1474 (Hain 7869). Described and printed in Albertotti (1897: 3–60).
H	Hannover, Niedersächsische Landesbibliothek, MS. IV. 339, ff. 244v–253v and 279v–284v. Fifteenth century. Described in Härtel/Erkowski (1982–1989: II, 121–27). Unpublished.
M	Metz, Bibliothèques-Médiathèques de Metz/Département Patrimoine, MS. 176, ff. 1r–16r. Fourteenth century. Described in Quicherat/Michelant/Raynaud (1879: 78–79). Printed in Laborde (1901) and this same volume.
P	Forlì, Biblioteca Communale Aurelio Saffi, Collezioni Piancastelli, sala O, MS. 111/49 (*olim* Boncompagni 507), ff. 165r–177r. Dated 1476 on f. 220v and 1479 on f. 162r. Attributed by the scribe Marco Sinzanogio to Jacobus Palmerius, but actually the work of Benvenutus, though

arranged in a different order. Described and printed in Albertotti (1906: 7–80).

VP1   Vatican, Biblioteca Apostolica, MS. Palat. Lat. 1254 ff. 245v–256v. Circa 1400. Described in Schuba (1981: 299–303). Unpublished.

VP2   Vatican, Biblioteca Apostolica, MS Palat. Lat. 1268, ff. 288r–314r. Dated 1434 on f. 314r. Described in Schuba (1981: 343–345). Unpublished.

VP3   Vatican, Biblioteca Apostolica, MS. Palat. Lat. 1320, ff. 97r–110r. Dated 1384 on f. 135v. Described in Schuba (1981: 418–423). Unpublished.

VR   Vatican, Biblioteca Apostolica, MS. Regin. Lat. 373, ff. 29r–63v. Sixteenth century. Described in Albertotti (1896: 9) and Wilmart (1937–1945: 364–369). Printed in Albertotti (1902: 11–147), in parallel columns with Al, N, and VV.

Wr   Wrocław (olim Breslau), Biblioteka Uniwersytecka, MS. III. Fol. 14, ff. 253v–267r. Dated 1461–1464 on f. 41v. Described in Albertotti (1896: 42–53). Printed in Berger/Auracher (1884–1886: II, 7–58).

Taking the two recensions together, we find that there are twenty-one manuscripts from the fifteenth century (seven dated), five from the fourteenth (one dated), and one from the sixteenth. If processes of time worked the way they should, we ought to be able to trace the decline of accuracy from the earliest to the latest manuscript, but the evidence does not support our expectations. It is true that manuscript VR, dating from the sixteenth century, omits the mountebank passage and the anatomy and goes directly to the diseases, beginning with the cataract. And this would seem to suggest that the later in time we go, the more the manuscript reliability deteriorates. But on the other hand both N and Mad, from the fifteenth century, seem to preserve an accurate text of the shorter recension, where Am, for example, from the thirteenth to mid-fourteenth century, omits several important parts and M, a fourteenth-century manuscript, includes much omitted from VR. On the whole I have found it best to take each manuscript as it stands and not to look for temporal trends but for completeness from manuscript to manuscript.

All the Latin manuscripts record the part of the treatise that deals with diseases of the eye and their treatments, §§15–55. Most of the manuscripts, whether of the long or the short version, record Benvenutus' anatomical section, where he defines the eye, describes its anatomy, and argues his theory on eye colour.[4] The exhortation at §56, always to have a supply of *Unguentum Alabastrum* at hand, is found in both the longer and the shorter recensions. This short recommendation concludes the common parts of the treatise, and following that paragraph each manuscript of the shorter recension adds a series of recipes and comments, few of which correspond with one another.

These additions often seem to suggest that a particular manuscript was used by a practicing physician or by a specialist ophthalmologist, and in fact the colophons to Clm1 and VV state that they were copied and evidently used by physicians. Most of the additions are recipes for various medicines which the copyist found useful, and in some places various experiences are recorded. For example on f. 179r VV tells how he cured an elderly man of a headache which had affected his sight, and on f. 179v he tells how the brother of the bishop of Verona was cured of an everted eyelid by an Arabic physician with a pair of remarkably fine sharp scissors (*forficellos tenuissimos et acutissimos*) with which he trimmed away the excess flesh. Another manuscript, Clm1, concludes on ff. 112r–v with thanks to God for his help in curing eye diseases and some eight recipes which he evidently found effective. Two manuscripts, Ric f. 292r and G f. 70r, record the same treatment for an eye that has been hit with a stick, and Clm3 f. 6r offers a dietary to promote good vision.

On the other hand the manuscripts of the longer recension, which include all the material on diseases from the shorter recension, also offer consistent agreement, in that all of them present very nearly identical additions to the text of the shorter version. These begin with the addition

---

4   A detailed description of some of these variations can be found in Eldredge (1993: 108–120).

of two melancholic diseases omitted from the shorter text, paragraph 57 dealing with an everted eyelid that may follow on from a badly healed stye and paragraphs 58–59 describing an infection in the corner of the eye nearest the nose. With a remarkable degree of consistency the additions then go on to add some fifteen accounts of injuries to the eye and their treatments (§§61–71). These injuries include various types of blow to the eye or to the bone around the eye, lacrimal fistulas, fragments in the eye such as might be an industrial hazard for a mason or a miller, and various bites from poisonous insects such as spiders and wasps.

From §72 to §81 the longer recension returns to diseases of the eye, specifically to a *Nebula*. It is difficult to say just what contemporary disease corresponds to a *Nebula*, but it seems to be a sort of film that develops over the conjunctiva, such that the patient sees everything as through a haze. The treatments that are prescribed generally include some sort of abrasive powder to be put into the eye, in an effort to erode the *Nebula*. The powders include the relatively innocuous sugar, which might scrape a bit but would eventually dissolve in tears. But some of the others, such as ground beryl or ground red coral, would seem at least at first glance more damaging than helpful.

The overall impression that the treatise, in both recensions, makes on the reader is that of a remarkably conservative text, where each manuscript describes pretty much the same diseases, the same diagnoses, the same treatments, the same warnings and cautions about what to do and what not to do. One might suppose that this agreement characterises, or ought to characterise, all medical manuscripts from the Middle Ages and Renaissance, for proper diagnoses and treatments depend on the accuracy and consistency of the texts upon which physicians depended – and the manuscripts of Benvenutus' treatise do in general meet our expectations.

4. Vision

In several places throughout the treatise Benvenutus uses the word *lumen*, most often to mean the sense of sight. For example in §35 he says, "... et patientes recuperabunt *lumen* usque ad plenum." Or again at §52, "... et rehabeat *lumen* suum sicut disiderat." Or at §72, "... corrodit nebulam, acuit *lumen*, pupillam constringit." It would serve little purpose to cite other instances, but the reader will note that there are many. Occasionally in the treatise, however, he uses the word to mean natural light outside the eye, such as sunlight or the light of a lantern. At §41 this meaning is evident: "... mittetis in oculis de puluere ... donec recipiat *lumen* usque ad plenum." Another instance of this usage in §51 is similar: "... et recipit *lumen* pacientis." One could argue that there is little or no difference in these two uses of the word, but there is, I would argue, a subtle difference which is clarified in the description of the anatomy of the eye, §§3–14.

In defining the eye in §3, Benvenutus says: "Oculus est callus concauus, plenus aque clarissime, positus in fronte capitis ut ministret *lumen* toti corpori, adiuuante spiritu uisibili cum maiori *lumine*." And he goes on to clarify the function of the visible spirit: "Et per medium illius claritatis apparet pupilla per quam spiritus uisibilis ueniens ad neruum concauum habet exitum suum." Again in §4 he repeats essentially the same information: "... spiritus visibilis ueniens per neruum opticum repleat totam concavitatem oculi, donec iungantur cum maiori claritate – et simul *lumen* corpori ministrent." Paragraph 7 ostensibly deals with the tunics of the eye and with eye colour, but Benvenutus sneaks in another version of the same information: "Tunica oculi est ille circulus clarus ... et per medium circuli est foramen, de quo foramine ducitur pupilla per quam spiritus uisibilis, veniendo per neruum concauum, habet exitum suum et recipit *lumen* a maiori claritate."

The rest of §7 and all of §8 and §9 deal with eye colour, and §10 describes the humours of the eye, although without much anatomical detail. Paragraph 11 offers an alternative definition of the eye, described as a hollow thing at the end of the optic nerve. Paragraph 12, arguing

Benvenutus' own theory of the number of tunics, is marred by a confusion of pronouns and some anticipation of the treatment of cataracts, but it too concludes with a summary of the notion of *lumen*: "Vnde dicimus quod per illud foramen exit spiritus visibilis et recipit *lumen* a maiori *lumine*." I suggest that there is more here than meets the eye, and yet Benvenutus does little to explain further the theory on which he clearly depends.

During late antiquity and the Middle Ages, there were essentially two explanations to account for the sense of sight, extramission and intromission.[5] Both theories recognised a phenomenon which we can still recognise today: sight directed at an object brings that object into focus, but objects seen with peripheral vision are not in focus. This phenomenon led some early students of both optics and ophthalmology to pose the idea that the eye itself produced a sort of cone of light, which in extending to the thing seen met with natural light and grew broad enough to accommodate the thing seen. These were the extramissionists. Intromissionists on the other hand theorised that natural light illuminated a given object, and when the eye focused on it the reflected light was transmitted to the lens of the eye, which Galen took to be the actual organ of vision.

Benvenutus does not argue one theory or the other, or even make mention of either, but he does presuppose the validity of the extramission theory of vision. Moreover, he also assumes that the optic nerve is hollow. This too is consonant with most anatomical descriptions of the body during the Middle Ages, and the account of it depends on Galen's idea of the animal spirits. These spirits are generated in the heart and are distributed from there via the veins and arteries to the various parts of the body where they are needed. The animal spirits reaching the brain are partly used there and partly converted into the visual spirit, which was in its turn transmitted to the eye by means of the optic nerve. Yet this was the only nerve in the body through which a spirit flowed, and in order to accommodate this variation, the optical nerve was thought to be hollow.[6] Thus all that may seem merely a confusion of terms and

---

5   For a full account of the development of theories of vision, see Lindberg (1976).
6   Avicenna (1556), III.iii.1.cap.1, describes the optic nerve more fully.

their meaning does in fact exemplify a theory of vision contemporary with Benvenutus, even if he assumes it instead of describing it.

5. Instruments and Pharmacology

Generally medieval medicine had at its disposal various types of procedures and compounds, and Benvenutus relies on several standard ones and some of his own invention. In his armory he could count on purges (as the name suggests, laxatives), powders (usually mildly abrasive, to put into the eye), electuaries (to be swallowed, usually sweet), *colliria* (compounds to go into the eye), and egg white, which figures in many recipes and is also used directly in the eye. In addition he often mentions phlebotomy, diet, and cautery – frequently he recommends to his students a book he has written on cautery, but it has never been identified. At §66 he mentions another book he has written, this time on fistulas, but again it has never been identified. When the occasion calls for it, he suggests using an *emplastrum* or bandage, sometimes with a medicine on it, and a *bombax*, which was probably a bit of cotton, either a boll directly from the plant or a bit of finished cloth, to administer a medicine. A synonym for *bombax* is *stuppa*, and a *piluillum* is a small cushion or pillow to prevent the loss of a medicine or to staunch a flow of blood.

Among the surgical instruments available to him, Benvenutus chooses relatively few: a needle (*acus*) or sometimes two needles, two types of cautery irons (*cauterium*), a hook (*uncinum*), and a razor (*rasorium*).[7] As an instrument for couching a cataract in 16, Benvenutus recommends a silver needle; and to remove a fragment of stone or metal from the eye in §69, he describes using the length of the needle as

---

[7] Illustrations of these instruments from medieval manuscripts can be found in Tabanelli (1973): hooks and needles, fig. 33 (following p. 32), cautery irons, fig. 56 and 61 (following p. 80), and razors (= scalpels), fig. 38 (following p. 48), figure 53 (following p. 72).

if shaving the fragment from the surface of the eye. In two places, §40 and §70, he describes using two needles, in §40 as a clamp and in §70 to catch the end of an awn, wind it round the needles, and roll it off the surface of the eye. For more surgical procedures he speaks of using a hook to lift a tumor or a bit of flesh (§§43, 52, 57) and a razor, as one might expect, to cut (§§42, 43, 52, 57, 58, 66). But wherever possible he avoids surgical procedures and prefers the use of the several types of compounds available to him.

Benvenutus generally does not rely on chemical or metallic medicines for the eye, although some contemporary physicians did. He does not say why this is the case, so we do not know whether he took a firm position against them or just did not know about them. Some of his medicines are *simples* – that is, medicines consisting of a single ingredient. The *Pulvis Benedictus* of §28, for example, consists of simply *Anzarut Album*, which he explains is the same as *Sarcolla* (more usually *Sarcocolla*), reduced to powder in a mortar, and administered directly into the eye as a cure for *Obtalmia*. Another single-ingredient medicine is *Virtus a Deo Data*, described in §61 and §69. This consists of the germ from a dozen egg whites beaten to an ointment. Other medicines are compounded of only two ingredients, such as *Pulvis Nabetis*, for which the recipe comes nearly at the end of the treatise at §76, though it is mentioned often earlier. It consists of powdered sugar and egg white. Another recipe of just two ingredients is called an *Emplastrum Gloriosum et Sanctissimum* and is made only of *Cardus Benedictus* or Our Lady's Thistle and egg white.

But Benvenutus's pharmacology consists chiefly of compound herbal medicines, whether a laxative or an electuary or a collirium, and often the ingredients for one of these will pile up to such an extent that the reader may wonder whether the complaint might not go away while the medicine is being made. Some of the compounds go by the name Benvenutus claims to have given them and others by formula alone. Often he refers to a compound before he gives a recipe for it, and presumably a prospective ophthalmologist would have to search the rest of the treatise to find how to make it. Below I list the ones he has named together with the number of the paragraph in which they are mentioned and the ingredients. For the most part these are listed in an oblique case, since that is how they occur in the manuscript.

- *Diaolibano Iherosolimitano*, an electuary, §22. *Olibani, gariofili, nucis muscate, nucis indice, croci, castorei, mellis.*
- *Collirio Iherosolimitano*, a collirium, §26. *Tutye alexandrini, vini albi, rosarum siccarum*, boiled over a slow fire until reduced to half its volume.
- *Puluerem Benedictum*, a powder, §28. Powered *anzarut album* or *sarcollam*.
- *Puluis Nabetis* and *Puluis Alexandrinis*, powders, mentioned without recipes, §§29, 35, and 41; §37 with recipe for *Puluis Nabetis* only. *Zuccaro nabetis or candi alexandrini* (i.e., sugar), ground to a fine powder.
- *Unguentum Alabastrum*, an ointment, §31. *Rubi, vini albi, rute, camomile*, alabaster, rose oil, wax – all ground together, then six egg whites added.
- *Emplastrum Laudabilem*, a plaster to put on the closed eye, §51. *Poma acerba et coque ... pistentur ... clara oui.*
- *Collirium Ruborum*, a collirium, §53. *Ruborum teneres ... vini albi.*
- *Virtus a Deo Data*, an ointment, §62. *Germina pullorum ... de oua recencia de gallinis albis.*
- *Pillulis Iherosolomitanis*, a laxative, §16. *Turbit, aloe epatici, macis, cubebe, masticis, croci ... cum succo rosarum.*

There are many more nameless compounds for various purposes in the text and although the variety of ingredients is striking, from soot and badger's gall bladder to roasted apples or roasted lily root, most of the ingredients seem harmless enough. But they probably would not have done much good either, although no doubt some patients responded to the placebo effect. A surprising number of recipes, however, especially those intended to go into the eye, contain egg white – in addition to those mentioned above, these are in the following paragraphs: §§35, 38, 42, 43, 52, 54, 55, 58, 61, 66, 69–71, and 76. No doubt Benvenutus knew nothing of the actual chemical properties of egg white and probably used and recommended it because its consistency resembled that of the humours in the eye, as he explains in paragraph §11, and he assumed that like cures like. But he could not have known that egg white helps to heal diseases and injuries to the eye because it contains large amounts of lysozyme, an enzyme also found in tears, saliva, mucus, etc. Its natural function seems to be to keep the eye healthy by acting against any infectious matter that enters through the dust and grit of day to day activity.[8]

This brief essay is not the place for a full analysis of either the theories or the medical compounds of *De Probatissima Arte Oculorum*, but I hope that these few remarks may help a reader at least to place the procedures and pharmaceuticals somewhere in the full spectrum of medicine during the Middle Ages.[9]

---

[8] See <http://en.wikipedia.org/wiki/Lysozyme> and <http://users.rcm.com/jkimball.ma.ultranet/BiologyPages/L/Lysozyme> (retrieved 14/12/2010).

[9] I should like to thank the following people for their help in writing this essay: Sylwia Bulat, Peter Murray Jones, Lea Olsan and David Moreno Olalla. As the editor of MS *M*, I am most indebted to Klaus-Dietrich Fischer and David Moreno Olalla for their careful reading and suggestions; to Emilie Savage-Smith for her comments on Benvenutus' Arabic transcriptions; and to Sylwia Bulat for help with the Polish in connection with the Wrocław MS. Any errors that remain are, of course, my own responsibility

Javier Calle Martín

Through the Looking Glass: The Palaeography of Benvenutus Grassus' English Vernacular Tradition[1]

1. Introduction

A man of parts, as the English often say, may be a suitable designation to the author of *De Probatissima Arte Oculorum*, both on account of his self-taught medical expertise and his vast humanist education as the speaker of at least four languages. According to Laurence Eldredge, the scholar who with more impetus has investigated the textual transmission of this ophthalmic treatise, the life of Benvenutus Grassus has traditionally been in a welter of confusion (1996: 1–5; 1998: 47–52; 1999: 149–163). Of uncertain provenance (plausibly from Salerno, Jerusalem or Montpellier), Grassus was a medical practitioner educated in the first half of the 13th century becoming a well-known ocular surgeon in Italy in the second and third quarters of that same century.[2] Apart from all this, everything has been a matter of pure speculation.

González has recently reviewed the state-of-the-art about this piece of *Fachliteratur* providing a comprehensive account of some of the contradictions, these having to do with the author and the language of the original text (Marqués/Miranda/González 2008: 1–17). From an

---

[1] The present research has been funded by the Spanish Ministry of Education (project FFI2008-02336) and the Autonomous Government of Andalusia (project P07-HUM–2609). These grants are hereby gratefully acknowledged.

[2] Even though the 13th century is widely accepted to date Benvenutus Grassus' life, González finds an earlier 12th-century dating according to the Health Sciences Center of the University of West Virginia and at the Eye Center at the University of Chicago (Marqués/Miranda/González 2008: 11).

authorial perspective, on the one hand, he pinpoints not less than six common names for the author in the relevant literature, although he concludes that Eldredge's proposal for Benvenutus Grassus seems to be more widely disseminated. More doubts arise when considering the ups and downs of Benvenutus himself as to how such a self-taught man could have acquired the bulk of his medical expertise, something which could have been learnt by heart and/or through his supposed visits to Egypt and other Middle Eastern countries.

The language of the holograph, on the other hand, also remains unsolved, being plausible to assume a Latinate or a vernacular original. González summarises the pros and cons of these two alternatives by reconsidering Grassus' professional activity as a practitioner. The vernacular composition of the piece may be justified on account of the social background of his patients, probably accommodated burghers with whom he communicated in everyday language, eventually transposing this medical lore into the vernacular – Provençal or Neapolitan Romance as the most likely candidates. As a mediaeval scholar, Grassus was yet surely proficient in Mediaeval Latin and the academic nature of the specific vocabulary, which was "ultimately Greek in origin via Latin and Arabic calques" (Marqués/Miranda/González 2008: 13), a fact which supports a likely Latinate composition. Other possibilities cannot be discarded beforehand, as his journeys still give substantial evidence that he was fluent up to a certain extent in Arabic, Greek and Hebrew (or Aramaic).

It is a fact that Grassus' work was widely known in the latter Middle Ages, both among general practitioners and laymen. The mediaeval appraisal of this work is corroborated by the number of handwritten copies, not only in Latin, but also in different European vernacular languages, Spanish also included (Marqués/Miranda/González 2008: 28). This scholarly interest in Grassus' work has persisted thereafter with the publication of several printed editions (Albertotti 1896; 1902; Berger/Auracher 1884–1886; Wood 1929). In the particular case of mediaeval England, the level of estimation was such that a saga of vernacular copies proliferated from the 15th century, where four different witnesses have been preserved, all of which accordingly reproduced in the present volume:

H503   Glasgow, GUL, Hunter MS 503 (V.8.6), pp. 2–137.
H513   Glasgow, GUL, Hunter MS 513 (V.8.16), ff. 1r–37r.
A   Oxford, Bodleian Library, Ashmole MS 1468, pp. 1–6.
S   London, British Library, Sloane MS 661, ff. 32r–46v.

While the three first witnesses are 15th-century copies, the Sloane manuscript is by an early modern hand. In light of this, the objective of the present contribution is to review the palaeography of the English versions of Grassus' *De Probatissima Arte Oculorum* in terms of a) the inventory of letterforms; and b) the scribal attitude towards line-final word division. According to the above premises, the study has been organised into four different sections. Section 2 describes the framework and the methodology used for the analysis of the different witnesses. Sections 3–4, in turn, concentrate on the palaeography of the witnesses in terms of the script and word division. Finally, Section 5 contains the conclusions deriving from the study.

2. Methodology

The present paper forms part of an on-going collaborative project of the universities of Málaga, Murcia, Oviedo, Jaén and Glasgow which contemplates the electronic editing of the mediaeval handwritten material, of a scientific scope, hitherto preserved in the Hunterian collection at Glasgow University Library. The task is therefore accomplished in two stages, necessarily sequential. The first consists in the graphemic transcription of the material, provided on-line together with the digitised images and some palaeographic/codicological information (see <http://hunter.uma.es>). The impetus here is the offering of a diplomatic transcription which may be used for research in a variety of disciplines, not only linguistic (Orthography, Phonology, Morphosyntax) but also extra-linguistic (History of Medicine, Palaeography, etc.). Second, the bulk of transcribed material is later taken as the input for the compilation of an annotated corpus. The particularities of the corpus as to genre (*Fachliteratur*), chronology (14th- and 15th-century English) and annotation (containing the lemma, word class and accidence of every corpus item) shape it as an ideal tool for research in late Middle English (Moreno Olalla/Miranda García 2009).

On methodological grounds, the present study exclusively rests upon the high-quality digitised images of the witnesses, with the exception of *A* which has been based on a microfilmed copy, all allowing the researcher to examine the scribe's handwriting in sufficient detail. Our approach to letterforms, on the one hand, relies on the accounts provided by the foundations of Palaeography, particularly Petti (1977), Derolez (2003) and Roberts (2005) for the mediaeval copies whilst Tannenbaum (1930), Denholm-Yong (1954) and Hector (1958) have been used as secondary sources for the early modern version.

The analysis of line-final word division, on the other hand, is modelled on Hladký's original scheme (1985a; 1985b) and later reformulated by Calle Martín (2009), proposing to study the phenomenon in light of the ultimate motivation for the break, distinguishing morphological, phonological and anomalous divisions (see also Powell 1984: 452–458). This aspect of Palaeography will be investigated across the four texts to determine the level of scribal variation and find whether the scribal practice is governed by a predetermined set of rules, a statement which is often discarded in the literature. For the purpose, an Excel spread-sheet has been used wherein all word-division instances have been allocated in terms of a) the manuscript; b) the type of division involved; and c) the rule used in each case.

3. Letterforms

The present section reports the inventory of letterforms found in the English vernacular tradition of this ophthalmic treatise, including both minuscules and figures, on the assumption that they are reliable clues to date handwritten documents. Marginalia and other inscriptions, however, have been systematically ruled out from our analysis for they constitute an alternative text, therefore alien to the scribe's hand.

3.1. Glasgow, GUL Hunter MS 513 (V.8.16)

Two different dates have been proposed for this witness. Young and Aitken's cursory glance at the manuscript led them spuriously to suggest a late 14th-century composition (1908: 421–422), an opinion which has been later disproved by other fresh approaches, such as those by Eldredge (1996: 27) and Cross (2004: 35), reconsidering it a mid-15th-century text. Although the most recent edition of this text reports that "the evidence that all of them use to support such a claim remains in the shadow" (Marqués/Miranda/González 2008: 27), a palaeographic approach serves here to corroborate Eldredge's and Cross' proposals.

The hand of *H513* has already been the object of palaeographic description (Marqués/Miranda/González 2008: 31–36) and, as far as the script is concerned, the volume overwhelmingly displays a pretty clear cursive 15th-century Secretary hand with sporadic tinges of the Anglicana, the latter skipped in Eldredge's account (1996: 27). Figure 1 below reproduces the inventory of the minuscules and the figures used by the scribe, numbered for reference purposes.

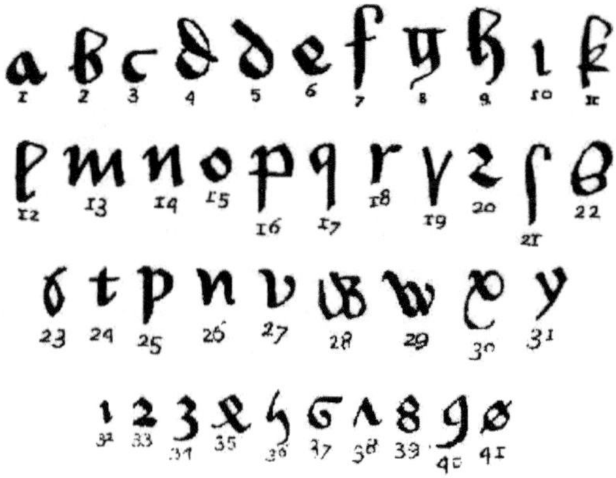

Fig. 1. Inventory of minuscules and figures in *H513*.

As illustrated, the Secretary script characterises by the use of distinctive letterforms, which sharply differ from the conventional cursive hand of the Anglicana. Among others, the following stand out: single-lobed ⟨a⟩ with a pointed head (1); two-lobed ⟨b⟩ (2); the letter ⟨d⟩ either with a looped stem (4) or with a shank and an oblique ascender (5); the single stroke ⟨e⟩ (6); the letter ⟨f⟩ showing a shaft with an arced headstroke (7); the 15th-century crossed ⟨g⟩ with a pronounced headstroke (8); the letter ⟨k⟩ with its characteristic right-arced headstroke (11); the letter ⟨l⟩ with a lobed arm (12); the right-shouldered ⟨r⟩, footed and sitting on the script line (18); the heavy ascender of the letter ⟨v⟩; and cursive ⟨x⟩ written with a single stroke (30). The letter ⟨þ⟩ consists of an infra-linear letter rendered by a vertical and clubbed stroke with a curved serif at the top of the backbone (25), thus preventing the likely association with the letter ⟨y⟩.

In light of the currency of these scripts in the 15th century, Petti argues that "*secretary* and *anglicana* often borrowed from one another both in features of general style and in use of graphs" (1977: 15). This is particularly the case of *H513* wherein three conventional Anglicana letterforms co-occur with the dominant script to such extent that many a time they eventually adopt specific contexts. The letter ⟨s⟩, on the one hand, is particularly illustrative insofar as the Anglicana grading is witnessed in the use of the double-length long ⟨s⟩ with its upright form (21), systematically in initial and medial positions, together with the diamond-shaped sigma-like form (23), which is the choice if word-finally. The Secretary beta-like ⟨s⟩ (22) is sporadically used in final position, particularly in the rendering of foreign words, thus co-existing with the Anglicana version (Petti 1977: 14). Similarly, the Secretary ⟨r⟩ predominates over the long-forked Anglicana version (19). Finally, a similar picture is witnessed in the distribution of the letter ⟨w⟩, consistently displaying double ⟨v⟩ (29) instead of the combination of two looped *l*'s and a *3* (28), a letterform which belongs to the late 14th-century *Anglicana* script.

To the letterforms must be added the scribal use of Arabic figures, which may be taken as reliable cues for a close dating of the text, there being sharp palaeographic discrepancies from one century to another (see Hector 1958: 43–45). In the particular case of *H513*, Arabic figures consistently point to a 15th-century composition: ⟨4⟩ resembling a pair of pincers wherein two curved lines are crossed near their bases (35); the G-like form of ⟨5⟩ (36); the sigma form of ⟨6⟩ (37) together with the characteristic form of ⟨9⟩, with a pointed head and the tail curved leftwards (40).

3.2. Glasgow, GUL Hunter MS 503 (V.8.6)

According to Eldredge's own inspection, this text was composed with a fairly legible *Bastard Anglicana* script (Eldredge 1996: 25), defined by Derolez as the result of the merging of two prior variations of the Gothic script, the Textualis and the Anglicana (2003: 140–141). On the whole, this emerging style agglutinates "the best features of text and cursive" (Petti 1977: 15). Thus, the size, beauty, angularity and spikiness are a direct influence of the Textualis whilst letterforms and the ease of writing becomes notably cursive in origin. On chronological grounds, this handwriting style spread in English documents from the second half of the 14th century reaching its climax one century later when the two composites were completely assimilated. As a result, this style eventually became a recurrent choice for the composition of luxury manuscripts.

H503 is a neat example of this late mediaeval English script, though at the same time incorporating some Secretary element. Roberts refers to this grading of Secretary influence by adding *hybrida* to *Formata*, thereby termed as *cursive anglicana formata hybrida* (Roberts 2005: 164). Even though the text has been traditionally dated as a 15th-century composition (Young/Aitken 1908; 411; Cross 2004: 34), it is Eldredge who further proposes the last quarter of the 15th century on account of its palaeographic similarity with Parkes' plate 8 (1979: 8). Fig. 2 below reproduces the complete inventory of letterforms used by the scrivener.

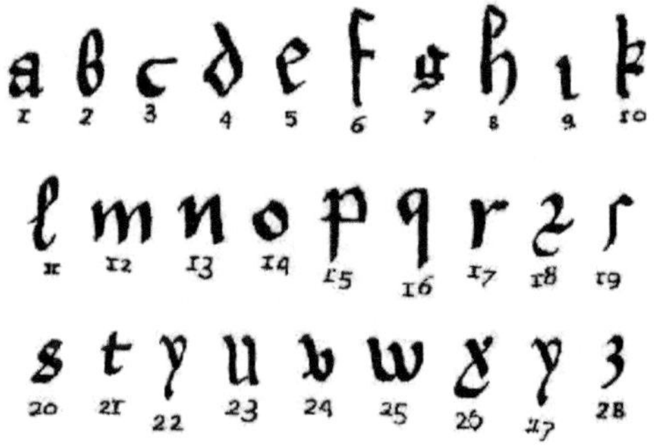

a b c d e f g h i k
1 2 3 4 5 6 7 8 9 10

l m n o p q r ɹ ſ
11 12 13 14 15 16 17 18 19

s t y u v w x y ȝ
20 21 22 23 24 25 26 27 28

Fig. 2. Inventory of minuscules in *H503*.

Fig. 2 allows the analyst to classify the letterforms from a threefold perspective. The textualis gradient, on the one hand, consists of a pre-defined set of letters common to the vast majority of manuscripts written under the shelter of this style, leaving then small room for the scribe to reshape the inventory. These items are the two-compartment ⟨a⟩ (1); the loopless ⟨d⟩ (4); the single-compartment ⟨g⟩, with occasional horns (7); the 8-shaped ⟨s⟩, exclusively word-finally (20); and the two versions of letter ⟨r⟩, *i.e.* the short and right-shouldered one (17) together with the 2-shaped alternative (18), the latter exclusively after vowel ⟨o⟩ and other letters with a bow (see Derolez 2003: 138; Roberts 2005: 164).

The cursive component, on the other hand, predominates in the text as a result of the larger contribution of the Anglicana Formata forms. The most distinctive cursive letterforms are the following: the loop at the right side of the letter ⟨b⟩ (2); the absence of infralinear ⟨f⟩ (6); the (occasional) hooked ascender of the letters ⟨h⟩ (8) and ⟨l⟩ (11); the three-stroke ⟨m⟩ (12) – a clue which sharply differentiates the Anglicana Formata from the single stroke Anglicana (Derolez 2003: 138); long ⟨s⟩ in initial and medial positions (19); the long-approach stroke of the letter ⟨v⟩ (24) together with the conventional form of the letter ⟨x⟩ (26).

The grading of the Secretary script is also witnessed in the use of two letters. First, the scribe abandons the looped and three-shaped final stroke ⟨w⟩ of the Anglicana in favour of the simpler version of the Secretary, thus resembling a double ⟨v⟩ (25). Second, as noted by Eldredge (1996: 25), the text shows the use of the three-stroke ⟨e⟩ (5) instead of the conventional Anglicana two-stroke form (see Derolez 2003: 137).

Of the special letters, it is significant to note that the author does not differentiate ⟨þ⟩ from ⟨y⟩, the latter also systematically undotted. Likewise, this picture is partially mirrored in the writing of the letters ⟨u⟩ and ⟨v⟩ insofar as the conventional distribution of these letters in mediaeval compositions is not always observed inasmuch as both can occur in word-initial and word-medial environments.

3.3. *Oxford, Bodleian Library, Ashmole MS 1468*

A is a long volume (378 pages) hosting three different manuscripts which contain, among others, some well-known pieces of the Middle Ages, both of scientific and literary merit, i.e. Guy de Chauliac's *Cyrurgia* (pp. 7–54) and William Langland's A version of *Piers Plowman* (pp. 307–378). Some of them are unfortunately abridged; this is the case of Grassus' treatise, which is the shortest witness of the tradition. According to Black's own collation, the volume was originally conceived in groups of ten pages and "it seems that not only

'Aj' (before what is now p. 7) is lost, but 7 leaves out of the first [...] set, namely, 6 leaves before p. 1, and 1 leaf after p. 6; which last seems [...] to have been vacant" (Black 1845: 1275).

Even though the hand of the text has been commonly dated in the 15th century (Black 1845: 1275), Eldredge, based on some palaeographic evidence, has recently proposed a more precise ascription to the first half of that same century (1996: 23). Eldredge's proposal is well-founded on account of the writer's hybrid script, which displays a 15th-century Secretary hand combined with some characteristic items of the Anglicana, this hybrid hand being a commonplace practice in the early phase of the 15th century (Petti 1977: 15). Still, the presence of the Anglicana is inadvertently skipped in Eldredge's description. The inventory of letterforms used by the writer is reproduced in Fig. 3 below:

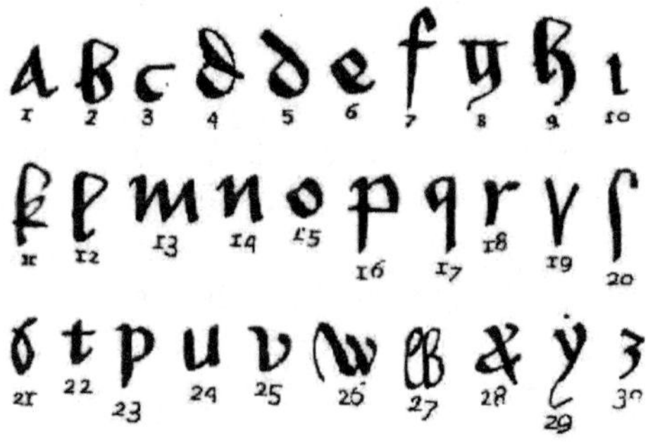

Fig. 3. Inventory of letterforms in *A*.

The cursive component of the Secretary, on the one hand, is characterised by two distinguishing features: the angularity of some letters – with loops and horns on the head and sides of letters (see the letters ⟨f⟩ and ⟨k⟩ for instance); and the combination of thin and thick strokes (as in the letters ⟨a⟩ and ⟨e⟩, for instance). In this fashion, the letters which mostly typify the Secretary hand are the following: the single compartment ⟨a⟩ with a pointed head (1), the double-compartment ⟨b⟩ (2); the letter ⟨d⟩, both looped (4) and loopless (5), irrespective of context; the tailed

⟨g⟩ with an *u*-shaped top and a headstroke (8), hence anticipating the Tudor and the Elizabethan forms; the letters ⟨h⟩ (8), ⟨k⟩ (11) and ⟨l⟩ (12) with the characteristic loop at the top of the ascender, the former also displaying a distinctive extension of the right limb below the baseline whilst the letter ⟨k⟩, in turn, presents the shortened form of the right limb (Clemens/Graham 2007: 167–168); together with the one-stroke versions of the letters ⟨m⟩ (13) and ⟨n⟩ (14).

There are three letters which deserve special attention. The first is the letter ⟨r⟩ insofar as it is rendered with a twofold representation in *A*, the right-shouldered ⟨r⟩ (18) with the typical angularity of the Secretary hand, and the long-forked ⟨r⟩ extending below the baseline, which stands out as a direct influence of the Anglicana (19). There is no trace, however, of the *v*-form of ⟨r⟩ which characterises the 15th-century version of the Secretary, a fact which may also witness the early composition of this copy.

A similar picture is observed in the rendering of the letter ⟨s⟩ to such extent that the typical forms of the Secretary and the Anglicana occur, more virtually than effectively, in particular contexts. In this vein, the long hooked ⟨s⟩ (20) of the cursive script is vastly preferred in initial and medial positions whilst the Anglicana sigma form of ⟨s⟩ (21) predominates word-finally. Still, the odds are not an exception and the reader occasionally finds word-initial instances, monosyllabic words in particular, as in *so* (p. 1), *sunne* (p. 2), *sonne* (p. 3). Likewise, the letter ⟨w⟩ also shows the parallel use of two writing standards: the Secretary form, resembling a double *v* (26), predominates word-initially while the Anglicana style, consisting of two looped l's (27), is the alternative if in the middle of a word.

Apart from the above contributions, the Anglicana grading is also noted in the writing of other letterforms, such as the letter ⟨c⟩, rounded and curved at the bottom (3); the letter ⟨e⟩, with three strokes and a pointed head (6); and the letter ⟨x⟩ (28) with the two distinctive 15th century strokes (Derolez 2003: 140).

Finally, the letters ⟨u⟩ and ⟨v⟩ are virtually indistinguishable from each other, except word-initially, where the latter presents a tall left limb curved to the left (nos. 24 and 25). Contrariwise, the letter ⟨y⟩ is consistently dotted in the manuscript, not in order to distinguish it from the letter ⟨þ⟩ – because they actually keep distinctive forms (see nos. 23 and 29 above), "but according to general medieval practice" (Derolez 2003: 140).

3.4. London, British Library, Sloane MS 661

Different dates have been proposed for this text in the relevant literature. Voigts and Kurtz, on the one hand, dated the witness in the 16th century, plausibly after a careful inspection of the original (Voigts/Kurtz 2000). The holder, on the other hand, reports it as a 15th-17th century English translation, a hitherto long time-span which is certainly in need of some kind of revision.[3] A cursory look at the palaeography of the text reveals that the translation kept in *S* is unlikely to be dated as early as the 15th century nor as late as the 17th century, the 16th being then the most likely candidate.

Even though similar to Petti's *Engrossing Elizabethan Secretary* in many respects (1977: 17), the wider range of minuscule forms found in *S* – letters ⟨a⟩, ⟨f⟩, ⟨h⟩ and ⟨s⟩ in particular, easily allows attributing a commonplace Elizabethan Secretary hand, plausibly from the last quarter of the 16th century on account of the use of particular letterforms, which help the analyst ascertain a likely date with some level of accuracy.

Fig. 4 reproduces the complete inventory of letters in *S*, where four items may be singled out for descriptive purposes. The letter ⟨a⟩ shows the conventional shapes of Elizabethan penmen, both with the oval body open at the top (2) and with an oblique supralinear descending stroke (1), the latter a recurrent scribal practice by the end of the century (Petti 1977: 17). Second, the letter ⟨e⟩ is rendered with the Greek (7) and with the open reversed form (8), there not being any contextual clues governing the use of one or the other. Third, the shape of the letter ⟨h⟩ is also twofold, with a reduced supralinear loop and an infralinear tail (13) and with a simple double-looped shaft (14), the former predominating

---

3   See <http://www.bl.uk/catalogues/manuscripts> (retrieved 18/05/2011).

in initial and medial positions while the latter is exclusively word-final. Denholm-Young describes a characteristic gradient of this letter for the purposes of identification in the sense that "in the first half of the period the letter *h* is still half above the line. As time wears on it sinks lower and lower" to such extent that three quarters of the letter are below the line in the later Secretary hands (1954: 71). In this particular case, the letter is conspicuously infralinear, which suggests a late 16th century composition.

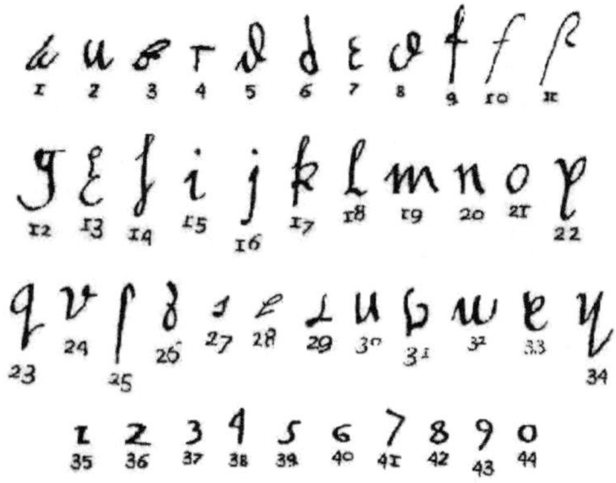

Fig. 4. Inventory of minuscules and figures in *S*.

Contrariwise, the letter ⟨s⟩ does not respond to any contextual variation, where four different types are observed, the long hooked form (25), the sigma ⟨s⟩ (26) and the two varieties of the small round ⟨s⟩ (27 and 28), the former sporadically found in *S* in the writing of foreign words.

There are other letters which also help typify the Elizabethan Secretary hand of *S*: the letter ⟨c⟩ characterised by the horizontal stroke at the top of the crescent with the absence of the foot serif (4); the ⟨g⟩ with its head converted into a semi-oval and the infralinear loop into a simple tail (12) (Tannenbaum 1930: 45); the v-like ⟨r⟩ (24); and the letter ⟨f⟩, which is markedly leant to the right among Elizabethan writers (10 and 11), the latter in final with the crossbar omitted, its place accordingly taken by a flourish at the lower end of the head loop.

Finally, as in the case of *H513* above, the scribal use of Arabic figures may provide the analyst with additional cues about the composition of the manuscript. In this vein, the shape of some distinct figures actually corroborates the conclusions obtained from the analysis of letterforms, thus pointing to a late 16th century hand. Of these, number one is a conspicuous example consisting of a simple stroke with the (conventional) head and foot serifs at the time (35). Number four, in turn, already appears with its present form, though slightly leant, which was, according to Petti (1977: 28), recently adopted throughout the second half of the 16th century (38). A similar point may be used to establish the chronology of number five, which develops from the mediaeval angular ⟨h⟩ to a lower-case printed ⟨s⟩ in the course of the 16th-century (39). Finally, the traditional acute angle form of number seven is also progressively modified to such extent that its left arm shortens while the right one moved vertically towards the end of that same century (41).

4. Line-final word division

4.1. Rationale

Following the line initiated in two other recent studies (Calle Martín, 2009, forthcoming), this section investigates line-final word-division practice in the English vernacular tradition of Grassus' *De Probatissima Arte Oculorum*. The relevant literature has been eye to eye as to the arbitrary character of line-final breaks in early English handwriting. Most palaeographic publications contain just brief notes about the topic where the only precept "seems to have been that not less than two completing letters could be carried over to the second line" (Hector 1958: 48; Denholm-Young 1964: 70). Even though true in many a scribal composition, the modern approaches have found the existence of recurrent patterns used by mediaeval scribes (Hladký 1985a: 73; Lutz 1986: 193; Burchfield 1994: 182).

From a methodological standpoint, Hladký's approach to the study of word division in English historical texts is partially adopted as a theoretical framework (1985a; 1985b). He proposes a functional classification of the phenomenon in terms of the two basic tendencies for splitting, *i.e.* Morphology and Phonology. The former recurs to word formation whereas the latter divides words in terms of its actual pronunciation, i.e. ⟨dri-ed⟩ (*H503*) vs. ⟨corrupt-cion⟩ (*H503*). Still, a third group has been added to account for those anomalous divisions which fall apart from this classification, and which seem to escape Hladký's attention, i.e. ⟨vpri-ght⟩ (*H513*), ⟨ab-undance⟩ (*S*), etc. The present paper also examines the distribution of the rules which seem to govern the breaking of a word, both morphologically and phonologically. The former necessarily depend upon word-formation processes and the latter are liable to incorporate different rules. In this fashion, Hladký (1985a; 1985b) observes the division after an open syllable (henceforth the CV – CV rule), the division between two consonants (the C – C rule), the division between two vowels (the V – V rule) and the division between the pairs *-st* and *-ct* (the ST rule and the CT rule, respectively).

In light of these premises, this section investigates line-final breaking devices in Grassus' copies with the following objectives: a) to evaluate the weight of morphological and phonological boundaries; b) to offer a taxonomy of word-division rules used by mediaeval scribes; and c) to find whether the chaotic situation referred to in the literature can be safely applied to the pieces under examination.

4.2. Analysis

The marking off of a line-final break is not orthographically conventionalized among mediaeval scribes and the use of one symbol or another will ultimately depend upon variables such as the scribal choice, on the one hand, and the space available at the margin of the folio, on the other. In this vein, up to three punctuation symbols may occur therein, i.e. the colon, the hyphen and the double hyphen (Calle Martín/Miranda García 2005: 32). In Benvenutus Grassus' vernacular witnesses, the four copyists opted for the double hyphen, slightly curved upwards whilst still horizontal in the Sloane version. Even though the double hyphen is consistent across the hands, the symbol is left out many a time when there is not enough room at the margin, particularly in the case of *H503*.

Table 1 below reproduces the distribution of line-final breaks in the four pieces. For comparative purposes, the figures have also been normalized to a text of 1,000 words. From a quantitative perspective, one can tentatively conclude that the phenomenon is irregularly distributed across the samples in the sense that *H503* amounts to 339 word-division instances in spite of having conspicuously less running words than the other Hunterian witness (13,306 vs. 15,655 words), the writer therefore being more committed to line-final boundaries than the other copyists. Setting aside *H503*, the phenomenon is observed to correlate in the other witnesses, ranging from 8.1 to just 13.5 occurrences every 1,000 words in *A* and *H513*, respectively.

On a qualitative perspective, on the other hand, the four manuscripts tentatively confirm an overwhelming preference for phonological boundaries to such extent that they exceed 80% of the occurrences across the samples, with the only exception of *A* that reaches just 60.52%, plausibly as a result of its fragmentary condition. Morphological and anomalous divisions, on the whole, are sporadic and one can tentatively conclude that they occur when there is little room available at the margin of the folio. In this same fashion, if compared with the other pieces, the figures for morphological and anomalous divisions are notably higher in *A* as it is the only text written in two columns, a fact which substantially constrains the scribe's act of writing.

MS	Instances	Morphological	Phonological	Anomalous	Total
H503	Absolute	39	285	15	339
	Normalized	2.46	18.42	0.96	21.84
H513	Absolute	30	206	14	250
	Normalized	1.62	11.14	0.75	13.5
S	Absolute	9	81	1	91
	Normalized	0.93	8.37	0.1	9.4
A	Absolute	12	23	3	38
	Normalized	2.58	4.97	0.64	8.1

Table 1. Word division instances (absolute and normalized figures).

The second objective of this survey is the assessment of the word-division rules used by mediaeval scribes in these MSS. Figure 5 below reproduces, in absolute figures, the distribution of the phonological rules in the witnesses under examination. As observed, the four copies reveal a major preference for the CV – CV rule, as in ⟨ca-teractis⟩ (*H503*), ⟨ma-lancoly⟩ (*H513*), ⟨uisi-ble⟩ (*A*) or ⟨disfi-gured⟩ (*S*). The only exception to this rule is consonant ⟨x⟩, which is systematically attached to the preceding vowel regardless of any other phonological consideration as in ⟨alex-andrinum⟩ or ⟨lax-atyff⟩ (*H503*). This orthographic convention often coincides with a morphological division, i.e. ⟨flex-en⟩ (*H503*).

Second, if the word at a line-end is not amenable to open syllable division, the scribe is therefore committed to divide between two consonants (the C – C rule) and to a lesser extent, between two vowels (the V – V rule), always on condition that the result is readable and that the consonants do not belong to the same syllable, i.e. ⟨mor-ter⟩ (*H503*), ⟨oc-casioun⟩ (*H513*), ⟨wor-mode⟩ (*A*) or ⟨begin-ninge⟩ (*S*). In the case of the V – V rule, in turn, the scribe is not particularly concerned about the phonological dimension of the split vowels, both diphthongs and monophthongs, being a visual rather than a strictly phonological rule in order to facilitate the reading of these groups, i.e. ⟨occasy-on⟩ (*H503*), ⟨no-ught⟩ (*H513*) and ⟨speci-allye⟩ (*S*) vs. ⟨se-ed⟩ (*H503*), ⟨wo-unde⟩ (*H513*) and ⟨glorio-us⟩ (*H513*).

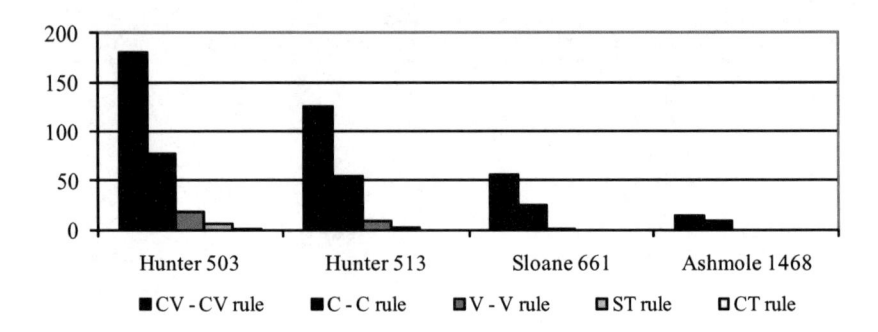

Fig. 5. Distribution of phonological rules.

In light of the above premises, the particularities of the word and the space available at the margin leave room for other rules like the division between the pairs -*st* and -*ct*, exclusively featured in the Hunterian copies. See, for instance, examples like ⟨auc-tor⟩ (*H503*), ⟨cris-tallyne⟩ (*H503*), ⟨was-ted⟩ (*H513*) and ⟨bris-till⟩ (*H513*).

Morphologically speaking, on the other hand, there is more room for variation, prefixation and suffixation in particular. Figure 6 presents the distribution of the three morphological boundaries in normalized figures so as to facilitate any subsequent comparison. Setting aside the case of *A*, where the three mechanisms are balanced, one can safely gather that prefixation outnumbers suffixation in MSS Hunter 513 and Sloane 661, respectively. The other side of the coin, however, is offered by *H503* insofar as suffixation outweighs prefixation. Note the following examples for each category: ⟨fore-seyd⟩ (*H503*), ⟨ouer-moche⟩ (*H513*), ⟨super-abundance⟩ (*S*) vs. ⟨hand-ful⟩ (*H503*), ⟨sotyl-lyche⟩ (*H513*), ⟨happ-eth⟩ (*A*), ⟨breefe-lye⟩ (*S*), etc. Composition, in turn, is generally the least frequent device with examples like ⟨there-to⟩ (*S*), ⟨eyʒe-liddes⟩ (*A*), ⟨wherso-euere⟩ (*H503*), etc.

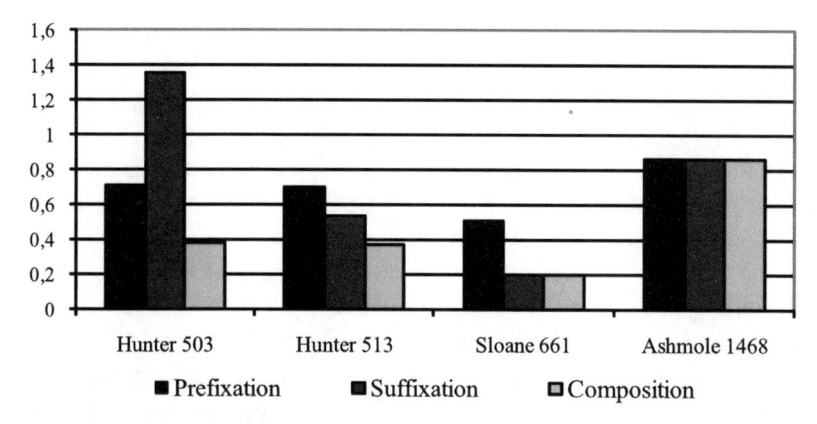

[Chart with bars for Hunter 503, Hunter 513, Sloane 661, Ashmole 1468 showing Prefixation, Suffixation, Composition]

Fig. 6. Distribution of morphological rules.

Finally, the set of anomalous divisions comprises the instances in which the scribe splits the letters of a same syllable and, consequently, the result becomes unpronounceable. On quantitative grounds, the number of anomalous breakings is sporadic, the four scribes being thoroughly committed to phonological and, to a lesser extent, morphological boundaries. Note, for instance, ⟨len-ght⟩ (*H503*), ⟨vncurab-le⟩ (*H513*), ⟨gry-nde⟩ (*H513*), ⟨Adaman-dston⟩ (*A*), ⟨ab-undance⟩ (*S*), etc.

5. Conclusions

The present study has been conceived as an introductory paper to the synoptic edition of Benvenutus Grassus' *De Probatissima Arte Oculorum*, which represents the major collaborative contribution of the present volume. Palaeographic in itself, this paper examines the handwriting of Grassus' vernacular tradition in English, hitherto preserved in four different documents, from a twofold perspective, i.e. script and line-final word-division.

Originally conceived to complement Eldredge's partial account of the topic (1996: 20–30), the objective here was to offer a detailed picture of the scribes' hands. The task has been accomplished in three stages, necessarily sequential: the first is the compilation of the complete inventory of letterforms, which subsequently leads to the other two, i.e. the taxonomy of the scripts and the establishment of a likely date of composition. In the particular case of Grassus' witnesses, though slippery it may be, there is empirical evidence to propose the following chronology. As for the mediaeval copies, *A* would be the oldest version, written some time in the first half of the 15th century under the shelter of the Secretary hand with a slight Anglicana grading. Of the Hunterian copies, *H513* would be the earliest witness, being plausibly copied towards the mid-15th century whilst *H503* is taken to have been composed in the last quarter of that same century, combining a Bastard Anglicana hand with some Secretary element. Finally, the Sloane manuscript is clearly a late 16th-century text penned with a distinctive Elizabethan script.

Line-final word division, on the other hand, has been surveyed on the assumption that there are underlying principles used by mediaeval and early modern writers. In line with other previous contributions to the topic (Calle Martín, forthcoming), the results come to corroborate the working hypothesis that the phonological outnumbers the morphological, the former generally exceeding 80% in the four witnesses. The scribal practice also points to the existence of a hierarchy of rules which, depending on the syllabic particularities of the word and the space available at the margin, is consistently applied, i.e. the CV – CV rule, the C – C rule and the V – V rule. If morphological, the motivation for breaking is found to vary across the samples, prefixation or suffixation tending to predominate depending on the scribe's choice. As a result of all this and setting aside the anomalous instances, it may be tentatively concluded that the picture is not that chaotic as frequently published in the literature. Contrariwise, Benvenutus Grassus' English tradition has been found to display a preconceived set of word-division rules, in our opinion, consciously and proficiently schemed by the writers.

Teresa Marqués Aguado

Depunctuating the Middle English Benvenutus Grassus: The Cases of GUL, MSS Hunter 503 and 513[1]

1. Introduction

The use of punctuation has been traditionally taken as a haphazard, inconsistent and erratic component of medieval manuscripts (Jenkinson 1926: 153; Zeeman 1956: 11; Lucas 1971: 19 and Mitchell 1980: 412, among others), but recent research on medieval treatises (Alonso Almeida 2002; Calle Martín 2004; Calle Martín/Miranda García 2005; Obegi Gallardo 2006; Esteban Segura 2009 and Marqués Aguado 2009b) has shown that this is not necessarily the case. Although not all texts share the same inventory of punctuation marks (or, if they do, this is not always employed in exactly the same way), certain regularity can be observed within individual texts.

As a matter of fact, Parkes argued that factors such as the nature of the text, the different forms in which it could be read or the ultimate use it would serve might bear an influence on the punctuation employed (1978: 132–133). In this case, we are facing the same text (an ophthalmologic treatise, written by Benvenutus Grassus), but preserved in two different witnesses (Glasgow, Glasgow University Library, MSS Hunter 503 [pages 1–137; *H503*] and Hunter 513 [ff. 1r–37r; *H513*]), which were, moreover, written at approximately the same period, i.e. the 15th century (Cross 2004: 34–35; see also Calle Martín's contribution in this volume). Yet, a passing look at both manuscripts allows us to

---

1   The present research has been funded by the Spanish Ministry of Education (project FFI2008-02336). This grant is hereby gratefully acknowledged.

observe that punctuation is used differently in each copy, and this may lead us to argue that punctuation was not authorial but scribal, and that the ultimate goal pursued with its use might be found in the type of text that we are dealing with.

In connection with this, it must be stated that one of the main issues of contention regarding medieval punctuation is to determine the function that it displays, that is to say, whether grammatical or rhetorical: on the one hand, punctuation could be used to mark the syntactic relations established between the components of sentences; on the other, it could indicate points of rest for a meaningful oral delivery. Lucas added a third function, the macro-textual one, which had to do with the marking of the layout and organisation of the text (1971: 5).

In this light, the aim of this chapter is to compare the punctuation marks employed, along with their specific uses, in the two Middle English versions of the ophthalmologic treatise written by Benvenutus Grassus held in *H503* and *H513*. For the purpose, a brief reference to the methodology followed will be made, and then the different punctuation systems will be explored separately with a view to ascertaining whether these are followed consistently, and whether there is any overlap in the use of specific punctuation marks. The conclusion section offers a table summarising and contrasting the punctuation marks used in both witnesses, so that the differences in the inventories and in the functions that these fulfil become evident. The analysis of the function that punctuation displays is also provided.

2. Methodology

The study of the punctuation inventories employed in *H503* and *H513* is based on the transcriptions of these treatises, which were later on pasted onto Excel spreadsheets. Then, they were lemmatised and tagged as part of a major corpus containing unedited Middle English *Fachprosa*, and all the instances of punctuation marks were retrieved. For this purpose, the data in the Excel spreadsheets containing the two treatises were arranged according to the lemmas, since all the punctuation marks had been previously lemmatised under the label 'punctuationmark'. Then, these were arranged according to the manuscript that the examples belonged to so as to be able to produce an individual analysis of each treatise. Finally, the different marks employed within each text were grouped with the aim of classifying each occurrence of the signs found into the four levels of analysis (explained in section 3). Therefore, a quantitative study has been carried out in order to provide a qualitative analysis of the functions performed by the different punctuation symbols.

3. Analysis of the punctuation systems of *H503* and *H513*

This study of the two punctuation repertoires is organised into two sections: section 3.1 focuses on the punctuation of *H503* and section 3.2. on that of *H513*. Within each section, the various functions performed at the different levels of study (macro-textual, sentential, clausal and phrasal) are explained. The classification into these four levels (which is also found in most recent research, such as Calle Martín 2004, Calle Martín/Miranda García 2005, Esteban Segura 2009 and Marqués Aguado 2009b) responds to the three levels into which grammatical constructions are classified (that is, sentential, clausal and phrasal), plus the importance that the macro-textual function is expected to have in the texts. Examples of the different marks employed for each use are supplied and are cited according to the folios or pages of the original manuscripts. The brackets { } are used to enclose the relevant sign and the context under discussion in the examples. Sometimes, an example may feature more than one pair of these brackets, which may point out at several functions of punctuation being shown at the same time, as with example (3), for instance.

3.1. Analysis of H503

The total number of punctuation marks employed in *H503* is 1,883 items, which means that punctuation is abundantly used in this text. Out of the total number of signs, the period is, by far, the most frequently used one, with 1,788×, followed by the combination of the period and the paragraph mark (95×).[2] Within this inventory, hyphens to divide words between two lines are also to be counted, but will be left aside in the study owing to their stable function throughout the text. Nevertheless, some of the examples below also contain instances of the hyphen.

It must be added that, sometimes, the period shows a descending stroke in the manner of a flourish, but this does not imply a different function or a different punctuation mark at all. Indeed, it usually appears after rubricated technical terms, which increases its ornamental value.

3.1.1. Macro-textual level

At this level, introducing a new paragraph (and, consequently, a distinct idea or topic) is commonly marked by the combination of the period plus the paragraph mark (39×) or by the period (16×), as in (1) and (2). Usually, this new paragraph starts with a decorated capital letter.[3] In some other cases (pages 9, 30, 40, 72, 93, 102, 112, 130, etc.) a line-filler is found at the end of the line and the next line begins with a decorated initial, so that the division into paragraphs is also visually marked, as shown in (3):

(1) and thyes happyn to be engendred more abowte the ende of august [...].
{.¶ Obtalmies}
comun̄ly haue þer domyne or power þat

---

2   Whenever this mark is employed, the period usually appears at the end of the line, the paragraph mark being then moved to the initial position in the following line. This can be observed on pages 33, 44, 62, 82 and 118 (*H503*).
3   This visual device obviously contributes to breaking the text into major sense-units, or sections, rather than simply marking new paragraphs.

tyme (*H503*:34.2–8)[4]

(2) And yn thys wyse ye shal
cure thys mane*r* of disease. yf it be a
plied. & vsed. At the begynnyng{.
Of} thys plaster thyes be vertues. (*H503*:78.12–15)

(3) callyd{. Vnguentu*m* subtile.} tyll it
{be hoole ———}
In the fyrst p*a*rtye of thys
tretys (*H503*:93.11–14)

Although *H503* is not very prolific in the use of chapter titles (as opposed to with *H513*, as explained in 3.2.1.), whenever they are employed, periods are used to mark their end, and consequently the beginning of the paragraph. This happens 4×. These headings are commonly rubricated so as to visually enhance their importance. This is shown in (4):

(4) so ha
ue I founde & manny haue I holpen.
{Off the infirmytees causyd of
Coolore.} (*H503*:65.12–15)

One of the most outstanding functions of the punctuation system employed at macro-textual level is to call attention to names of authorities, other proper names (especially place names), names of works and various technical terms (such as those referring to substances, parts of the body, etc., whether in Latin or in English). Usually, these sections are rubricated, a device that again contributes to highlight the importance of these words for the intended recipient of the text. The specific mark employed to fulfil this function is the period (188×). It often comes in pairs, and, especially in the case of technical terms rendered in Latin, the second period introduces the translation,

---

4   The reference system used throughout the volume is as follows: '*MS*:page/folio. line'.

definition or paraphrase of that concept into English, too. Examples (5), (6) and (3) illustrate these uses:

(5) The first tunicle or Cote ys cle
pid {. Rectina.} The secunde {. Secundina.}
The thirde {. Scliros.} The iiijth {. Aranea.}
The vth {. Vuea.} The vjth {. Cornea.} The
vijth and the last {. Co*n*iu*n*ctiua.} (*H503*:3.13–4.1)

(6) Take and hand
ful of an herbe callyd {. Cardus be
nedictus. Sowthystyl yn englych.} (*H503*:57.8–10)

The introduction of an alternative course of treatment, of the next step in the curation of a disease, of a new phase in the preparation of a remedy, etc. are all likely to be marked by punctuation. This occurs mainly with the combination of the period and the paragraph mark (19×), as in (7), and with the period on its own (19×), as in (8). Likewise, the introduction of recipes is occasionally overtly marked by means of the period (16×) or of the period plus the paragraph mark (9×), as in (9) and (10), respectively:

(7) and it shall
frete it wythoute peyn or vyolence.
an claryfie the sy3te {.¶ Also take}
the dragons roote. and. scrape a
wey (*H503*:125.8–12)

(8) and they
were sone spede {. wherfore} rawe onions
be noyows to the sy3te {. And} yn winter
lett nat the pacyent drynk hoote wynes. (*H503*:23.12–15)

(9) Fyrst he must porge his
brayn wyth pelett*is* callyd. Pillule ihero-
solimitane. wherof thus is the maky*n*g {.
Take} turbite. aloes. epatica. (*H503*:15.3–6)

(10) as for the
   medycyne callyd. Virtus a deo data.
   that knyttyth and sowdeth the tonycle a geyn yf it be brokyn. and it
   is made on thys wyse {.¶ Take}
   xij. stren*us* of new freshe leyd egg*is* (*H503*:98.1–6)

At this level, punctuation may also be used to mark that what follows in the text is either the conclusion or the explanation of what has been previously stated (and here the introduction of the explanation of a treatment, for instance, as been included, as shown in (12)). In the former case, the period is the only sign used (17×) – as shown in (11) and in (8) above, whereas in the latter there is an overlap of marks, although the period is still the most common sign (31×), as shown in (12), followed by the combination of the period and the paragraph mark (10×):

(11) And neiþ*er* yn
   the eyon. nor wythoute. ys no spot .
   aperyng {. and þ*er*fore .} the defaute of thys
   ys not yn the eye. but i*n* the
   stomake (*H503*:66.14 – 67.3)

(12) Off thys dysease {thus ys the
   cure.} yf the pacyent be yong . lete
   hym blode on the veyne yn the myddys of the forhede (*H503*:82.12–15)

Another function displayed by the period (59×) at macro-textual level is to signal the beginning – and in many occasions the end as well – of parenthetical comments (for instance, those including the quantities of each ingredient in recipes, but they may also be whole sentences) and of examples, as shown in (13) and (14):

(13) sarcacolle. spykenard. Sa
   fron {. of eche a drame.} suger candy
   an*e* {vnc*er*.} (*H503*:131.7–9)

(14) & occasyonyd of the
iiij hum*ers* {. as blode. flewme. color.
& malyncolye} (*H503*:30.12–14)

3.1.2. Sentential level

At sentence level, punctuation fulfils four main functions. First, it is used to mark independent sentences, and for this purpose two different signs may be used: the period (173×) (see (15)) or the period and the paragraph mark together (13×):

(15) Also take totye and
sarcacolle of eche halfe an*e* vnc*er*. roses sedys .ij. vnc*er* camphyr .ij. dra*m*-
mys {. poud*er* } thyes to ghed*er* {. and bo-
yll} them (*H503*:134.6–10)

Second, juxtaposition is also sometimes marked, and in this case there is no overlap of signs, since the period is the only symbol employed (31×), as illustrated in (16):

(16) and stampe
them wele to geddyr wyth wo-
mans mylke {. mollifi yt}. (*H503*:85.9–11)

Third, coordinate clauses are also signalled by means of periods most of the times (387×), as shown in (17) and in (15), although the combination of the period and the paragraph mark is occasionally employed (1×). It must be added that many times these coordinate clauses could eventually work as independent sentences on account of their length or of the fact that five or even six coordinate clauses may follow:

(17) {Take} sarcacollu*m* album {.
and bete} yt wele to pouder yn a bra
sym mort*er* {. And of pouder put} the eye
ful {. and lette} hym ley wydeopyn (*H503*:35.12–15)

Finally, subordinate clauses are frequently marked off from main clauses by using the three signs featuring in *H503*: the period (332×) and the period plus the paragraph mark (3×). Subordinate clauses of cause, condition and purpose, together with relative clauses, are the most frequent types encountered, as shown in examples (18) to (20). In the case of direct speech, the period is employed 5×, as in (21):

(18) be ware þat yt boylle not
after but lytle {. for} þan shal the spy
cys lese theyr wertu & her might (*H503*:68.10–12)

(19) so thys vertu youen of god co*n*
sowdyth the tonycle of the eye {. yf}
it be hurte and purified the eye (*H503*:99.2–4)

(20) lete
hym blode on the veyne yn the myddys of the forhede {. whych} so doon.
cure hym w*ith* a colerie clepid. Cole-
riu*m* rubor*um*. (*H503*:82.13–83.2)

(21) hume*r*s lyke teres. whych leches cal-
len festeles. wherfore {q*uo*d Benny-
micius.} of them oure lorde ihe*s*u yaue (*H503*:103.10–12)

3.1.3. Clausal level

At clause level, punctuation marks relate clause components, a function that is fulfilled by the period (193×), as shown in (22), where this sign is placed between the subject and the main verb, and by one instance of the period and the paragraph mark together:

(22) Also {cri-
stall sotylly powderd. doth} the same (*H503*:121.9–11)

Similarly, the period is employed to relate the two particles of correlative constructions (3×), such as PDE *neither… nor* or *so… that*, as in (23):

(23) that fro
thens foreward. the concaue or the holow synewys {be so stoppyd & ouerlayd.
that the vysyble spiryte may nomore
passe downn} by them. (*H503*:29.1–5)

Also, the period is employed to mark the coordination of phrases (138×), whether nominal, verbal or prepositional, as illustrated in (24) and (25):

(24) and it ys comunly gendryd {of exces
meete and drynk yndegest. and also
of gret labour} (*H503*:11.14–15)

(25) and for cowes fleshe {.
ghetys fleshe. and eelys. and such oþer} (*H503*:23.5–6)

Likewise, the enumeration of phrases (again, nominal, verbal or prepositional) is sometimes marked by using the period (22×), as shown in (26), and also in (25). Example (26) evinces that there is not consistency in the use of punctuation marks for particular functions (i.e. 'esule myrabolanys cytryne'):

(26) Take {poly-
podye. esule} myrabolanys {cytryne.
rubarbe. ana. ʒ. 1. Masticys. Cubibys.
saferon. spygnarde. Nucys Indicem.} (*H503*:38.14–39.2)

Vocatives are rarely employed, but these instances are marked with periods (5×), as in (27):

(27) But hyer fynally I
wyl ʒe knowe {. ʒe þat wyll be
practyfe yn the acurye crafte.} þat (*H503*:25.10–12)

Finally, it may be added that the period is employed twice before a pleonastic pronoun (see Mustanoja 1960: 123, 137–138). In other words, this mark signals that the word that follows is the subject of the clause under the form of a pronoun, while being preceded by a long subject. For instance, the long multiple subject in (28), extending from lines 8 to 12 is summarised by way of 'thei' to continue with the explanation of diseases:

(28) And
 the Colo*ur* of the eyon ys meueable blak.
 that we call grey. but often*n* yt ys seyn
 þat i*n* þis man*er* of eyon. obtalmie. þat
 is derknes of sy3t. And. Panniclus.
 that is smale webbys. and oþ*er* dyue*r*se
 dyseasis. whych shald be declaryd here
 aft*er* {. thei} grow rather þan yn oþ*er* man*er*
 of eyen*n* colourid (*H503*:6.5–13)

3.1.4. Phrasal level

Punctuation symbols are very frequently used to mark off numerals (both Roman and Arabic ones, whether ordinal or cardinal) and abbreviations of apothecaries' weights and measures from the surrounding text. They often come in pairs, even if the first sign falls at the end of the line and the numeral or abbreviation appears in the first position in the next line. The period is the only sign employed (99×), as shown in (29), and also in (26):

(29) And sum tyme for
 oon*n* growith {.iij. or iiij.} (*H503*:51.6–7)

The relation established between the different constituents of a phrase (for instance, between the noun head and the following *of*-phrase) may also be overtly marked by means of the period (24×), as in (30):

(30) tyll þei be incarnate. vpon
 the {tonycles. of} the ey (*H503*:113.8–9)

Finally, coordination between the elements of a phrase may eventually surface (marked with the period 22×), especially with the PDE correlative structure *neither... nor* in the case of prepositional phrases, as shown in (31):

(31) lete hym not goo a broode
 {yn the wynde. nor in the soon.} (*H503*:137.2–3)

3.2. Analysis of H513

Although a preliminary description of the punctuation marks in this treatise is already available in Marqués/Miranda/González (2008: 39–40), no detailed reference has been made to the specific uses and functions that the inventory of punctuation marks has. There is a total of 808 punctuation marks in this text, a figure that can be broken down into the following symbols: 414× periods, 277× paragraph marks, 81× virgules, 21× of the sign consisting of a period plus a virgule plus another period, and 15× double virgules. As with *H503*, hyphens (used to divide words between lines) and carets (employed to mark insertions) will be left aside from this study owing to their straightforward uses (see for this purpose Marqués/Miranda/González 2008: 40).

Two remarks must be made regarding this punctuation system. On the one hand, although some doubts might occasionally arise regarding the position of the period (that is, whether a slightly raised period or one placed at the baseline is being intended), no differences in terms of their uses have been noted. On the other hand, double virgules sometimes co-occur with paragraph marks, but in these cases it seems that the former are an indication left for the rubricator to insert a paragraph mark when adding colour to the manuscript, as explained in section 4.

3.2.1. Macro-textual level

At macro-textual level, a variety of uses are found. First of all, chapters usually end with the combination of a period, a virgule and another period (21×), a sign that marks the end of large sense-units according to Petti (1977: 26), as in (32) and (33):

Depunctuating the ME Benvenutus Grassus 67

(32) ¶ The 4 kynd of catarract*es*
is that that is in colour citrine and hit comethe of
moche drynkyng and of ouer moch etyng and of grete trauell in many folke {it comethe thorowe ma-
lancoly humour ·/·}
Of the Cure of the· 4· kindes of Cate-
ractus curabill & of worching w*ith* nedill (*H513*:4v.6–12)

Occasionally, periods (16×) are employed to mark the end of chapter titles, as shown in (33):

(33) that {precious oynement ·/·} {Of ·2· secunde
pannicle and the cure of it.}
Of the ·2· pannicle is that the whiche appe=
rethe on the tonicle in the maner of a·
vecche or in the maner of a scale of a·fissh (*H513*:12r.6–10)

It is also possible for punctuation symbols to mark the introduction of relevant information from the medical standpoint (for instance, a recipe, the description of the pattern of symptoms, the different courses of treatment for a disease, the steps to be followed when preparing a remedy, etc.). This is very frequently conveyed by means of paragraph marks (207×), but also by means of periods (13×), virgules (9×) and double virgules (7×), as shown in (34) and (35):

(34) w*ith*oute none poudres ne colleries ben for suche
maladies {¶ And ther for} this is the Cure for
soche maladies {¶ ffirst it behouethe} to purgen (*H513*:19r.16–18)

(35) And yif thou doste thus thou shalte departe of þ*at*
pece of stone fro the tonicle {/ And yif} that hole be
moche putte therin than vertu of god y yeue (*H513*:32r.16–18)

In this line, punctuation may also serve to introduce the conclusion or the explanation of what has been previously stated, as it happens with paragraph marks (12×), virgules (5×), periods (4×) and double virgules (1×), as shown in (36) and (37):

(36) is in the water that is stondyng in many lakes //
      {¶ Wherfor} knowell that this maner of cataractes (*H513*:8r.1–2)

(37) ye shull do as we
      haue saide in the ·2ᵉ· pannicle as ye haue afore {/ þat
      is to saye} w*ith* atuterye in the templis (*H513*:13r.11–13)

Parenthetical comments are rarely marked, but this happens once with two virgules, which enclose this comment, as shown in (38):

(38) beside the nose beside that ey3e lidde and that
      other {/ and they do this cure worste /} they hauen a·
      glowyng yren (*H513*:30r.13–15)

Finally, punctuation may be employed to add an element to an enumeration, a function that is conveyed by the paragraph mark (27×), the virgule (1×) and the double virgule (1×), as shown in (39):

(39) westis that ben in the ey3en
      {// The first spice} is curable the whiche is white
      as clerist chalke {¶ The secunde} is white and
      is liche to the whitnes of firmament {¶ The ·3ᵉ·}
      is white and is liche a·skyn ·i· cuue*rs* colours (*H513*:4r.13–17)

3.2.2. Sentential level

Many independent sentences are marked by means of punctuation signs, namely: virgules (21×), paragraph marks (8×) and double virgules (6×). It must be added, though, that many of these independent sentences are headed by the conjunction *and*, a phenomenon that is also observed in *H503*. Examples (40) and (41) illustrate these uses:

(40) and bynde it to a
      nother morwe {/ In the morwe} putte ther the
      poudre (*H513*:30v.19–21)

(41) till the heres be don all away and y pluc=
ked a·way with smalle pynsours ·i· whynders {¶ But
vnderstonde} that by suche heres the state (*H513*:15r.17–19)

Likewise, coordinate clauses are sometimes marked by the virgule (24×), the paragraph mark (11×) or the period (4×), as shown in (42) and (43). Asyndetic coordination, whereby the coordinating conjunction is omitted (Fischer 1992: 289), is not commonly marked, although two exceptions are found with a paragraph mark and a virgule, respectively, as in (44):

(42) and kepe it for thyne store {/ and} erliche and
late at euyn dothe it in the sore ey3en (*H513*:37r.3–4)

(43) and they sein nought clerely {¶ But} they haue
her ey3en full of smoke (*H513*:10r.21–22)

(44) it constraynethe and stoppethe teres it dis=
troieth fleume {/ it hetethe} the brayne (*H513*:18v.19–20)

Marking off main from subordinate clauses is another function commonly fulfilled by punctuation, especially in the case of subordinate clauses of cause, but also in relative clauses. Periods (20×), virgules (13×) and paragraph marks (8×) are used for this purpose, as shown in (45), (46) and (47):

(45) But
vnderstonde that {whan} ye putten yn the forsaide
spices with the zucre {· it shall} sethe but alitell (*H513*:19v.3–5)

(46) and it is comen to hem
for her euyll kepyng {/ for whi} they wole ete (*H513*:10r.22–23)

(47) we
make poudre nabatis {¶ The whiche} poudre
doithe many grete merueiles to the pannicles (*H513*:13v.21–23)

3.2.3. Clausal level

At clause level, punctuation is used to relate clause constituents, as in the case of the period (4×), as in (48), and of the paragraph mark (1×):

(48) withe medecyns
      {I· added} afterward wreten (*H513*:12v.16–17)

Other uses at clausal level are to mark coordinate noun phrases (4× of the virgule and 1× of the period) and to mark the enumeration of noun phrases (only once, with the virgule), as shown in (49) and (50), respectively:

(49) and hauen {one vertue / and one sauour} (*H513*:35v.9)

(50) as from {oxe flesshe / Cowe flessh} (*H513*:36r.21)

3.2.4. Phrasal level

The most frequent function of punctuation at phrasal level is to mark off numerals (whether Roman or Arabic ones) and abbreviations of apothecaries' weights and measures from the rest of the text. For this purpose, the period is consistently used throughout (269×). In most cases it features in pairs (196×, as in (51) and (52)), but it can be found in isolation (28×, as in (53)) or in strings of numerals and abbreviations together (46×, as in (54)):

(51) The {·5·} vuea ¶ The
      {·6·} cornea ¶ The {·7·} coniunctiua (*H513*:2r.12–13)

(52) twies in a day ther of in
      the ey3e {.s.} erly at morwe and late at euene (*H513*:8v.18–19)

(53) And the {3ᵉ·} humours were y sey (*H513*:28r.8)

(54) lactuce acorie basiliconis {ana. ℥ .1.} alle (*H513*:22r.8)

Another function displayed at phrasal level is to relate the different components of a phrase (mostly the determiner and the noun head within noun phrases), performed by the period (82×), as in (55). The paragraph mark is employed in this way only twice, as in (56):

(55) putte theron {a·litill} pilwe of lynnen
 clothe and bynde it well with {a·clothe} (*H513*:30v.8–9)

(56) we token {a ¶ Rasour} and we kutte (*H513*:25r.14)

4. Conclusions

A number of conclusions can be drawn from the individual study of the punctuation systems displayed by *H503* and *H513*:

FIRST. The number of punctuation marks found in *H503* is outstandingly higher than that in *H513*, although the range of symbols is more reduced. Although the punctuation of *H503* may seem at first chaotic and somewhat random (much more than that in *H513*), the research carried out has allowed for the finding of a certain regularity in the functions that punctuation fulfils in this text, despite the overlapping of marks and a lack of total consistency in the use of punctuation symbols. As for *H513*, overlapping does exist, as with *H503*, although again there is regularity in the functions displayed by punctuation signs.

If we delve more into the system of *H503*, it can be observed that the paragraph mark never appears isolated, but rather in conjunction with the period, even if they appear on different lines. It might be speculated, hence, that the period was here intended as a mark for the rubricator to insert a paragraph mark, as they appear so close as to be barely distinguished in some instances of penwork surrounding the paragraph mark.

As regards *H513* (see 3.2) and already explained in Marqués/ Miranda/González (2008: 40), double virgules also seem to act as an indication for the rubricator to insert a coloured paragraph mark, rather than constitute an altogether different sign. Examples (36) and (39), where a faint double virgule is still perceived, may be used as examples of this.

Table 1 below shows graphically which marks are used for each function in each manuscript, along with their corresponding frequencies. If no mark is found for a particular function, then the symbol ∅ is employed:

LEVEL	FUNCTION	H503	H513
Macro-textual	To indicate a new paragraph	.¶ (39×) . (16×)	∅
	To mark the end of chapter titles	. (4×)	. (16×)
	To mark the end of a chapter	∅	·/· (21×)
	To indicate names of relevant authorities, technical terms, etc.	. (188×)	∅
	To indicate relevant medical information	.¶ (19×) . (19×)	¶ (207×) . (13×) / (9×) // (7×)
	To indicate that a conclusion or explanation follows	. (48×) .¶ (10×)	¶ (12×) / (5×) . (4×) // (1×)
	To indicate parenthetical comments	. (59×)	/ (2×)
	To add an element to an enumeration	∅	¶ (27×) / (1×) // (1×)
Sentential	To mark off independent sentences	. (173×) .¶ (13×)	/ (21×) ¶ (8×) // (6×)
	To mark juxtaposition	. (31×)	∅
	To mark coordinate clauses	. (388×) .¶ (1×)	/ (25×) ¶ (12×) . (4×)
	To mark off main and subordinate clauses	. (337×) .¶ (3×)	. (20×) / (13×) ¶ (8×)

		. (193×)	. (4×)
	To relate clause components	.¶ (1×)	¶ (1×)
	To relate particles of correlative expressions	. (3×)	∅
Clausal	To coordinate phrases	. (138×)	/ (4×) . (1×)
	To enumerate phrases	. (22×)	/ (1×)
	To mark off vocatives	. (5×)	∅
	To indicate that the following subject repeats the previous idea	. (2×)	∅
Phrasal	To mark off numerals and abbreviations	. (99×)	. (269×)
	To relate phrase components	. (24×)	. (82×) ¶ (2×)
	To coordinate phrase constituents	. (22×)	∅

Table 1. Punctuation inventories and functions in *H503* and *H513*.

As shown in Table 1, in both manuscripts a certain hierarchy can be observed regarding the uses of particular punctuation marks; for instance, paragraph marks rarely appear at clausal or phrasal levels, whereas the period is used for all kinds of functions at all levels, especially in *H503*. At the same time, it becomes evident that there exists a certain overlap in the uses of the specific symbols, although the attempt on the part of the scribes to mark various types of syntactic relations can be also appreciated. As a matter of fact, the range of functions signalled by punctuation in *H503* is wider than that in *H513*, especially concerning the clause and phrase domains. Yet, *H503* seems to be more concerned about marking gramatical relations at sentential level, whereas *H513* focuses more on the macro-textual and phrasal levels.

SECOND. Despite the differences regarding the inventory of punctuation marks and the particular uses that each of them performs, the general function that punctuation fulfils in both manuscripts remains the same, as the symbols mark grammatical relations rather than contribute to a meaningful oral delivery. Yet, these marks primarily show a macro-textual function (along with the grammatical one), since marking chapter titles, important concepts (especially medical terms, such as names of substances or preparations), names of authorities, etc. implies a deep concern on the part of the author / scribes for the specialised content of the treatises. Likewise, it also reveals an interest in the correct reception of the information by the recipients of the text, medical practitioners in need of manuals to check remedies, courses of treatment and so on to heal their patients.

Moreover, in the case of *H503*, the use of colour (i.e. rubrications) and of decorated initials (including gilding) contributes to the macro-textual function of punctuation, insofar as new sections, names of authorities or of parts of the body are visually highlighted on the page.

THIRD. The present research has also shown that the same text may feature several punctuation systems (that is, different signs and different functions) according to the copy in which it is found. In other words, punctuation appears in these cases as a scribal fingerprint, rather than an authorial trait. This might also be connected to the quality of the manuscript. On the one hand, *H503* seems to be a much more polished copy, probably intended for display rather than for being carried and consulted by the medical practitioner, as evinced by the use of gilding and colour to decorate initials, of line-fillers and of a clear handwriting which are features that point out to the high-quality of the manuscript. On the other, *H513* shows a cursive script and a partial concern for colour as an organising device.

Laura Esteban-Segura

Syntactic Aspects of MSS Hunter 503 and 513: Relatives and Negation[1]

1. Introduction

The present contribution deals with two syntactic features from the Middle English copies of Benvenutus's work contained in Glasgow, Glasgow University Library, MSS Hunter 503 and 513 (*H503* and *H513* hereafter). The approach followed takes into consideration those aspects which are a source of divergence, that is, attention is paid to noteworthy differences between the texts. It begins with a discussion of relative clauses, focusing mainly on the relative markers employed in each of them. Although variation in the choice of relativizers in the English language has been a widely researched topic, quantitative diachronic studies have been exclusively centred on the history of the modern relative system, with a resulting examination of data from the Early Modern period onwards (Dekeyser 1984; Ball 1996; Lezcano 1996).

Different ways to convey negation in the texts are analysed next. The study of negative constructions in Middle English from a syntactic and sentential point of view has also been tackled using quantitative methods (Frisch 1997; van Kemenade 2000; Iyeiri 2001) and with a diachronic perspective in mind (Tieken-Boon van Ostade/Tottie/van der Wurff 1999; Iyeiri 2005).

This paper does not claim to provide an exhaustive syntactic description of relatives and negation; the aim, as mentioned before, is to give an account of the most significant aspects on which the two

---

[1] The present research has been funded by the Spanish Ministry of Education (project FFI2008-02336). This grant is hereby gratefully acknowledged.

texts differ, an objective which has motivated the selection of these two specific areas, since syntactic changes are particularly easier to find in them. The variation of linguistic issues is also reflected in non-linguistic dimensions, such as the geographical and chronological ones, for "texts from different areas are different, and later texts differ very markedly from earlier ones" (Milroy 1992: 156). By contrasting two versions of the same text, these types of diversity will be very likely accounted for.[2]

The analysis of data is quantitative in the sense that frequency of each occurrence of the words and structures concerned is checked. In order to do this, the texts have been previously transcribed, lemmatized and morphologically tagged,[3] a process which has allowed the retrieval of figures for examination and contrast purposes.

2. Relative clauses

In Present-Day English, two parameters are associated to the choice of relative marker (*who*, *which*, *that*), namely the animacy parameter and the 'information' parameter (Fischer 1992: 295). The former refers to whether the antecedent is personal or inanimate (*who* and *that* if personal, *which* and *that* otherwise), whereas the latter distinguishes between restrictive (defining) and non-restrictive (non-defining) clauses, depending on whether the information provided about the antecedent is essential (restrictive) or additional (non-restrictive). The relative marker which shows a greater difference of usage in *H503* and *H513* is *which*.[4]

---

2   The dialectal provenance of MSS Hunter 503 and 513 has been analysed by Moreno Olalla (2006) and Marqués Aguado (2009a) respectively. For discussion of dates of composition, see Calle Martín in this volume.

3   The tasks of transcription, lemmatization and morphological tagging have been carried out by Moreno Olalla (*H503*) and Marqués Aguado (*H513*). The stages of this work are explained in Moreno Olalla/Miranda García (2009).

4   Due to multiple spelling variants, the form in Present-Day English is employed when referring to pronouns, adjectives and prepositions in general; this form represents, accordingly, all the possible spellings.

In *H513* there are 44 instances of *which* as a relative pronoun; of them, 40 are preceded by the definite article *the*. The combination *the which* spread from the north, where it first occurred at the beginning of the fourteenth century, towards the south throughout that century (Fischer 1992: 303). According to this scholar, it typically introduces a non-restrictive clause, being more common for its antecedent to be inanimate rather than animate and to be frequently placed at some distance from the relative. Reuter (1937: 158, 161) explains that "*the* is to be regarded as a kind of demonstrative used to emphasize the antecedent and at the same time pointing to the following relative clause". Therefore, the two elements (*the* and *which*) "were regarded as forming together a unit, functioning as a relative but preserving some demonstrative force". The origin of *the which* has generally been ascribed to French influence, corresponding to Old French *liquels*; however, the analogy of the construction with the Old English composite relative *se þe*, as well as other syntactic features, has led some scholars to reject the theory of French influence and to consider it a native development instead (see Reuter 1937).

The examples provided hereafter on *the which* show that the clauses containing this structure are generally non-restrictive, since the information given is additional. They also confirm that the antecedent tends to be inanimate (cf. examples (8), (18) and (19)). However, although the structure is separated from its antecedent in several cases, the general rule is for *the which* to follow right after it (cf. Reuter 1937: 173–176).[5] Examples (1)–(8) illustrate the usage of *(the) which* in *H513*.

(1) ... all these sotilliche shull be grounde to right sotill poudre and with a sotill sarce hem ontaken olibanum **the whiche** shall be ysoden in good clene skemed hony... (*H513*:18v.8–11)

---

5 Fischer (1992: 303), following Curme (1912) and Reuter (1937), argues that *the* in *the which* developed from an Old English demonstrative and this may explain the fact that *the which* "occurs in Middle English in places where there was need for a relative capable of recalling the antecedent more strongly, i.e. in non-restrictive clauses, particularly in clauses separated from their antecedents".

(2)　Also the gumme dothe of soure plumme treis **the whiche** growen amonge vyne treis (*H513*:34r.21–22)

Which is also found – following Mossé's terminology (1952: 62) – as an adjective and, when functioning as such, all the instances, which amount to 5, are accompanied by *the*:

(3)　... and by the myddell of the ei3e ther is an hole **the whiche** hole is saide pupilla anglice. (*H513*:2r.21–22)

(4)　... of these 3ucre candi of Alisaunder we make poudre nabatis ¶ **The whiche** poudre doithe many grete merueiles to the pannicles of the ey3en... (*H513*:13v.21–14r. 1)

A preposition is encountered before the construction *the which* in 8 instances (*of* in 6 and *by* in 2) when working as a pronoun, as shown in examples (5) and (6), and in 2 instances (with prepositions *in* and *of*) when it is an adjective, as in (7).

(5)　Of the thre maner of kyndes that be vncurable of cataractis **of the whiche** maystirs of saleren clepen guttum cerenam anglice a · shere goute (*H513*:7r.15–17)

(6)　the appell of the ey3e **bi the whiche** the visible spirite comyng by þe holwe nerffe hathe his outegoyng and takethe lyght of a · grete clerete (*H513*:2r.22–2v.1)

(7)　... and therfor the ey3en ben made white in soche maner þat neuer efte may come ayene to her former helþe ¶ **In the whiche** maner humours of the ey3en ben dissoluid for her grete anguysshe and sorowe and for her contrarie medicynes (*H513*:10r.6–11)

While the information parameter is always complied with (*which* is the relativizer employed in non-restrictive clauses having an inanimate antecedent), there is an instance in which the animacy parameter is overruled, since *which*, as can be seen in (8), makes reference to a personal antecedent.

(8)　And whiles he lyethe vpryght with the medecine for that houre after thou shalt see wonder and meruelous thing ¶ That **the pacient the whiche** myght afore this medicyne nought slepe ne reste anone ryght he shall begynne to reste and to slepe for his penaunce (*H513*:9v.12–17)

In *H503*, there are 63 instances of *which* as a relative pronoun, but only 6 of them are preceded by *the*. The presence (or absence) of the definite article does not change the type of clause, which is non-restrictive:

(9) and oþer dyuerse dyseasis . **whych** shald be declaryd hereafter . thei grow rather þan yn oþer maner of eyene colourid. (*H503*:6.10–13)

(10) Fyrst the stomake and the brayn must be porged wyth oure pelatis of comforth . **whych** are made on thys wyse. (*H503*:76.11–14)

(11) But yn þem that haue þer humurs depedowne **the whych** causyth the ey to seme blak as I sayd before better þan oþer seyn. (*H503*:8.4–7)

With regards to *which* as an adjective, in this text there are 16 instances, 2 of which are preceded by the definite article:

(12) Thys spyce of Cateractis is as the aucter seyth easely and sone cured . but yit þei þat ben cured seene not ryght wele for as much as the humor yn the eye ys yn party dysgregat and dyssoluyd by the stroke . and be bruser therof . **whych** stroke was cause of the Cateractis. (*H503*:20.12–21.4)

(13) And entitled thys boke . and clepid it, Deus oculorum . Of the **which** boke yn the fyrst Chapitre he declarith what ane eye ys. (*H503*:1.13–16)

Restrictive and non-restrictive clauses are formally distinguished in Present-Day English by a break in intonation, which is indicated in writing by the use of a comma. It is remarkable to point out that in *H503*, a punctuation mark is employed before the relative pronoun (*which* and *the which*), or the construction preposition plus relative pronoun, on 47 occasions (period, 45 instances; comma, 2 instances) to mark the relative clause. A period appears before the relative particle (which may be preceded by a preposition) when it functions as an adjective in all the instances. In *H513*, the only punctuation mark found before the relative is the paragraph mark, which occurs in 3 instances, in 2 of which a preposition precedes.

As for prepositions, they forego relative constructions in 8 cases (*of*, 5 instances; *in*, 2; *among*, 1) when they include a pronoun (examples (14) and (15)), and in 10 instances (*of*, 4; *in*, 3; *after*, 1; *to*, 1; *with*, 1) when an adjective is used instead (examples (16) and (17)).

(14) And lyke as blode arne gendryd obtalmyes and pannycles . ry3te so by occasyon of flewme arne gendrid oþer dyuerse sekenes . and specyally . iiij . **Of whych** the fyrst ys habundance of terys. (*H503*:50.2–8)

(15) and with thys ryght vertuous medycyne many one haue I cured and holpen . men . women . and chyldren . yn dyuers placys . **Amonge whych** yn a cetee callyd . Messana . was brought to me a chylde whos eye was oute yn the myddys. (*H503*:99.4–11)

(16) And thys Incysionn or kuttyng shal be but oonly þorugh the skyn in lenghtwyse . **In whych** yncysion . put the grane of a fecche . (*H503*:107.3–6)

(17) And thys sekenes ys gendred of superhabundance of salt flewme . **To whych** sekenes . do thys cure fyrst . 3e must pourge the stomake and the brayn of the pacyent . with þis resceyte . (*H503*:60.1–5)

Regarding the animacy parameter, in the case of *H503*, it is also flouted on two occasions with pronouns, as reference is made to personal subject antecedents, as shown in (18) and (19), and none with adjectives.

(18) Thys sayd lectuarye ys not oonly good for thys sekenes . but also for all **tho whych** see not clerely . but haue yn maner a myste yn þer eyon. (*H503*:75.3–6)

(19) Benuemicius . spekyth to hys dysciplis concludyng thus . O 3e my **dyscyples whych** wyll be practysers yn cures off sore eyon. (*H503*:135.11–14)

In most cases, *which* and *the which* occupy subject position; this fact does not seem to be significant in the choice of one or the other structure. As for the relation with the antecedent, this usually appears next to both relative markers, but *the which* is also found in continuative relative clauses, i.e. relative clauses that are loosely linked to what precedes them and frequently function as a summing up of ideas, whereas *which* is not found in this context.[6] It has been remarked that, as a consequence, the structure *the which* is more common in texts of a didactic nature, as this type of texts often employ non-restrictive and continuative clauses (Fischer 1992: 304). This holds especially true for the two texts under study, since they are medical treatises whose main purpose is the transmission of knowledge. An example of a continuative relative clause is supplied in (20) where *the which* refers back to "cauterye".

(20) And the cure of it is this ffirst late shaue all his hede and with a longe cauterye as we haue ysaide in oure cauterijs do to hym **the whiche** y do putte into his ey3e of oure poudre of Alisaunder onys in the day till the pacient take is sight at the ffull... (*H513*:16r.21–16v.3)

There is yet another notable aspect on which the texts differ. In *H513*, two relative markers, *(the) which* and *that*, occur together. There are two instances of *the which that*, as illustrated in (21) and one of *which that*, example (22), whereas none is present in *H503*. This co-occurrence is ungrammatical in Present-Day English, but normal all through the Middle English period, especially in poetry, where it was a useful metrical device. The combination became infrequent by the end of the fifteenth century (Fischer 1992: 302–303), and this decline is seen in the scarce number of instances found in the text. Fischer also indicates that, as opposed to *which that*, *the which* is more recurrent in prose, particularly in the fifteenth century.

A possible explanation for the use of *(the) which that* in *H513* might be a wish to place more emphasis on the relative meaning of the clause, where *(the) which* is felt to reinforce the antecedent and *that* to properly introduce the relative construction.

(21) ... and that with our cure **the whiche that** folwithe neuer after it worthe helpen ne cured at the full that they euer shall see wele after (*H513*:12r.13–16)

(22) Of coliries of diuerse infirmite3 in the ey3en Go we nowe to coleries for diuerse infirmitees **whiche that** fallen into the ey3eliddes that otherwhile defenden

---

6 Note that in Present-Day English *which* is usually the preferred relative pronoun when complex phrases or clauses are interposed between the antecedent and the relative pronoun (Quirk *et al*. 1985: 1252).

lyght and wasten the tonicles and they suffren nought the pacient to haue reste (*H513*:36v.10–15)

In the rest of instances in both texts, the relative marker *that* appears alone. The development by means of which this relativizer became confined to restrictive clauses started in Middle English, although it came about mainly in later periods (Fischer *et al.* 2000: 91). The use of *that* with restrictive clauses can be ascertained from evidence taken from the texts analysed, as most of the instances are of this type:

(23) And þerfore yf colerie be made wyth wyne and be put yn the eye **that** hath a webbe . the pacyent shall neuer be hoole . nor holpyn þerewyth . but rather and appayred. (*H503*:134.1–6)

(24) But many apostomys **that** me clepun obtolmeys comon in soche eiȝe more than in any othir eyȝen (*H513*:3r.2–4)

One point of agreement between the two texts is the fact that prepositions are not found in front of the relative particle *that*,[7] the relative *(the) which* is preferred for this, as it has been described above.

3. Negative constructions

Sentential negation in Old and Middle English is to a large extent indicated by preverbal *ne* right before the finite verb (van Kemenade 1999: 148). This typical practice of negating a verb by placing *ne* (or

---

[7] It seems that the inability of *that* to take a preposition in front of it assisted in the rising of WH-forms, as the latter did allow to be preceded by prepositions (Fischer 1992: 300). In Old English, the dominant pattern is *that* (*þæt*) followed by prepositions, although there are occasional examples in which they appear before (Mitchell 1985: 153–154). The Middle English trend continues in Present-Day English: *that* cannot be preceded by a preposition – WH-pronouns are used instead – and, as in the previous periods, *that* can be the complement of a preposition only if postposition with deferred preposition takes place (Quirk *et al.* 1985: 1252–1253).

no/na) directly in front of it continued throughout the period. In order to reinforce the negative, another negative word could be found along with *ne* in the sentence, being the commonest *nouʒt*[8] (Burrow/Turville-Petre 1996: 52–53). The occurrence of two or more negative particles is known as multiple negation or negative concord. Negation is conveyed by means of preverbal *ne* together with *nouʒt* in *H513* on four occasions, an example of which is shown in (25).

(25) Wherfor knowe that this **ne** fallethe **nouʒt** but hem in whom that colre hathe dominioun vpon (*H513*:19v.18–20)

Nevertheless, *ne* is more commonly employed in *H513* as a connector in coordinate or correlative constructions (26 instances), in which both the initial and the second clause are negative:

(26) ... Of diuerse restoryng of lyght after dyuerse kyndes of cataractes for why they be **nouʒt** euen **ne** parfitely yseyn as thus verbi gracia (*H513*:6v.14–17)

(27) ... ffor the forsaid paniclos they helpen and **neuer** offenden **ne** trespassyn (*H513*:34v.1–3)

No instance of *ne* is encountered in *H503*, where the usual negator is *not* (*nat*) with 87 occurrences. This particle alone negates the verb following it, the common practice from the fourteenth century onwards (Burrow/Turville-Petre 1996: 53). Two examples are provided as illustration of this usage:

(28) And also yt ys rownder . wherfore yt may **not** be leyd ryghtdowne yn the ey . (*H503*:25.2–4)

(29) And wyth a rasur cutt it so discretly þat ȝe touché **not** . the parte of the eylede that the here growyth . (*H503*:91.13–92.1)

In *H513*, *not* (*nat*) is sparingly found (9 occurrences), whereas *nought* (*nouʒt, naught*, etc.) is much more frequent (100 occurrences):

---

8 Spelling variant of *not* (also *noht, noʒt, nauht, nawht*, etc.), termed "reinforcing negator" by Fischer *et al.* (2000: 314).

(30) And Also whan thou haste putte that nedyll in the ey3e thou shalt **not** drawe her oute till the cataracte be all ygadered as it is said aboue (*H513*:5v.15–18)

(31) Wherfor vnkunning leches and foles that knowen **nought** that place Where that rothed comethe out and... (*H513*:30r.10–11)

(32) ... and they suffren **nought** the pacient to haue reste (*H513*:36v.14–15)

The negative elements employed in coordinate negative constructions also differ in the two texts. In 503, there are 24 instances of *nor* as a constituent (examples (33) and (34)), whereas no instance of this particle occurs in *H513*.

(33) And abstene he from commenyng of women . **nor** let nat hym com in no bath **nor** stew and yff he wyll algattis bath hym . (*H503*:24.1–4)

(34) wherfore yf 3e wyll not dysteyne your name **nor** hurt your pacyentis in cure of thys maner of fystyl . leue thys foreseyd lewde craft . (*H503*:106.4–8)

Neither, on the other hand, is found in both texts:

(35) and hir syght is not right goode, **neþer** yn yowgth nor age . (*H503*:6.15–7.2)

(36) The ffirste it makethe the pacient to resten nyght and day from ache As though he hadde none spot **neither** webbe ne penaunce in his ey3e ·/· (*H513*:25r.3–6)

Negation can also be expressed by means of indefinite pronouns: *nothing* is employed on one occasion in each of the texts. The difference is that in *H513* another negative particle precedes the pronoun, whereas in *H503* it negates the clause on its own:

(37) ... and none blake ys ther yseyn **neyþer nothinge** of the tonicle of the ey3en neither of the sight (*H513*:14r.17–18)

(38) for it shuld **nothyng** avayle . (*H503*:56.1–2)

Adverbs such as *never* or *no more* are also found in both texts to express negation but, in this case, the usage is similar; multiple negation is not attested, since the adverb does not appear combined with other particles:

(39) ... and therfore yiff þer be yputte a collerie ymade with wyne on a webbe of the ey3e the pacient shall **neuer** haue his sight (*H513*:37r.20–22)

(40) the concaue or the holow synewys be so stoppyd and ouerlayd . that the vysyble spiryte may **nomore** passe downe by them. (*H503*:29.2–5)

4. Conclusions

From the analysis carried out, several conclusions about syntactic differences between the texts *H503* and *H513* have been reached. The first issue tackled, that concerning relatives, indicates a variation in the number of clauses employing the pronouns *which* and *the which*. Even though both structures are employed in Middle English – wh-relatives (*(the) which (that)*, *whom*, *whose*) were used from the beginning of the Middle English period, although they became truly frequent in the early Modern English period (Fischer/van der Wurff 2006: 128) – *H503* prefers to employ *which* without the article, whereas *H513* favours the construction *the which*. The explanation for this may lie in scribal practice, as the combination *the which* was preferred by some writers (Burrow/Turville-Petre 1996: 44), but dialectal provenance could also justify the selection of one or the other. Concerning this last point, the occurrence or absence of *the which* has been taken by some scholars as an indicator of the place of origin of a text (see Reuter 1937: 151).

The restriction on the use of *that* for restrictive relative clauses is said to have become felt to some extent in later Middle English, although without any clear-cut rule (Mustanoja 1960: 197); the use of *that* for restrictive relative clauses and of *(the) which* for non-restrictive is generally consistent in both *H503* and *H513*. This may be valuable evidence to prove that the regularising tendency to confine the use of *that* to restrictive clauses was well under way in the period (cf. Lezcano 1996: 66), as well as to demonstrate that non-restrictive relatives favour WH-forms, a preference similar in standard Present-Day English (Quirk et al. 1985: 1257).

Another type of constraint is that imposed by the type of antecedent, whether animate or inanimate, which can explain the choice of relative marker. In both *H503* and *H513*, *(the) which* has, but for a few exceptions, non-personal antecedents, in accordance with the animacy parameter discussed. Although *which* is common as an alternative to *that* in later Middle English for both animate and inanimate antecedents (Burrow/Turville-Petre 1996: 44; see also Fischer 1992: 297), the development of *which* as a relative marker referring back to inanimate antecedents seems to have already started.

Punctuation is a further aspect in which the texts are at variance, this having to do mainly with the inclusion of a punctuation mark in order to signal a relative clause. Punctuation marks before relative constructions (*the which* and *which*) are almost non-existent in *H513*, whereas in *H503* the insertion of a mark therein is the normal practice. A deep analysis of the punctuation system employed in each of texts is undertaken by Marqués Aguado elsewhere in this volume and, although it is customary for manuscripts to present a different system and inventory of symbols depending on factors such as scribal practice, the use of punctuation marks before relativizers can denote awareness on the part of the scribe of the presence of a non-restrictive clause and the means to indicate it accordingly.

Syntactic features can provide clues to help date and locate the texts. Thus, the absence of the negator *ne* and multiple negation at sentence level in *H503* may suggest a later date of composition of this text to that of *H513*, since *ne* starts to disappear in the course of the Middle English period, thus accelerating the decline of multiple negation (Fischer 1992: 283). The employment of *ne* for negating the main verb in *H513* is not high, which may be proof that it was being dropped; the fact that it still appears (together with multiple negation), however, can indicate a less developed stage of the language in that text or else imply a south-eastern origin.[9] On the other hand, the absence of *ne* in *H503* could be a sign that it was, as it has just been argued, later composed or from a different geographical area.

---

9   In Late Middle English *no(gh)t* had become the rule, but there were some texts from the south-eastern region in which the combination *ne* ... *not* was still often used (Fischer 1992: 281); see also Ingham (2006).

Alejandro Alcaraz Sintes

A Textual Analysis of MSS Hunter 503 and 513[1]

1. Introduction

This essay is a textual analysis of Glasgow, GUL, Hunter MS 503, pp. 1–135 and Glasgow, GUL, Hunter MS 513, ff. 2r–37r (*H503* and *H513* henceforward), more specifically of their Thematic structures.[2] The analysis is conducted at various levels: clause, sentence, paragraph, and whole text. The theoretical tenets on which it rests are summarized in section 1.1. This is followed by a brief description of the two texts under analysis. Section 2 is devoted to the analysis proper. We move from a description of the Thematic structure of the work as a whole, through major and minor-sections, down to sentences and clauses. In section 3, we illustrate meaning reference chains and grammatical complexity in Themes and Rhemes in two types of sections in *H513*. Finally, conclusions are presented in section 4, followed by the References.

1.1. Textual meaning

One of the meaning components of clauses in Systemic Functional Linguistics is *textual meaning*. This meaning is conveyed basically by the manner in which a clause is organized or configured as a message, that is, the Theme system of the clause. This system is made up of

---

1   The present research has been funded by the Spanish Ministry of Education (project FFI2008-02336). This grant is hereby gratefully acknowledged.
2   For our analysis we have used the annotated editions of *H513* and *H503* in this volume.

two components, the *Theme* and the *Rheme*. Semantically, the Theme is the point of departure for the message, while the Rheme is usually the new information about this point of departure (see Eggins 2004: 296). To organize a clause thematically is simply to decide how to package the information so that it fits the purpose and context of the text (*ibid*: 298). In other words, textual meaning is conveyed through the ordering of the clause's constituents. Therefore, structurally, the Theme is the constituent appearing first in the clause, while the Rheme is all other constituents placed after the Theme. Choosing what goes as Theme, the starting-point of the message (Halliday & Matthiessen 2004: 64), is most important from a communicative point of view, since it affects the meaning of the clause as a message. For example, the second clause in the clausal sequence *I bought a book. There are many illustrations in the book* is grammatically correct, and yet somehow unnatural. The listener or reader would have expected its starting-point to be *the book* or a pronoun referring to the book: ***The book/It*** *contains many illustrations.*[3] The reason for this is that speakers or writers normally move from what they know their listeners or writers are already familiar with (in our example, they would already know about the book, mentioned in the first clause) to what is new to them (the great number of illustrations). Therefore, the first constituent of the Clause, the Theme, normally contains known or given information.[4] This information, in the case of written texts, is easily retrievable from the immediately preceding context or, more generally, from previous textual material. The Rheme simply develops the point expressed in the Theme. To signal what is new, writers sequence the information "so that readers have the relevant background information in their attention as they read each new sentence" and "they tend to sequence the information presented in each sentence so that, where possible, the New information is placed

---

3   Or else *There are many illustrations in **it**,* avoiding the repetition of and focus on the noun.
4   Or *presuming* information, to use Fries's (2002: 122–3) term, that is, "participants whose identities are familiar to the audience." This contrasts with newsworthy information, or *presenting* information (*ibid.*), that is, information presented as new.

[...] toward the end of the clause, thus strengthening the correlation of New with Rheme" (Fries 2002: 125).

Up to three constituents may make up a clause's Theme. The most important one is that which conveys experiential meanings and refers to the processes, participants and circumstances involved, that is, those having to do with the Transitivity function.[5] These are called *topical Themes* (Eggins 2004: 301). For example, *travelling* in ***Travelling** is not expensive nowadays*. However, there are other words found in initial position which do not convey experiential meaning. For example, words that create structural cohesion by relating the clause to its context, such as conjunctions or conjuncts. These are *textual Themes* (Eggins 2004: 302). The word *but* in the following clause is a textual Theme: ***But** travelling is not expensive nowadays*. A second type of constituent that does not add to the propositional content of the message has to do with a Mood function. They are called *interpersonal Themes*.[6] The word *luckily* in *But,* ***luckily***, *travelling is not expensive nowadays* is an interpersonal Theme. Table 1 shows these three types of Themes.

	Theme		Rheme
Textual	*Interpersonal*	*Topical*	
But,	**luckily,**	**travelling**	*is not expensive nowadays.*

Table 1. A multiple Theme.

This example shows that all three types of Theme may be used in the same clause (multiple or complex Themes), but only the topical Theme is capable of ending or exhausting the Thematic stretch: whatever comes to its right is the Rheme (*is not expensive nowadays* in our example). Choosing what to place in initial position is not always an option. A textual Theme like *but* is structurally constrained to appear first, while others, such as *however*, are more mobile: **Travelling is not expensive **but**; **However**, travelling is not expensive; Travelling,* ***however***, *is not*

---

5   See Eggins (2004: 206 ff.).
6   See Eggins (2004: 141 ff.).

*expensive; Travelling is not expensive, **however**.*[7] The same holds for interpersonal Themes. Some are mobile: *luckily* in the above example may also be found in clause-final position, but operators in *yes/no*-questions must come first, as in ***Do** you like travelling?* It is, therefore, constituents expressing experiential meanings that are really the most mobile. Speakers can choose whether to use them as topical Themes or as part of the Rheme.

Normally the choice made by the language user is the *default* option, the most usual one according to the type of clause. In declarative mood clauses, the Theme is realized by the Subject, as in ***Books** are expensive*. In *yes/no*-questions, the Theme is the auxiliary and the Subject, as in ***Do you** like reading?* In *wh*-questions, it is the *wh*-element: ***What** did you buy?* In imperative mood clauses, it is the Predicator and the preceding auxiliary, if any: ***Come** here!*, ***Do sit** down!* All these are *unmarked Themes*. Any other experiential constituent chosen as Theme is an atypical or *marked Theme*, that is, a Theme which the user has selected for some communicative reason. Adverbials or Objects are the most usual constituents chosen for promotion to Theme. Table 2 illustrates this. In row **a**, *after lunch* has been fronted so that the clause is shaped optimally to allow progression from known to new information. In **b**, the speaker simply wishes to establish a contrast by emphasizing the element on which the contrast rests. It is these choices that make a text sound natural and hang together. The fronted elements do not provide new contents, but internal cohesion.[8]

---

7   In this last example, *however* has been made part of the Rheme.

8   When a marked experiential Theme precedes the Subject, a number of authors within Systemic-Functional linguistics consider that the Theme also includes the Subject. Since textual meaning is realized by Theme (given information) and Rheme (new information), the area between them should be seen as a continuum in which the Theme effect diminishes as it draws near the central section and the Rheme effect increases as it moves away from the centre. See Cummings (2005: 131).

	Previous clauses	Theme	Rheme
a	I took a day off and had lunch in a shopping centre.	**After lunch,**	*I went to the cinema.*
b	She wrote a novel and a play. The play is good, but	**the novel,**	*I still haven't read.*

Table 2. Marked Themes.

The Rheme, then, expresses the newsworthy part of a message, that which the writer wants to impress on the reader. For this reason, as Fries (2002: 126) argues, the content of the Rheme[9] correlates with "the goals of the text as whole, the goals of a text segment within those larger goals, and the goals of the sentence and the clause as well." For example, in a paragraph dealing with a problem and its solution, the problem will tend to be included in the Theme and the solution in the Rheme. The Theme will present different aspects of the problem or its causes, while the Rheme will deal with notions such as temporal order of the actions taken "to solve the problem" (*ibid.*).

Just as clauses have a textual meaning expressed through its Thematic structure, so do units larger than clauses, such as *clauses-complexes*, that is, a concatenation of clauses (Cummings 2005: 130; Eggins 2004: 314 ff.). The language user can start a sentence with a dependent or subordinate clause and finish with the main clause. The dependent clause acts as Theme to a sentence. Thematic expectations are thus created in the reader concerning the rest of the sentence: a dependent clause indicates that another clause follows. This is illustrated in Table 3.

	Theme	Rheme
CLAUSE	**After lunch,**	*I went to the cinema.*
SENTENCE	**After I had finished my lunch,**	

Table 3. Marked Theme at clause and sentence levels.

---

9 Or rather, the last constituent of the clause, which he calls *N-Rheme* and defines as that part of the clause that contains what is newsworthy, that is, what "the writer wants the reader to remember" (Fries 2002: 126).

Textual meaning is therefore expressed by the user's selection of Thematic patterns. These patterns depend to a great extent on the text's mode, that is, on where it stands in the continuum between a purely spoken interactive text and a purely written monologic text. For example, Themes in written texts contain more lenghty topical nominalizations and fewer interpersonal constituents than oral texts. Nominalizations of prior information become the points of departure, the Themes in the writer's next piece of information. Alternatively, dependent clauses may be used as topical Themes in clauses-complexes. They permit the writer to opt for another textual style, in which lexical density gives way to grammatical complexity. This use of fronted dependent clauses, instead of lexical nominalizations, is also quite common in written texts, but still allows the writer to keep them close to spoken language – see Eggins (2004: 323). The circumstancial elements susceptible of promotion to Theme usually convey time, place, manner, reason, contingency, concession and respect meanings. Table 4 illustrates this fronting of a time expression.

Previous clause: I had my wisdom tooth extracted.

	Theme	Rheme
NOMINALIZATION	**After the extraction,**	*the pain remained for some time.*
DEPENDENT CLAUSE	**After the tooth was extracted,**	

Table 4. Nominalizations and dependent clauses in (Marked) Themes.

The manner in which Themes succeed one another in a series of single clauses or in clauses-complexes also contributes significantly to the coherence of a text. There are three main types of Thematic progression patterns: *reiteration* (the same Theme is used in a number of clauses), *zig-zag* (an element in a clause's Rheme – or simply material from previous Themes and Rhemes in the same paragraph or text – is promoted to Theme in the next clause, and *multiple-Rheme* (each of a series of elements in a clause's Rheme is promoted to Theme in successive clauses). These patterns are summarized in Table 5. The

Theme reiteration pattern is used to keep the textual meaning well focused, particularly in short oral conversational texts, where the method of development is not planned beforehand. The other two patterns involving a Theme shift are more common in written monologic texts. The zig-zag pattern is often found in written texts, where it forwards the argument smoothly from given to new information, particularly through nominalizations and fronting of dependent clauses. Finally, the multiple-Rheme pattern is common in long expository texts, where it provides the "underlying organizing principle for a text, with both the zig-zag and Theme reiteration strategies being used for elaborating on each of the main Thematic points" (Eggins 2004: 325–6).

	Reiteration		Zig-zag		Multiple Rheme	
CLAUSE 1	Theme	Rheme	Theme	Rheme	Theme	Rheme1, Rheme 2
CLAUSE 2		Rheme	Theme	Rheme	Theme	Rheme
CLAUSE 3		Rheme	Theme	Rheme	Theme	Rheme

Table 5. Thematic progression patterns.

From what has just been said, it is understandable that the meaning of Theme has changed since Halliday's (1967: 212) original definition as "what is being talked about, the point of departure for the clause as a message". For Fries (1995: 55) the main function of Themes is precisely to structure a text. As Cummings (2005: 131) explains, within a "unitary stretch of text, successive clause and sentence Themes convey framing concepts for the texts." For Fries (2002: 120), the Theme is "a framework within which the Rheme […] can be interpreted." Depending on the Thematic progression pattern chosen, the Theme will convey local consistency or variation and development. Consistency explains the frequent correlation between Theme and given information. From a rhetorical point of view, the Themes are recurring *motifs* that help identify the field of a text or a part of a text.[10]

Just as these "waves of information" operate at clause and sentence level, they may also be seen in operation at higher level units. A paragraph may also have its own Thematic clause. (A *paragraph*, for our purposes here, is a portion of a text whose semantic contents have been discoursively announced by a sentence or clause acting as Theme – see Martin (1992: 271). This clause is the Hyper-Theme and allows the reader to predict what is likely to be found in the paragraph. Above that, an entire text may be headed by a Macro-Theme, which orients the overall expectations of the reader, as regards the whole text – see Martin (1992: 436 ff.) and Fries (2002: 120).

	Clause	Sentence	Paragraph/Short section	Work/Long section
TYPE OF THEME	Theme	Thematic clause	Hyper-Theme	Macro-Theme

Table 6. Themes at various text levels.

All these layers of textual structure (Clause Theme, Sentence Theme, Hyper-Theme and Macro-Theme) contribute to the textual meaning in different, but comparable, ways. Their function is basically to allow ideational and interpersonal meaning to be realized cohesively and coherently (Eggins 2004: 326).

Finally, as already pointed out, Themes tend to be consistent as regards the Field and thus they concentrate on a limited collection of objects, while Rhemes, because they express new points, tend to have more varied grammatical structures and greater lexical variation (Cummings 2005: 135–6). This is so because of the different functions Themes and Rhemes perform. There is no room in this chapter to present an in-depth quantitative analysis of the differences in the distribution

---

10 We are fully aware that this introduction is short and general, and scores of authors are missing. Starting with Aristotle's distinction between *onoma* and *rhema*, *hypokeimenon* and *kategoroumenon*, and their subsequent re-interpretations in the history of linguistics would have been beyond the purpose of our practical analysis and the scope of this book.

of forms and features between Themes and Rhemes in our two texts. However, a few observations will be made in section 3.

1.2. The medical treatises

Our two works are adapted translations from the same Latin medical work of the late ME period, a time when a double (or perhaps the same) development was under way. On the one hand, Latin was being replaced by the vernaculars in many areas of science, particularly in medicine and medical practical treatises such as these (Taavitsainen and Pahta 1997: 212–3). On the other hand, in the case of English, it was the period when the creation of a standard English was starting (Taavitsainen 2001: 196–8). This double development means that the English used in the works is still not modern or standard and that the syntax of the Latin original is often faithfully imitated.[11]

The two works contain several sections[12] which differ in contents and style. These differences are also found in the original, which was probably a conflation of various writings. Basically, the works have two types of sections. Some are more academic, such as the anatomical description of the eye, the physiology of the humours and the descriptions of the cataracts and other diseases, for example. These belong to a tradition of medical writing going back to ancient Greece. Other sections seem to derive from manuals for practising professionals, either surgeons or lay ophtalmologists or doctors, such as those dealing with surgical treatments and medicinal cures. The last section of the work, a short pharmacopoeia, looks almost like an appended work and, like the medicinal cures prescribed for each

---

[11] As, for example, the literal rendering of Latin absolute participles or resumptive relative pronouns. However, for practical purposes, no comparison of the English works with the presumed Latin original is attempted in this chapter.

[12] Misplaced sections or sections that are not exactly parallel in *H503* and *H513* are explained by Moreno Olalla in the Foreword.

disease, is similar to OE leechbooks[13] or even ME cookbooks.[14] These differences in contents and purpose between the various sections are also reflected linguistically. In the anatomo-physiological descriptions and explanations, which basically convey information, there are long periods, declarative clauses, subordination, and a Thematic organization that contributes to structuring the works, to organizing taxonomies and to developing the author's arguments smoothly. In the other more practical sections, though, where the author basically tells the readers what to do and how to proceed, we find many directives (imperatives and modals of obligation), shorter periods, but still the same type of Thematic organization to speed information processing by the reader, particularly as regards sequencing in medical protocol stages. However, within all types of sections we find a lot of variation or inconsistency in grammatical complexity and lexicalizations.

Throughout, the author addresses his readers at regular intervals, often by means of interpersonal vocative Themes. Even though he invests himself of authority from the beginning (he refers to the original author and work, to Greco-Roman and Muslim physicians, with all of whom he differs slightly at some point, and to his own successful experience), he does not look down on his readers. He uses emotive adjectives in the vocative phrases and shows concern about their professional and financial success, and reputation. More interesting linguistically is the use of the first person for the author and the second person for the reader, though with many departures from this norm, particularly in *H503*, as we shall see. All these create the effect of a dialogic text, even in the descriptive-explanatory sections. Yet, the treatises do not follow the scholastic tradition of turntaking discourse and deductive argumentation. Rather, they stand somewhere in the middle between monologic and dialogic texts, between formality and informality in this respect, and present arguments inductively and in an instructive form for a non-academic audience.

---

13   See Taavitsainen (2001: 188).
14   See Austin (1964).

2. Thematic organization

In this section we first describe the way in which the titles of the works and of the different sections, subsections, and paragraphs actually convey Themes, macro-Themes and Hyper-Themes. Then we take a closer look into the choice and progression patterns of Themes and Rhemes in the different types of sections, according to the linguistic functions they perform.

2.1. The title

The most important and succinct summary of a book's contents is the title, particularly if non-fictional, because it informs about what may be learned by reading it. This title simply points forward to what is very likely to be new information to the reader. However, neither *H503* nor *H513* are initiated by a title summarizing the whole contents of the work, although *H503* does contain an introductory sentence giving the name of the author and the title of the book, reproduced in example (1). The whole of this anticipatory sentence is to be considered as the text's Theme. Being placed at the very beginning of the work, this Theme contains no previously given information. At intrasentential level, the second clause is the Rheme, where the new information is to be found: first, the contents – *the sekenes of eyon* – and, second, the title of the book – *Deus oculorum*.

(1) A grete phylosopher and a profunde phycycyane clepid. Benuomicius Grapheus [...] compilyd and made a boke of the sekenes of eyon. and of her curys. And entituled thys boke. and clepid it, Deus oculorum. (*H503*:1.1–14)

2.2. Sections, subsections and macro-Themes

Each of the major sections in which the book is organized is introduced by its own Macro-Theme. However, this is achieved differently in the two works.[15] *H513* systematically gives a title to each section, but with no differences in the wording that might show where each section belongs in the hierarchy of levels. In *H503*, on the other hand, there are no titles,[16] but each section is signalled by two statements recapitulating and anticipating contents.[17] From a macrotextual or discursive point of view, these two statements act as a Macro-Theme for the following new section. Since they are syntactically expressed by means of a single sentence, the sentence may also be analyzed internally. Thus, at clause-complex level, the first clause is Thematic and recapitulates given (or inferred) information, while the second clause is Rhematic and anticipates the new information that follows.[18] The contents of this anticipatory Rhematic part is what actually corresponds to the title in *H513*, but the whole statement or sentence must be viewed as the Theme of the following section. Examples (2) and (3) illustrate this.

---

15   As explained in Marqués/Miranda/González (2008: 41–2), "this could be put down either to different scribes supplying different text organisations or to different textual traditions being involved."
16   With two or three exceptions: *H503*:50, 65–66 and 71, at the beginning of the sections on phlegm-, choler- and melancholy-related diseases.
17   At one point (blows on the forehead, brows, eyelids…), instead of an anticipatory segment, *H503* has a short summary of the section, for, as is explained in the text itself, the chapter was missing in the original Latin manuscript: "*But here it ys to be noted and vnderstonde that yn my latene apy lacked an hoole Chapytere. In whych tretys of hurtys taken aboute the eyon as by strokys of the forhede and the browys the ey lyddes. the boyth lacrymall. the temples. and such oþer of their cures*" (*H503:*102–103). This summary corresponds to a title in *H513*:29r.
18   See the sections on cataracts (*H503*:9 and *H513*:4r), humour-related diseases (*H503*:30 and *H513*:8r), phlegm-related diseases (*H503*:54, 55 and 59, and *H513*:16r, 16v and 17v), the second choler-related disease (*H503*:69 and *H513*:19v), all the melancholy-related diseases (*H503*:75, 79, 82, 85 and 92, and *H513*:21v, 22v, 23r, 32v and 16r), turned-up eyelids (*H503*:88–89 and *H513*:25r), stone chips lodged in the eye (*H503*:112–113 and *H513*:31r), awns lodged in the eye (*H503*:115–116 and *H513*:32v), insect bitings (*H503*:118 and *H513*:33r), the cure of the nebulae (*H503*:120 and *H513*:33v), other medicines for the nebulae (*H503*:123 and *H513*:34r) and advice on diet (*H503*:136).

	Theme	Rheme
(2)	Of the which boke yn the fyrst Chapitre	he declarith what ane eye ys. and the makyng þerof. (*H503*:1.14–16)
		Of tonicle of the ey3en and the humours and cataractus. (*H513*:2r.1–2)
(3)	In the fyrst partye of thys tretys [...] I declared to yow what ane eye is. And how it ys maid [...] And after yn the secunde partye I tau3t yow of the infirmitees of eyon that be caused Inwarde. by occasyon of distemperance of the iiij humers. þat ys to wyt. blode. Color. flewme. and malyncolye. and þeir cures.	And now yn thys thyrde partye and last of my tretys. I wyll tel yow of þies hurtis and diseases causyd yn eyon from wythouteward. as wyth smytyng of stekkys and stonys and staues. or ony such oþer. (*H503*:93.13–95.8)
		Of smytyng and hurtyng of þe ey3e and brekyng of the tunicle and the cure therof (*H513*:26v.18–20)

Table 7. Macro-Themes.

What is more, the macro-Themes are connected to one another in *H503*, notwithstanding the distance between them by means of a zig-zag Thematic progression pattern. The point expressed in the Rheme segment of one Macro-Theme is retaken, in an expanded form often, in the Theme segment of the next Macro-Theme, as in example (4) in Table 8.

	Theme	Rheme
(4)	Now after he hath tau3t what an eye is. and how it ys mayd. and of the colour and of the humors of eyon.	he consequently bygynneth to trete of the infirmytees of an ey. and after of the curys. And fyrst he begynnyth to trete of cateractis. (*H503*:9.4–11)
	Now after the doctryne and knowlege of Cateractis and the nombre of theme. and whych be curable. and whych nat. And the cures of the curable. and the knowlege of the causes of vncurable.	Now I wyll QUOD HE speke of oþer sekenes causyd and occasyonyd of the iiij humers. as blode. flewme. color. and malyncolye. (*H50*.30.5–14)

Table 8. A zig-zag macro-Theme.

At the next level down, that of sub-sections, *H503* uses short transitional passages (with internal Theme and Rheme), as in example (5).[19] *H513*, on the other hand, often repeats the point of the title in the very first text segment of the section, by way of Thematic summary or double macro-Theme. However, the title is often more specific than this summary: it may point forward to both the following section in general and the first sub-section in particular, as in example (6).[20]

(5) **Now I haue shewed quod he the knowlege of corrupt terys. wherof bene caused fystyllys. and the cures of them.** *Now I teche yow the verry knowlege of verry terys. and yn what place they veryly spryng.* (*H503*:110.5–11)

(6) TITLE: Of 4 sikenesse þat comeþ of flume and þe cure of þe first · ANTICIPATORY SEGMENT: Nowe in the name of criste begynne we of the sekenesse that comethe thorough the accasioun of fleume. (*H513*:15r.3–7)

2.3. Paragraphs and hyper-Themes

The usual way in which the lower sections, or paragraphs, as we defined them in section 1.1, begin is by means of a Thematic clause or sentence. This is the Hyper-Theme of the paragraph, its point of departure, as in (7) to (9).

(7) And now I wyl teche yow practysers a merveilous and a prescious lectuarye for the forsayd terys. (*H503*:63.2–4)[21]

(8) Off whych disease thys is the cure. (*H503*:85.5–6)

(9) thus sayth Johannicius; But. Benuomicius. varieth from hym in cotys and yn Colours. For as he seyth. an ey hath but ij tonycles or cotys. […] (*H503*:4.9–12)

---

19 Other similar passages may be found in *H503*:40, 112–113 and 130–131.
20 Other similar repeated Themes in *H513* are found at the beginning of the sections on choler-related diseases (19r), blows on the eye (26v and 27r, and *H503*:95), blows to the temples and lacrimals (29r and *H503*:102–3), blows to brows and nose and fistulas (29v and *H503*:103) and eye-drops (36v and *H503*:130–1).
21 See *H513*:18v for the equivalent segment.

In symmetrical relation to this, a paragraph may contain a Hyper-Rheme, that is, a summary of the new information conveyed in the central part of the paragraph. It is just a shorter rewording of the important new information, as in example (10). However, while the vast majority of paragraphs do have a Hyper-Theme, not many have a Hyper-Rheme.

(10) HYPER-THEME: **And lyke as blode arne gendryd obtalmyes and pannycles. ry3te so by occasyon of flewme arne gendrid oþer dyuerse sekenes. and specyally. iiij.** (*H503*:50.2–6)
RHEME: *for when the cristallyne humor ys nyght the tonycle of the ey. than the ey semyth of oone colour. And whane yt ys in the myddys. þan it semyth of another colour. and whene yt ys depe wythyn. þan it semyth of the iijde colour.*
HYPER-RHEME: ***wherof he concludyth þat the ey of ytselfe ys discolurd and hath no colurne propurly.*** (*H503*:5.6–14)

As we just saw in section 2.2, the Hyper-Themes or paragraph-Themes themselves contain a Theme and a Rheme, at both complex-clause or clause levels. The topical Theme is often preceded by a cohesive textual Theme, such as *and*, *now* or *here*, establishing the transition between the preceding material and what is to come.[22] Or else it is marked Theme, such as time or comparison clauses containing given information which thematically fits in frontmost position, as in (11) and (12).

(11) **thus þan bryefly shewid by this auctor what euery eye is.** *consequently he shewyth how an ey is made.* (*H503*:3.4–7)

(12) **And lyke as blode arne gendryd obtalmyes and pannycles.** *ry3te so by occasyon of flewme arne gendrid oþer dyuerse sekenes. and specyally. iiij.* (*H503*:50.2–6)

2.4. Themes and Rhemes

We have already seen in section 1.1 and in the analysis of examples so far that clauses normally start with *given* information and finish with *new* information, and the canonical *Theme + Rheme* structure tends to

---

22 But also indirectly pointing to this preceding material (*and* means "in addition to", *now* and *here* imply a *before* and a *there*).

coincide with the word-order *Subject* + *predication*, as shown in Table 9 (for declarative clauses).

Informative value	Given	New
Thematic structure	Theme	Rheme
Syntax	Subject	Verb, Object, Complement, Adverbial…

Table 9. Unmarked correlations.

This is not always the case and the writer very often departs from the unmarked syntax by fronting elements from elsewhere in the clause, thereby replacing the unmarked Theme (clause Subject) by a marked one (any other clause element), as in Table 10. In our texts this is almost always done in order to preserve *given* + *new* informative structure.[23] At the same time, of course, new information appears at the end. If the known information has been given in the Rheme of the immediately preceding clause, a Thematic progression is created which contributes to a smooth informative flow.

Informative value	Given	New
Thematic structure	Theme	Rheme
Syntax	Object, Complement, Adverbial…	Subject, Verb

Table 10. Marked correlations.

In this section we analyze the choice and progression of Themes and Rhemes and correlate them with the type of of language function in the different sections of the two medical treatises. The major linguistic functions observed are: **classifications**, **descriptions/definitions**, **explanations**, **directives**, **persuasion** and **meta-textual indications**.[24] Language used for these purposes may be found in any section in the

---

23 As Quirk *et al*. (1995: 1377–8) have also observed for Present-Day English.
24 This is an *ad-hoc* classification of functions serving our purposes for these two works.

works studied. For example, classifications are found in sections on anatomy, diseases or medicines. In general, the internal structure of each major section or chapter corresponds to these functions.

2.4.1. Classifications

Classifications are normally found at the beginning of each section, whether low or high in the internal hierarchical structure, particularly the anatomy of the eyes and the various subtypes within each type of disease. Depending on the object of classification, different methods are used. However, what all classifications have in common is the multiple-Rheme progression pattern, since no argumentation or explanations are developed. Once the taxonomy has been created, it is re-used as Theme in the sections or paragraphs on each individual item.

When the objects of classification constitute a closed set of items, such as the anatomical parts of the eye, we find, in both witnesses, a Thematic clause heading the taxonomy, as in (13). This is followed by second-level classifications observing a multiple-Rheme Thematic progression pattern, whether the Theme is unmarked (Subject) or marked (Object), as in examples (14) and (15) in Table 11.[25]

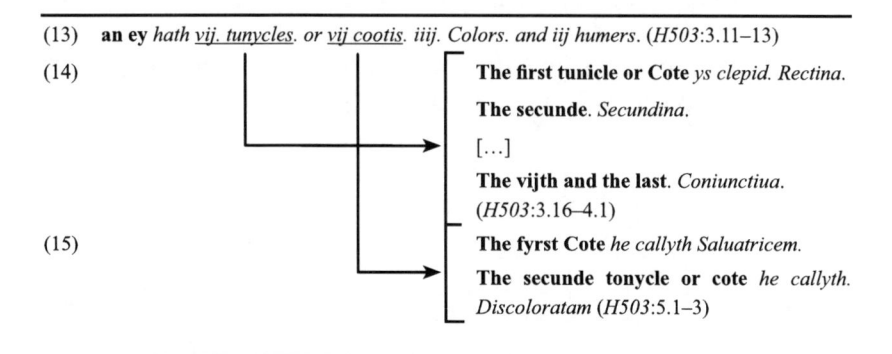

(13) **an ey** hath *vij. tunycles*. or *vij cootis*. *iiij. Colors*. and *iij humers*. (*H503*:3.11–13)

(14) **The first tunicle or Cote** *ys clepid. Rectina.*
The secunde. *Secundina.*
[...]
The vijth and the last. *Coniunctiua.*
(*H503*:3.16–4.1)

(15) **The fyrst Cote** *he callyth Saluatricem.*
The secunde tonycle or cote *he callyth. Discoloratam* (*H503*:5.1–3)

Table 11. Multiple-Rheme progression in classifications.

---

25   The equivalent segments in *H513* are in ff. 2r and 2v.

Classifications of diseases are presented differently in the two works. For example, in the section on cataracts[26], *H503* has an opening Thematic clause, as in (16). On the other hand, *H513* has a section title informing about the overall number (example (17)), followed by a short paragraph made of clauses informing about their colour. In either case the precise number of cataract types is stated. After that, both works continue with sections on each individual group and sub-group of cataracts, which in *H503* start with a Thematic clause, as in (18).

(16) **And of this maner of cateractis** *þer be vij. maner of dyuers spices.* **wherof.** *iiij. be curable. and. iij vncurable.* (*H503*:10.2–5)

(17) Of the · 7 · spicis and kyndes of catarractis · id est · of westis that ben in the ey3en (*H513*:4r.12–13)

(18) **And fyrst he tretyth of the iiij curable.** (*H503*:10.5–6)

When the object of classification is a set with an unspecified group of items, the structure is different from what we have seen. For example, *H503* does not say how many melancholy diseases there are, but *H513* does, whence (19) and (20). For this reason, the sections dealing with each individual type of melancholy disease start differently in each work. *H503* does not use ordinal numbers or thematically unmarked clauses, but rather existential and impersonal constructions with indefinite reference, as in (21) to (23), while *H513* does, as in (24) and (25).

(19) Off the Infyrmytees of Malencolye (*H503*:71.14–15)

(20) Of · 6 · infirmitees of malencoly and the cure of þe first (*H513*:20v.10–11)

(21) Ther ys also anoþer sekenes causyd of malyncolye. (*H503*:75.12–14)

---

26 The rationale for the taxonomy of cataracts is the aspect and presumed etiology. Other taxonomies are also created on account of the external symptoms of the disease and follow the same scheme, such as the types of panicles (*H503*:40 and *H513*:10v), phlegm diseases (*H503*:50 and *H513*:15r) or coler diseases (*H503*:66 and *H513*:18v–19r).

(22) Also superhabundance of the humor of malencolye is often gendryd yn the ey a dysease callyd. vngula. a nayle. (*H503*:79.6–9)

(23) It happyth sumtyme þat the malencolyous humor habundant yn the brayn [...] (*H503*:82.1–3)

(24) and we wolle tell you of the first (*H513*:20v.17–18)

(25) Secunde infirmite that comethe thorwe the accasioun of melancolie and we sayne that (*H513*:21v.15–16)

At the end of the treatises, in the short pharmacopoeia, medicines are broadly classified into two types, powders (ointments) and eye-drops. *H503* and *H513* differ sharply in this respect. *H503* has a Macro-Theme, whose Rhematic section presents a taxonomy of the different classes of medicines, as in (26), but *H513* has an apparently misleading section title which seems to refer to something altogether different, as in (27). However, the contents of the following sub-sections are the same. Each of the three broad sections in both treatises start with a macro-Theme, as in (28) and (29).

(26) Now here yn the laste ende of thys booke he techeth **generall medycyns**. and fyrst he techyth *powders*. and after *coleryous*. and fynally he techyth a general *dyatorye* for al maner of pacyentis (*H503*:120.10–15)

(27) Of þe cure of nebula þat is þe clowde in the ey3e (*H513*:33v.11)

(28) Fyrst as **towchyng powders**. (*H503*:121.1)

(29) Go we nowe to **coleries** for diuerse infirmitees (*H513*:36v.11)

As for the paragraphs describing each medicine, because there are so many of them in the pharmacopoeia, ordinals are not used in either MS. Instead, after the first item (example (30)), we find a list of clauses normally starting with summative conjuncts as textual Themes, particularly *also*, as in example (31),[27] which seems to function as an eye-catcher in a running text.[28]

(30) Fyrst as towchyng powders. I sey to yow. [...] that powder mayde of the margaryte. (*H503*:121.1-3)

(31) **Also** cristall sotylly powderd [...] **Also** a saphire powderd [...] **Also** powder of the berall [...] **Also** gumme of bitter almondis [...] And the bitter plumbes gumme. [...] **Also** take suger candy [...] **Also** take tutie of alexandre [...] **Also** take the strenys of eggis [...] **Also** take the dragons roote.[...] **Also** ane vnce of spyce callyd. Lignum aloes [...] **Also** the gall of a beste callyd. Castor [...] **Also** take the galle of a bere. [...] **Also** take the galle of an Eglee [...] **Also** the oyle of Olyfe [...] **Also** Jowus of a sowre crape [...] (*H503*:121.9-130.1)

2.4.2. Definitions, descriptions and explanations

Language used for descriptive purposes is mainly found in those sections dealing with the symptoms and etiology of diseases or injuries. These sections normally start with a description of the symptoms of the medical condition, continue with an explanation of the cause of the problem and derived consequences, and finish with a series of directives for treatment. As we shall see, the derived consequences are chained to one another, each being the cause of the next one. These concatenations are expressed lexico-syntactically (conjunctions and conjuncts) and very often thematically (a consequence found in a clause's Rheme re-appears as a cause in the next clause's Theme). This means that there is a clear progression from given to new information and that Themes, either marked or unmarked, unfalteringly point back to preceding material. Three broad patterns may be established as far as both Thematic choice and progression, and rhetorical structure are concerned.

■ **Pattern 1**. When diseases have been taxonomized and numbered from the beginning, Themes are unmarked, i.e., the clause element chosen as Theme is the Subject, which conveys known information. The clause is normally copulative, so that the Rheme conveying the

---

27 This example is made up of segments from different paragraphs.
28 *Also* corresponds very systematically to *Item* in the Latin source.

newsworthy information is a Complement. This Complement may be an adjective (example (32)), a prepositional phrase (example (33)) or a nominal relative clause (example (34)). In many cases, a result clause follows the Complement and informs about the final consequence. Example (34) illustrates the rhetorical structure "cause 1 > consequence 1 = cause 2 > consequence 2" (phlegm > troubled/venous eyes > deficient vision).[29]

(32) **The secunde cateractte curable** *ys sumwhat white.* (*H503*:10.11–12)

(33) **And the iiijth spice of cateracctis curable.** *ys of sytrynne color* [...] (*H503*:11.12–13)

(34) **The second sekenes cawsyd of flewme in the eyon.** *ys when þei appere trobled and ful of venys closed with a pannycle so that the pacyent may not wele se.* (*H503*:54.2–7)

(35) **Ther ys also anoþer sekenes causyd of malyncolye.** *and yt ys when the payne sodonly ascendyth ynto the eyon. and so greuousiely þat it semyth the eyon wolde stert out of theyr places. And þei aperyn passyngly bollen.* (*H503*:75.12–76.4)

Within this pattern may also be included descriptive paragraphs in which the original taxonomy is used to inform about the likelihood of success of the surgical and medicinal treatment. The topic is not the type of cataract, but the cure applied. Still, the unmarked Theme chosen refers to the type of cataract, not to the type of cure, as in example (36). For this reason, there are instances in which the Theme looks as if it is going to be the Subject, but turns out to be a marked one, an adjunct of respect, as in (37). The clause is ill-formed, for the Thematic NP performs no syntactic function in the clause and a preposition seems

---

29 This basic pattern may have variants: no consequence is expressed (*H503*:55, 70, and *H513*:16v, 18v), the consequence is repeated (*H503*:76–7), the result is conveyed by means of a coordinate clause (*and*) instead of a subordinate result clause (*so that*) (*H503*:70), or even two different causes are given for the same consequence (***The forth sekenes causyd of flewme yn the ey.*** *is when the eyon apere bolleyn. and be allweys wepyng. and the pacyent may not opyn hys eyon. for the ponderosyte and the heuynes of the ouerlyddys.* (*H503*:59; cf. *H513*:17v)).

to be missing.[30] A similar syntactic problem is also found in the section dealing on the vision quality that may be anticipated from the colour of the eyes, both in *H503*:6–8 and in *H513*:3r–3v). In example (38), from *H513*, the syntax is corrected once the sentence has started, by means of a repetition of the Thematic NP as a fronted Prepositional Phrase. In this and similar examples, it is clear that the writer attaches more importance to placing given contextualizing information in Thematic position, and therefore to facilitating the reading process, than to complying with the end-weight principle.[31] Complying with this principle would produce this clause: **But the syght lastethe longe tyme in tho that hauen her ey3en sumdell blake.*

(36) **Thys spyce of Cateractis** *is* [...] *easely and sone cured.*
 but yit þei þat ben cured *seene not ryght wele* (*H503*:20.12–15)

(37) **The secunde spyce of Cateractis curable**
 yf it be *welle cured with the nedyl as it is seyd before*
 the ly3te *turneth ayene to hys fyrst bryghnes.* (*H503*:21.4–7)

(38) **But tho that hauen her ey3en sumdell blake**
 in hem *the syght lastethe longe tyme* [...] (*H513*:3r.14–16)

■ **Pattern 2**. When diseases have not been taxonomized from the beginning, the Theme tends to be marked, a fronted adverbial referring to the origin or the ultimate cause of the disease. Since the Subject is the element conveying the new information, it is conveniently placed in Rhematic position by means of a passive or a *there*-existential construction. At left-most position there is often a textual Theme, e.g., an additive conjunct. Unlike pattern 1, the first consequence is not the cause of any subsequent ones. These other consequences originate in the same cause, expressed in the Theme. For this reason, the addition of further consequences is achieved through coordinate clauses or through

---

30 Another such instance of anacoluthon is found in *H503*:21–2. The equivalent segments in *H513* show similar syntactic, Thematic and rhetorical structures: see *H513*:3r.
31 Quirk *et al.* (1995: 1361–2).

relative postmodification of the Rhematic NP in the first consequence (*a sekenes, a corupte humor*), as in examples (39) and (40). In either case, the unmarked Subject Themes in the Rhematic part of the sentence refer to the preceding NP. In other words, the Theme is repeated and the Thematic progression is reiterative, as shown in Table 12.[32]

	Rheme		Thematic reiteration pattern
(39)	sekenes	→	that + it + it + it
(40)	corupte humor	→	whych + it

Table 12. Reiterative progression of Themes.

(39) **And also of the malencolyus humor quod the autor**
ther is gendrid yn many men <u>*a sekenes*</u>
that *growyth betwene the nose and the ey.*
and it *apperyth lyke the pece of a long.*
and it *grauelous and wydyth allway fylth.*
*and communly **it** towchyth withyn the ouereuelede. and also the neper.*
(*H503*:92.8–15)

(40) **Moreoure of such suprefluyte of malencolie.**
sumtyme þere grouyth <u>*a corupte humor*</u> *wythoute the eye betwyxte the place. where the here growyth. and the eyelydde.*
whych *bolnyth not oonly the eyelydde. but all the eye. wyth halfe the face.*
but it *hurtyth not the eye.* (*H503*:84.1–8)

A variant in this pattern is illustrated by example (41). Syntactically we find embedded consequences (*so...that* result clauses) and coordinated consequences. Also, right in the middle there is a marked Theme that re-uses given information and allows a new point of departure before the final consequence or new information is given. Finally, the correlation *when-then* also contributes to this zig-zag Thematic progression,

---

32 Again, the corresponding segments in *H513* (22v, 23v and 26r) are syntactically different at the beginning, but they basically coincide in the way the various consequences (not necessarily as many) are added to the first as coordinate clauses.

since Thematic *then* points back to the whole preceding Theme. It also triggers *Subject-Verb* inversion, which allows the long Subject to be placed rhematically and comply with the end-weight principle. The rhetorical structure is this: cause 1 > consequence 1 = cause 2 > consequence 2 = cause 3 > consequence 3 + consequence 4 + examples (abundant melancholy > brain disorder > blocking of the nerve > visible spirit cannot pass + polyopia).

(41) **sumtyme for the habundance of malencolye.**
the brayn ys so troublyd. þat the nerfe obtyk ys so opylate and stoppide. þat the vysyble spyryt may not passe the ryght wey.
And when thys nerfe. ys opylate and ouerleid.
þen aperen afore the pacyentis eyon. as yt were fleyng flyes yn the ayre on the day lyght. And of a lanterne of lyste. or of the moone. yt semyth þat yt were iiij. And yf he loke yn the face of a man. yt semyth to hym the same. (H503:72.5–73.3)

Within pattern 2 may also be included, on account of their Thematic progression pattern and rhetorical structure, a few paragraphs which belong to sections containing directives for surgical treatments. Occasionally the author explains why a certain procedure in the protocol should be followed. Again a zig-zag Thematic progression pattern is used, as in example (42). The topical Theme in this subordinate clause – *fire* – is unmarked and points back to the cauterization itself. In the second coordinate clause, there is a fronted manner adverbial – *by drawyng. dyssoluyng and consumyng* – placed topically since it is given information, a Thematic nominalization of the verbs in the previous clause's Rheme.

(42) make a Cauterye in the templys
for fire *drawyth and dissoluyth and conseruyth. and suffryth no pannycle to be Incarnate vpon the tonycle.*
And so by drawyng. dyssoluyng and consumyng by þat place cautery3ed.
thys maner of pannycle ys consumyd. wasted and dystroyed. and the ey able to be claryfyed with the medycyns folowyng (H503:47.13–48.11)

■ **Pattern 3.** This pattern, found in a few descriptive paragraphs, contains an *it*-impersonal sentence with the verb *happen*, as it were, an empty Theme. Like pattern 2, the diseases described have not been classified at the beginning of the section, whence this imprecise beginning. Since the information conveyed by *happen* is of little semantic import, we must turn to the following *that*-clause to establish what the Theme of the paragraph is. This Theme, like that of pattern 1, is unmarked, a Subject NP providing given information. The rest of the sentence is made up of several clauses, whose Thematic progression belongs to the zig-zag pattern. Each clause's Theme deploys material from the previous clause's Rheme, sometimes by nominalizing process verbs. This may be seen in example (43),[33] where *to wexe drye* becomes *þat drynes*. Alternatively, the known information expressed by the clauses' Themes does not point back to any linguistic material, but to contextual information, as happens with *pacyent* and *payn* in example (44).[34] Or else, as in example (45), the Rhematic information of the first clause is conveyed by the textual conjunctive *wherefor* in the second clause, which also serves to connect cause and consequence in the rhetorical structure.

Finally, example (46) illustrates a variant, in which a pattern of argumentation is also introduced by the author in order to present his final conclusion. After the final consequence, a new Theme is introduced (clear eyes with no spot) which explains the logical conclusion introduced by the textual Thematic conjunct *perfore*. This rhetorical structure, as illustrated in examples (43) to (46), is summarized in Table 13.[35] The effect of all this is to slow down the explanation, to make it easier to follow and understand.

---

33 This example is also interesting for its rhetorical structure, asymmetrical as regards the causes: the itching and burning is the consequence of both eyelid dryness and lack of purgations, and of a proper diet, which seems contradictory as it stands.
34 In *H513*, again, the syntactic, Thematic and rhetorical structures are very similar (see 23r and 31r), except that, at the very beginning, instead of the impersonal *it happens that*, the writer uses *we say that* or nothing at all.
35 Another example following this Thematic progression and rhetorical structure patterns is *H503*:50, the only difference being that there is no empty Theme of the type *it happens that*. It also contains a Thematic nominalization of a Rhematic verb (*prik > of which prikking*).

	Cause 1 Theme → Rheme	Conseq. 1 = Cause 2 Rheme → Theme	Conseq. 2 = Cause 3 Rheme > Theme	Conseq. 3 Rheme
(43)	excess of melancholy	→ eyelid dryness	→ itching and burning (← no purgation, bad diet)	
(44)	stone chips →	pain →	tears	→ inability to open eyes
(45)	biting + foul air →	swelling of face →	inability to open eyes	
	→	→	→ sorrow	→ inability to rest
(46)	excess of choler →	troubled eyes →	shadow	

Table 13. Rhetorical patterns in examples (43) to (46).

(43) It happyth sumtyme þat *the malencolyous humor habundant yn the brayn begynnyth to haue hys course by the eyon.*
 And for the superhabundance þereof. *it makyth the eyledys to wexe drye.*
 And þat drynes *tornyth after to an ycche. and to brynnyng*
 and the cause of thys brynnyng and ycche. *ys. for that he tooke no purgacion yn the begynnyng of the sekenesse nor absteyned from contraryous metys.* (*H503*:82.1–11)

(44) For yt happyth þat
 sum of here fragmentys *sterte ynto there eyes. vnwysyli and rechelesly be left þeryn. tyll þei be incarnate. vpon the tonycles. of the ey.*
 and the payn *causeth contynually þer eyon to water.*
 so that the pacyent *may no wele opon hys eye.* (*H503*:113.5–12)

(45) Also it appethe sumtyme that
 sum ben ybite of summe venemous beste as with waspes or of spidres or suche other or of summe aer ycorrupt or infecte
 wherefor *all the face is forswollen in soch maner*
 that the pacient may nought open his eyȝen
 and many of soche bitynges *wonderfulliche sorwyn*
 and for akthe *mowe nat haue reste* (*H513*:33r.5–12)

(46) **wherof.** [= the two coler-related diseases] **the first** *ys causyd of superhabundance of coler yn the stomake.*

Of the whych *ys resoluyd a corrupte fumosytie þat ascendyth vp to the brayn with greete furowre and pyne.*
wherof *the eyon be so troublyd þat betwene þem and their obiecte. þat ys the thyng. ys yn the maner of a shadowe or a clowde.*
and yit the eyon *apere ferre and bryght. And neiþer yn the eyon. nor wythoute. ys no spot. aperyng.*
and þerfore. *the defaute of thys ys not yn the eye. but in the stomake.*
and þerfore *no medycyne schal be put yn the ey. but in the stomake. (H503:66.4–67.6)*

■ **Pattern 4.** Finally, at the end of the sections dealing with medicines and recipes, the author lists their properties and beneficial effects. These are conveyed syntactically by means of very short syndetic and asyndetic coordinated clauses, both finite and non-finite. The Theme is always unmarked and the Thematic progression pattern is reiterative: the same Theme is repeated over and over again, expressly or elliptically, as shown in (47) and (48).[36]

(47) **And thys lectuarye.** QUOD HE **ys callyd meruelous and prescious.**
For yt doth many prescious merueleus.
hyt *dystroyth the teres and flewme.*
yt *warmyth the brayn.*
it *puttyth awey the peyne of the mygreyme.*
It *openyth the eyon.*
It *releuyth the eylyddys and clarifyth the syght. (H503:64.14–65.7)*

(48) **for the propurte of the sponge** is
to distroye waste flech
to drawe and to quyken the spiryt of the blode.
and to consowdyn and knit the wounde.
and to bryng yt to good astate. (*H503*:90.13–91.3)

---

36 Other examples are found in both treatises in the final pharmacopoeia (*H503*:120 ff., and *H513*:33v ff.), and in the final section of the work, on powders and colliria (*H503*:73 ff.).

2.4.3. Directives

The mode of our medical treatises, as we saw in section 1.1, is monological at times, but also dialogic to a certain extent, the writer being a teacher addressing his students and giving them instructions on how to treat eye-diseases and injuries. Therefore, directives are found particularly in the sections about medical treatments, whether surgical or medicinal. Surgical treatment sections may be divided into three sub-sections, actually corresponding to three chronological stages, namely, pre-surgical treatment, surgery itself and post-surgery or medicinal treatment. The third of these stages itself is also sub-divided into ingredients, recipe procedures and derived benefits.

Each of these sections prescribing the actions to take is normally headed by a short Hyper-Theme clause expressing the topic of the following paragraph, that is, the cure, as in examples (49) and (50).[37]

(49) **In whych craft** [Ars acuaria] **who so wyll procede artyfycyally. he must begyn thus.** (*H503*:15.1–3)

(50) **And þus it** [a lectuary] **schal be made** (*H503*:73.15)

Syntactically, the directives are expressed by means of different structures, often within the same paragraph:

- declarative clauses containing a modal verb of obligation (*must* and *shall*), with second or third person Subjects, referring to the reader-student, if in the active voice (passive clauses are also found);[38]
- imperative clauses; and occasionally
- infinitives.[39]

---

[37] Other examples are found in *H503*:59, 82 and 115.

[38] A variant of declarative-clause instructions is occasionally found: the instructions are given in a first person narrative, with verb in the past tense, as in *H503*:115–8. The Thematic progression of the clauses is the same, though. See section 3 too, where we use one such narrative text.

[39] For example, first **to pourge** the brayne withe oure pillull of Jerusalem (*H513*:5r).

Two types of Thematic progression patterns are used in directives. One pattern, illustrated in example (51),[40] follows a zig-zag pattern: the Rheme of one clause re-appears as Theme in the next clause. What is interesting is that this pattern clearly calques the chronological sequence of the treatment prescribed. The effect achieved is to impress on the reader that all the actions in chronological protocol are necessary and that each depends on the succesful completion of the previous one. For this reason, the transition between two groups of instructions or between the instructions themselves is very often indicated by a marked Theme, an adverbial denoting time or, rather, the completion of the previous instruction. This is achieved in several ways:

- a nominalization of a verb in the previous Rheme: *clense the stomake* > *purgacion*;
- a time clause (repetition of the Rheme):
  - finite clause: *tyl it be* [...] *dryed* > *And when the place ys dryed*;
  - non-finite clause: *clense the stomake* > *whych purgacion made*; *ley of the* [...] *powder* > *whych powder put yn*;
- a time adverbial (adverb or prepositional phrase): *þan, after thys*.

(51) **Fyrst** *clense the pacyentys stomake wyth the peletys of ierusalem* [...] **whych purgacion made.** ÞEN ȝe shall make *a lytle Insysyone* [...] **In whych yncysion.** put *the grane of a fecche.* **and yn the hole that it hath made.** ley *of the coresey and mortificat powder* [...] **whych powder** *put yn.* do *the pacyens shyt hys eye* [...] **and þan** anoynte *yt. or* ley *þerto clene freshe swynes grece* [...] **and after thys** take *a lytle pece of a sponge* [...] *and* ley *yt yn the hoole that the powder mayd tyl it be pourgyd and dryed.* **And when the place ys dryed** THAN leue *the sponge* [...] (*H503*:106.9–109.11)

However, very often we find sets of instructions that lack the Thematic progression observed in (51) because hardly any Rhematic material is recycled. Imperative clauses follow one another connected only by the textual Theme *and*. This is illustrated by example (52).[41] It contains

---

40 See *H503*:30r–30v for the equivalent segment.
41 See *H503*:5r–5v for the equivalent segment.

as many as fourteen clauses coordinated by *and* (except for one with *but here*, whose verb, though still an imperative (*be*), does not refer to yet one more step in the medical protocol). In fact, the real instruction is given more forcefully in the noun clause through negative deontic obligation: *you schalt no more wrythe*. The stylistic effect achieved by so much explicit coordination is different: the reader is told to perform one action after the other and practically all the information is new: the unmarked Theme (the imperative verb), the Rheme, and any marked Themes that may precede the verb, such as instrument, place, manner, time or contingency adverbials "supply first-time information necessary to interpret the remainder of the clause or sentence message", as Cummings (2005: 132) puts it. This fronted material is indicated in small capitals in the example. Many imperative directives contain time adverbials in right-most position, particularly those indicating the time length of the procedure or the manner in which it should be conducted. These tend to be weighty clauses never found in marked fronted position: clauses starting with the conjunctions *till* or *as long as*, and manner clauses. Besides, these time-clauses belong to the message, that is, they are new information, and thus their position is Rhematic, unlike other time clauses which are used to locate the clause temporally in the medical protocol sequence.

(52) **do** *hym sitte ouerthwhart rydyngwyse.*
    and sytte *you also on the stoke yn lykwyse face to face.*
    And do *the pacyent to holde the hole eye cloos with hys oon hand*
    And charge *hym that he syt stydfastly styl and styre not.*
    And THEN **blysse** *the.*
    and begyn *thy craft in the name of ihesu cryste.*
    and WITH THY LIFT HAND **lyft** *vp hys oon eylyd.*
    and WITH ÞIN OÞER HANDE **put** *yn thy nedyl made þerfore on the forþer syde from the nose.*
    and SOFTLY **thyrl** *the tonycle. Saluatrice*
    And ALWEY **wryth** *thy fyngers to and from tyll you touche wyth the poynt the corrupte water the whych ys the cateracte.*
    and THEN **begyn** *to remeue downward from aboue wyth the poynte the sayd corrupte water fro beforne the syȝth.*
    And dryue *yt down beneth as long as you mayst sey. iij. or. iiij. tymes. Pater noster.*

> **Than remeue** *esely the nedyl therfro.*
> **And** IT HAPE TO RYSE VP AYEN. ***bryng*** *it downe ageyne to the corner of the ey to the erewarde.*
> **But here** *be ware þat*
> **after tyme the nedyl hath towchyd the Cateractis.** *you schalt no more wrythe thy fyngars to and fro. tyl þat be set yn hys place. as it ys seyd before.*
> **And** ÞAN SOFTLYE ***drawe*** *out thy nedyl as you put it yn. Always thyrllyng thy fingurs to and fro. tyl yt be all owte. (H503:15.14–17.14)*

Recipe instructions[42] are almost always given by means of imperative clauses, usually coordinated to one another by *and*, and occasionally linked by a short time adverb phrase. Normally, the clauses start with the imperative verb (unmarked Theme), but very often we find fronted material, particularly the Complements of the verb. This occurs when one particular action must be applied to a number of already-mentioned ingredients. Thus, given information is presented first, as in (53) and (54), where *all thyes thyngys* and *to all thyes* anaphorically point back to medicinal ingredients.[43] Of course, examples with no fronted material are also found in our works, as in (55). In order to keep given material in Thematic position without fronting, passives are also fairly frequent used, as in (56).

(53) **all thyes thyngys saue roses ponderd.** *put yn a Erthen pote wythe iij pyntys of whyte wyne boyllyng wyth soft fyre* (*H503*:132.14–133.2)

(54) **And to all thyes.** *put iiij. vnce of drye floures of Camamyl. and of wexe. ane vnce* (*H503*:43.10–12)

(55) **Bete** *all thyes* *to powder.* (*H503*:22.10)

(56) **All thyes** *muste be betyn* *togyddyr to smal pouder and wele sarsed.* (*H503*:74.11–13)

---

42 See examples in *H503*:22–23, 36–36, 39–40, 43–44, 68 and 83.
43 Similar examples for dosage and application of medicines are found in *H503*:60, 74–75, 85 and H503:11r, 12v–13r.

Only in one example of a medicine recipe, (57), have we found a zig-zag Thematic progression pattern, with long adverbials very conspicuously fronted as marked Themes recycling given information.[44]

(57) **And on that other side**
haue ye a moche clene basyn [...]
And that fume yreseyued *than haue ye a nabiatis · 2 · quarter · poudred*
and in that bacyn where that the fume of Aloes ys receyued *medle hym theryn hym theryn* [sic] *with a · brasyn pestell* [...]
with that forsaide fume of the poudre *medle hem well togiders*
Whan this poudre ys ymade þus as y haue asayde than do of this poudre twyes a · day naturall [...] into the ey3e (513.13r.22–13v.9)

Between sets of directives or between two different medicinal treatments, a couple of conspicuous discourse markers are used in *H513*. The first is the Latin word *recipe* (frequently abbreviated into ⟨R⟩ in the MSS), which contrasts in *H503* with a clause whose most Rhematic part points forward to the recipe, as in (58) and (59). In both cases, we have a hyper-Theme for the following paragraph.

(58) when suche ben founde ye shullen helpe hem with oure coleri of ierusalem
R tutie of Alexandre · ʒ iii [...] (*H513*:8v.6–8)

(59) yt may be curyd QUOD HE with my Colery. that ys clepyd. Colerium iherossolimitanum.
that ys mayd yn thyse wyse.
Take tutie of alexandrye ane vnce (*H503*:31.10–14)

The second conspicuous marker is a phrase meaning "on the other hand", such as *on that other partie* or *on that other side*, whose equivalent segments in *H503* are *yn the meane tyme*, or else the usual

---

44 The same features (short imperative clauses coordinated by *and*, sentences starting with a fronted adverb *then* or a fronted dependent time clause conveying given information as marked Theme) are found in cookery books of the 15th century. An example will suffice: "[...] **an let** boyle to-gederys, **an whan þey haue boyle a whyle, take** pouder of gyngere an caste þerto, an a lytyl venegre, an a lytyl safron; **an loke** þat it be poynaunt an dowcet" (London, British Library, Harley MS 279, f. 6r). See Austin 1964.

fronted adverbials employed as marked Themes, as in (60) and (61). Thus, while in *H503* the writer exploits Thematic ordering, in *H513* he uses discourse markers.

(60) when thys Cauterye ys made lyke as I seyd.
 anoon put Into the pacyent ey [...] of the powder callyd. Puluis nabetus. [...]
 And whyle lyeth wyth the powder yn hys ey.
 take iiij. crabbys and rost þem. (*H503*:48.11–49.3)

(61) Whan the cautarie ys made
 putt withyn the ey3e of poudre-nabatis ir 3uccre-candi
 And on the other partye
 take 4 applis yrosted vnder hote euery (*H513*:12v.17–20)

Finally, we come to those parts giving the ingredients used to prepare the medicines. They are normally grouped together at the start of each paragraph. Again, we find fronting of Rhematic material: since quantities are usually given after each ingredient or sub-group of ingredients, these are moved to Thematic position and point back to the immediately preceding ingredients, the Rheme simply informing about the quantities. Again, a zig-zag progression pattern is used.

(62) **Take** *turbite. aloes. epatica.*
 of euerych *an ownce.*
 Macys *quibyb. Masticis. and. dylle.*
 of eche of þem *a dram.* (*H503*:15.6–8)

2.4.4. Persuasion (authorial statements)

Authoritative or authorial statements may be found throughout the text in various places. Whatever their specific contents, the syntax of the sentence is made to fit the requirement of placing the known information in Thematic position. It should be noted that this topical Theme is often preceded by a textual conjunctive word. Surgical or medicinal treatments almost always end with very short paragraphs or sentences, the section's coda, which serves not only to indicate the end of section, but also to allow the writer to assert his authority. He does so in several ways.

- USE OF EVALUATIVE TERMS to describe or name medicines, often followed by an explanation, as in (63) and (64). In these cases, the Theme is normally unmarked (Subject).

(63) **Thys powder** *ys goode and syker to hole al sekenes of eyon.* (*H503*:54.1–2)

(64) **And thys lectuarye.** QUOD HE *ys callyd meruelous and prescious For yt doth many prescious merueleus.* (*H503*:64.14–65.2)[45]

- CLAIMS REGARDING SUCCESS are provided after the directives and prescriptions. These clauses may be passive (with either the patient or the disease as Subjects), as in (65) to (67), or active (with either the author or the reader as Subjects, and either the patient or the disease as Objects), as in (68) to (70). Alternatively, imperative or third-person commands are used, often with fronting of a verbal Complement or of an adverbial clause, as in (71) to (74). Or else prediction with future *shall*, as in (75). In most examples there is a marked Theme recycling information and facilitating comprehension.

(65) **and so** *shall the* [the patient] *be delyuerd* (*H503*:109.14–15; see *H513*:31r.15)

(66) **and yn thys wyse** *be curyd all the cateractis curable.* (*H503*:19.7–8; see *H513*:6r.15–16)

(67) **with thys gracious plaster** he shall ben holpen (*H503*:120.2–3;[46] see *H513*:24r.14)

(68) **And on thys wyse** quod he. *I cured all that hade þere eylydys. turnyd by the same cause.* (*H503*:91.3–5;[47] see *H513*:25v.18–20)

---

45 See *H513*:18v for equivalent segment.
46 See also *H503*:89.
47 See also *H503*:32 (*H513*:8v), *H503*:62, *H503*:99 (*H513*:27v), *H503*:58 (*H513*:17r); *H503*:37 for an example with no fronting (*H513*:9v); *H503*:65 with fronting of direct Object. *H513*:16r, with fronting of A and O.

(69) **And yn thys wyse** *ye shal cure thys maner of disease (H503:78.12–13;*[48] see *H513:22r)*

(70) **On thys wyse** *shall ʒe cure all tho þat arne hurte in the ey wyth stroke or smytyng. (H503:100.7–9; see H513:18r)*

(71) **And of thys** *lete the pacyent ete* [...] *and he schal be hoole (H503:74.15–75.2)*[49]

(72) **þus do ʒe yn lyke wyse** *yf ʒe wyll gett your worschyp and your pacyent helth (H503:117.15–118.2; see H513:33r)*

(73) **And yf yt** [a colirium] **be takyn betymes.** *the pacyent schal be curyd (H503:32.9)*

(74) **and the pacient shall vsen therof erliche and late** *and he shall receyue his sight aʒeen. (H513:21v.3–5)*

(75) **And anoon thow** *schalt see þat he schal begynne to rest. and to sclepe. (H503:36.6–8)*[50]

- **WARNING AGAINST OTHER PROCEDURES** which are noxious, especially those practised by ignorant leeches; *H503*:14, *H513*:4v, *H503*:37, *H513*:10r, *H503*:106, *H503*:110, *H513*:30v.

(76) **On thys wyse** *shall ʒe cure* [...] *and not os lewde leches arne wont to doo (H503:100.7–11; see H513:28r)*

(77) **And who wyll cure hem oþer wyse shall dysceyue þemselfe** *ignorant of the true craft of curyng. (H503:19.8–11; see H513:6r.18–19)*

- **APPEALING TO HIS PAST PROFESSIONAL EXPERIENCE**, normally in other lands.

(78) **Al thyes** *I haue preuyd QUOD HE (H503:65.11–12)*[51]

---

48   See also *H503*:49 (*H513*:13r).
49   See also *H503*:45 (*H513*:11v, with a declarative clause), 71 (*H513*:20r), for examples without fronting.
50   See *H513*:9v, with terms of appraisal.
51   See *H503*:15 (*H513*:7r); *H513*:7v.

(79) **And wyth thys sekenes of eyon** QUOD MY AUTOR *I founde moo ywoxen yn Calabur. þen yn ony oþer prouynce.* (*H503*:53.7–10;[52] see *H513*:16r)

- **TEACHING THE DISEASES' OR MEDICINES' NAMES**, including his or other authors'; (*H513*:20v–r)

(80) **And thys crafte aforesayde** *ys callyd the nedyll crafte.* (*H503*:19.11–12; see *H513*:6r)

(81) **And thys sekenes** *we calle. Pannum vitreum.* (*H503*:54.7–8; see *H513*:16r)

(82) **Thys maner of infirmyte.** *the grete lechys of salerne clepyd. Obtalmyam.* (*H503*:36.8–10; see *H513*:9v)

- **VOCATIVES**. The writer often attempts to involve his readers by addressing them directly, sometimes in a very affectionate and respectful way, by means of vocatives. These vocatives are found at regular intervals in both works, as though the writer wished to maintain a friendly *rapport* with his readers. In *H503* this vocative is the word *practisers*, while in *H513* it is *friends*. It is found as an unmarked Rheme, in apposition to a Subject or an indirect Object, as in (83) and (84). If the appositive vocative NP is heavy it is moved to post-verbal position, with repetition of the Object, as in (85). Alternatively it may be found in marked Thematic position, having greater rhetorical strength, as in (86) and (87), where we find 'textual Theme + interpersonal Theme'.

(83) Moreoure quod. Benemicius, I wyl þat ʒe **practysers** that many of þem þat [...] (*H503*:88.12–15)

(84) I wyl teche <u>yow</u> **practysers** a merveilous and a prescious lectuarye (*H503*:63.2–4)[53]

(85) I wyl ʒe knowe. **ʒe þat wyll be practyse yn the acurye crafte.** þat [...] (*H503*:25.10–12)

---

52   See also *H503:55* (*H513*:16v), *H503*:58–59 (*H513*:17r–17v), *H503*:62 (*H513*:17v–18r), *H503*:83–84 (*H513*:23v), *H503*:92 (*H513*:16r).
53   See also *H503*:115.

(86) **wherfor the practysers** when ʒe se such a pacyent [...] (*H503*:73.7–8)[54]

(87) **Wherfor dere-worthi frendes** knowe ye that [...] (*H513*:10r.2–3)[55]

- **PRESCRIPTIVE VERBS.** The writer also urges his readers' attention to some particular issue by using directives not just to take some action, but to exercise their intellectual skills professionally: verbs of cognition and observation.[56] The predicates used in both *H503* and *H513* are: *be ware*, *know* and *wit*. These are used in the imperative (examples (88) to (90)) or else belong to an Object *that*-clause complementing a volition verb, as in (91). Being a directive, the most usual alternative (a modal verb of obligation) is also found, as in (92).

(88) But here **be ware þat** [...] (*H503*:17.7)[57]

(89) And **knowe thou well that** [...] (*H513*:5v.13)[58]

(90) Wherfor **wete the well that** they that seen somdell (*H513*:7v.2–3)[59]

(91) But hyer fynyally **I wyl ʒe knowe**. ʒe þat wyll be practyse yn the acurye crafte. **þat** [...] (*H503*:25.10–12)[60]

(92) wherfore my dere frendes **ye shull wetyn that** it happethe of the habundaunce of salte-fleume (*H513*:17v.13–15)

Alternatively or simultaneously the writer, particularly in *H513*, also asserts his claims by means of predicates of saying (*say* and *tell*), of showing (*show* and *teach*), of warning (*counsel* and *amonest*), or of ordering (*command*). One particular example shows a combination of

---

54 See also *H503*:91 and 93.
55 See also *H513*:10v, 12r, 17v and 26r. In all these examples in *H513* the vocative in Rhematic position.
56 Cf. Taavitsainen & Pahta (1997: 218–20).
57 See also *H503*:19, 68; *H513*:12v.
58 See also *H503*:34, 37; *H513*:10r, 12v, 21r, 22r, 29r, 29v.
59 See also *H503*:123; *H513*:14r, 20v, 21r, 27v, 28r.
60 See also *H503*:38, 46, 97.

two verbs, as in (98). Three of them (*take heed of, look* and *understand*) are used in the imperative, as in (100) to (102).

(93) Wherefor **we saye you that** [...] (*H513*:7r.5)[61]

(94) But **we telle you that** he haue with oure vnguentum de Alabastro nostro (*H513*:24v.16–18)[62]

(95) **we shull teche you** of the maladies of ey3en (*H513*:26v.26)[63]

(96) wherfore **I counsel yow that** when 3e se thys maner of pannycle. [...] (*H503*:47.2–4)[64]

(97) wherfor **we amoneste you that** in what-euer wey that the ey3e ys ysmete [...] (*H513*:28v.15–17)

(98) wherfore **I counsel you to be ware** of all suche plasters. (*H503*:102.5–6)

(99) wherfor derworþe frendes **we comaunde you** whan ye sein any suche pannicles [...] (*H513*:12r.20–22)

(100) **vnderstonde that** whan ye putten yn the forsaide spices with the 3ucre · it shall sethe but a litell (*H513*:19v.4–5)[65]

(101) And **loke that** ye do none othir medicyne into the ey3en but this (*H513*:23r.6–7)

(102) But **take good hede that** [...] (*H513*:27v.20–21)

- PRONOMINAL REFERENCE TO THE AUTHOR. The choice of personal pronouns is not exactly the same in the two texts. As regards pronominal references to the author of the treatise, *H503* uses both third and first person reference, while *H513* uses only the first person. The reason for

---

61   The clause *I say that* is especially frequent in *H513*, but not in *H503*. The force of this clause is sometimes rendered in *H503* by other means, such as truly used as a disjunct (see the equivalent segments *H513*:9r and *H503*:33).
62   See also *H503*:95.
63   See also *H513*:9r, 15r, 15v, 17v and 27r (with *show*).
64   See also *H503*:88.
65   See also *H513*:34r–v.

this is the manner in which the book is presented. *H503* opens with a long sentence about the author (*Benuomicius Grapheus*), the subject matter of the book that physician has written (*the sekenes of eyon and of her curys*) and the title of the book (*Deus oculorum*) (see example (1)), while *H513*:2r starts straight with the title of the first part, on tonicles. This sets the convention in *H503* of the copyist or physician-copyist referring to this author in the third person: the first ten tokens of explicit authorial comment contain a third person pronoun and/or verb, as in (103). Third person reference to the author may also be assumed in those cases in which the reader is addressed indirectly by means of a third person pronoun or verb, or a passive occasionally, as in examples (104) to (106). However, *H513* is written throughout in the first person.[66]

(103) [...] **he** declarith what ane eye ys [...] after oþer opynyoun. and also after **his** owne seying. (*H503*:1.15–2.2)

(104) In whych craft **who so** wyll procede artyfycyally. he must begyn thus. (*H503*:15.1–3)

(105) or **the practyser** begyn. **lete hym** make the pacyent [...] to blede. (*H503*:32.13–14)

(106) þis dyssease **must be cured** oþerwyse þan thus. (*H503*:51.13–15)

This use of the third person in *H503* is not kept consistently. As the text progresses, authorial comments in the first person begin to appear, used in two ways: either the first person pronoun only as the narrative voice (normally in the singular, but occasionally in the plural, as in examples (107) and (108), as in *H513*), or else the first person in direct speech segments is anchored in clauses such as *quod he* or *quod*

---

66 Except this segment: *fforsothe **Benemitus saye** that ther ben two tonicles of the eiȝen onyly* (*H513*:2v.3–4). However, it is also possible to interpret that *Benemitus* simply stands in apposition to a missing *I*. This interpretation is likely since the form *saye* is never used in *H513* for the third person and because a similar construction is found elsewhere in the text: *But **we Beneuenutus of Jerusalem say** that they comen oute by the poyntes palpebrarum* (*H513*:31r.24–31v.1).

Benuomicius, as in examples (109) and (110), which are never found in *H513*.[67]

(107) as **I** schal shew you afterwarde among my Cautaryes (*H503*:47.15–48.1)

(108) with **oure** electuarie that **we** calle Diolibanum salernitanum (*H503*:22.2–3)

(109) **I** made hem QUOD HE to ete rawe onyons (*H503*:23.11)

(110) But **I** QUOD BENUOMICIUS calle yt. Torturam tenebrosam. (*H503*:36.10–12)

- **PRONOMINAL REFERENCE TO THE READER.** We have seen in directives that the writer/author addresses his readers directly very often, by means of vocative interpersonal Themes, imperatives or clauses containing a modal verb of obligation. Pronominal references are found both in the singular (*thou, thy*) and in the plural (*ye, you, your*). However, in both works, plural pronouns are much more frequent than singular ones (a little less than 90%). In a very large number of examples, because these persuasive segments appear at the conclusion of a descriptive or explanatory section, they are very often introduced by the textual marker *wherefore*, both in *H503* and *H513*. This conjunct connects one

---

67 There are 22 tokens of direct speech in all sections of *H503*:23, 27, 31, 32, 36, 53, 58 (twice), 59, 62, 65, 66, 69, 83–4, 88–89, 91, 92, 93–94, 103, 112, 130 and 135. The reader is repeatedly reminded of who the real author is, which means that the phrase *quod he* may be considered as elided in those instances, illustrated by examples (107) and (108), in which it is not used. *H513*, as is expected, contains no direct speech chunks at all, since the author speaks in the first person, not through the intermediation of the copyist. However, the frequency of first person tokens in *H503* is much higher than that of third person if we include all those segments in which the author addresses his student readers or practisers directly by means of vocatives, second person pronouns or imperatives. If we take all these into account, the use of the third person becomes clearly insignificant in *H503* despite the initial convention of a copyist reporting the author's original treatise. The choice of number (*I, my* versus *we, our*) in self-references by the author is different in *H503* and *H513*: in *H503* the singular is found in the vast majority of all first person usages, while in *H513* it is the plural that is used in almost all cases.

paragraph to another, as in examples (86), (87), (90), (92), (93), and (96) to (99) above.

2.4.5. Metatextual indications

Both in *H503* and *H513*, reference to previous or subsequent contents is often made by means of the participial adjectives containing *said* (which perform an anaphorical reference function similar to the demonstratives *this*, *these* and, often, *that*, in our texts) or a clause containing the verbs *say*, *tell* or *write* and time or locative adverbs, such as *before*, *above*, *after*, or similar formulas, as in examples (111) to (114).[68] However, apart from these non-specific references to other contents in the work, the author (whether this be Benuomicius or the copyist-physician) also makes recurrent references to specific sections of the work itself. *H503* and *H513* contain a similar number of such metatextual references,[69] but they need not coincide at all: in equivalent segments both works may be specific or vague, or just one of them, or else one work does contain a reference, while the other does not give any at all. Examples (115) and (116) illustrate unlike referencing.[70]

(111) The Cure of these foure kyndes of catarractes **forsaid** is [...] (*H513*:4v.13–14)

(112) the whych causyth the ey to seme blak **as I sayd before** (*H503*:8.5–6)

(113) And wyth good dyet **as yt schal be tolde after** (*H503*:22.4–5)

---

68 At many places in *H503*, metatextual reference is made to the very place in the book where he is writing. This is normally done by the time adverb *now* and occasionally the locative adverb *here*, as in **here** *wyll I teche yow practysers a crafte to take out an hawe from the eye* (*H503*:116–117).
69 See *H503*:39, 47–48, 56, 61–62, 69, 92, 93, 94, 95, 100, 107, 120, 130 and 135; and *H513*:33r, 14v, 18r, 19v, 28r, 30v, 31r and 32v.
70 An interesting metatextual comment is also found in *H503* when the physician-copyist admits that there is a chapter missing in the original book he is copying or translating, and is specific about that chapter and the beginning of next one: *yn my latene apy lacked an hoole Chapytere. In whych tretys of hurtys taken aboute the eyon* [...] *And moreouere the nexte chapytre folowyng in the begynnyng lakked sumwhat* (*H503*:102–103).

(114) and claryfiethe the ey3en withe medecyns **I · added afterward wreten** (*H513*:12v.16–17)

(115) yeue hym [...] of the electuarie. Dyolibanum. or salernitanum. **os yt ys sayd beforn in the cure of the. iij. curable cateractis** (*H503*:39.6–9)

(116) yef hem [...] de olibano nostro ierusalitanus **the whiche was saide afore** (*H513*:10v.8–9)

These metatextual comments are systematically found in Rhematic position, even though they are not new information. This end position may be attributed to the fact that these comments are clauses and that the end-weight principle applies. However, we have seen many instances of fronted clauses as marked Themes (see examples (51), (52) and (57) for instances of such fronted clauses). The reason why certain clauses are fronted while others are not has to do with their capacity to forward the argumentation. Time and contingency clauses clearly mark the transition from one phase of a medical protocol or a medicine recipe to the next, while metatextual comment clauses are parenthetical disjuncts[71] not semantically relevant from the point of view of a paragraph's Thematic progression since they do not contain given information. In other words, they fall outside the *Theme-Rheme* structure in clauses complexes, particularly if another clause has been fronted already.

3. Grammar and lexis in Themes and Rhemes

Theme and Rheme complement each other. The Theme is basically the foundation upon which new information is added and the Rheme is the new informative point being made. Since they have two different meanings, it follows that they must be worded differently, according

---

71 See Quirk *et al.* (1985: 1112).

to their function. Fries's (2002) analysis shows that grammatical complexity is greater in Themes than in N-Rhemes, and Cummings (2005: 136 ff.) studies how Theme and Rheme differ in the distribution of forms and features. In particular, he quantifies the distribution of presuming reference[72] items in Theme and Rheme by comparing reference chains items in several short texts. Our findings here coincide in the main with their conclusions.

We have analyzed two sections from *H513* to show how texts with different functions are not alike in these features either: a short descriptive-explanatory section on the causes of some obtalmy-related diseases (*H513*:10r–10v), reproduced in Table 14, and a narrative section on the treatment for upturned eyelids[73] (*H513*:25r–25v), reproduced in Table 15. Both sections are well delimited from the previous and following sections by a Hyper-Theme (*H513*:9v.23–10r.1: *Nowe tell we of the kyndes of maladies* [...] *engendred* [...] *thorowe* [...] *obtolime*; *H513*:25r.6–7: *Of the turnyng of eyʒe-liddis and of þe same infirmite and of the cure*) and a Hyper-Rheme (*H513*:10v.3–5: *Wherfor yif any such come to oure cure ffirst we purge hem with these pillis that purgeþ her brain*; *H513*:26r.13–15: *and we haue cured so many at the full in Tusken and aboute boleyne we founden moo than aure elles*). Since these types of analysis are based on clauses (not on clause-complexes or sentences), each line in our tables contains a different clause. Small capitals are used to indicate the Theme, roman type for the initial portion of the Rheme and italics for the N-Rheme (the portion containing the newsworthy piece of information which we believe the writer wants the reader to remember).

	Theme	Rheme	N-Rheme
i	NOWE TELL WE	of the kyndes of	*maladies þat ben engendred in the eygen thorowe accacioun of obtolime* ·

---

72 That is, reference to participants whose identities are already known to the reader because they have appeared earlier in the text. See Martin 1992.
73 This narrative is in fact an alternative to the more usual imperative directives.

ii	FFOR SO MOCHE THAT IT	was nought cured	*at begynnyng*
iii	AS WE	haue saide	
iv	WHERFOR DERE-WORTHI FRENDES KNOWE	ye that	*for wycked and euyll kepyng and for euyll cure of vnwise leches that ben nought knowyng in this crafte*
v	AS MANY	doun	
vi	AND THERFOR THEY	may sorowe	*on sorowe*
vii	AND THERFOR THE EY3EN	ben made white	*in soche maner þat neuer efte may come ayene to her former helþe*
viii	IN THE WHICHE MANER	humours of the ey3nen ben dissoluid	*for her grete anguysshe and sorowe and for her contrarie medicynes*
ix	AND THE EY3EN	shewen hem	*with all the holowenes with-outen the ey3en-liddes*
x	AND THE PACIENT	is ben	*so dissowlid and for-blemysshed and nought mowyn see*
xi	WHERFOR WE	sayne	*of suche pacientes*
xii	AFTER THAT THEY	ben brought into	*soche state /*
xiii	NO MEDICYNE	may	*helpe hem ne delyuer ther afterward*
xiv	AND THAT THE EY3EN	is	*separat and departed fro his noursshynges and ymortified with all his substance*
xv	ALSO THORWE THE ACCASIOUN OF OBTOLMIE	the ey3en of many ben	*trubled*
xvi	AND THEY	sein nought	*clerely*
xvii	BUT THEY	haue her ey3en	*full of smoke*
xviii	AND IT	is comen to hem	*ete and drinke for her euyll kepyng /*

xix	FOR WHI THEY	wole	*all that is to hem contrary*
xx	WHAN THE PENAUNCE	was comen	*to hem*
xxi	AND THIS VICE	leuyþ	*with hem*
xxii	THAT HER EY3EN	always	*teren and wateryn*
xxiii	WHERFOR YIF ANY SUCH	come	*to oure cure ffirst*
xxiv	WE	purge hem	*with these pillis that purgeþ her brain*

Table 14. Structural complexity and reference chains in Themes and N-Rhemes in a descriptive/explanatory section in *H513*.

	Theme	Rheme	N-Rheme
	Of the turnyng of ey3e-liddis and of þe same infirmite and of the cure		
i	MANY THAT WERE [with] SUCHE INFIRMITEIS	comen afore vs	*with her ey3e-liddes ouer-turned Saynige we hauethe apostome that is clepid benedicta*
ii	AND WE	were	*not well ycured therof*
iii	WHERFOR THE KEPING OF THAT HELED WOUND	tho ey3e-liddes were	*so ouer-turned outward*
iv	IN THIS CAUSE	we token	*a Rasour*
v	AND WE	kutte and demde the ey3e-lydde from the heled wound	*so sotilliche and so curiousliche that the ey3e-lydde turned vp*
vi	AND WHAN THAT THE KUTTYNG	was ydone	
vii	THAN WE	layden	*a litell pelwe ymade in the shap of a fynger of lynnen clothe*
viii	AND WE	watte it	*in the white of an aye*
ix	AND WE	leide it	*on the wound tille that other day ybounde with a · bounde*
x	AND FROM INFORWARDE WE	chaunged	*that pilwis*

xi	DOYNG	so as it is saide	*till fiftene dayes*
xii	AND THAN WE	chaungid	*this cure*
xiii	AND WE	made	*an oynement of hennes grece and of white wexe*
xiv	AND WE	anoynted ther-with	*the litill pilwe*
xv	AS WE	did first	*with the white of an ay*
xvi	AND WE	layde on the wounde	*thoo litill pilwes*
xvii		as it is saide	
xviii	TILL THAT THE WOUNDE	was	*yheled /*
xix	AND AFTERWARD	that eyȝe-lidde [was] lefte	*in good state*
xx	AND AFTERWARD NEUER-THE-LESSE WE	dide to that wounde	*of a · sponge ymade in the maner of a litill pilwe*
xxi	FOR IT	shuld kepen	*kepen the wounde*
xxii	AND		*do away the superfluyte that the wounde hadde ymade*
xxiii	FFOR THE SEE SPONGE	is	*gode for iii · skeles /*
xxiv	FFIRST FOR IT	distroiethe	*þe fflesshi hede and the lunge that the drie wounde hade ymade thorugh his consowdyng.*
xxv	SECUNDE FOR	draweþ and quckethe	*the spirite and blode /*
xxvi	THE III^DE FOR IT	makethe the wounde to conseuden	*in soche maner as it may fayrist stonde*
xxvii	AND SO WE	heled all thoo that hadden her eyȝeliddes ouer-turned of what-euere cause it come out	*take thoo of whom the eyȝe-liddes were ouer-turned thorugh occasioun of berthen of moche flesshe or liche to hem*
xxviii	AND ALSO THORUGH OCCASIOUN OF OUER-HABUNDAUNCE OF BLOD AND OF ȜEICHE OF THE EYȜELIDDES	as ye haue	*in the ffirst tretise of yeȝche of eyȝen*

xxix	THE WHICHE	is	*thorugh the habundaunce of blode*
xxx	WHAN THEY	ben nought	*in a yere ycured*
xxxi	THAN THE EYƷELYDDES	ben	*ouer-turned*
xxxii	WHERFOR MY DERE FFRENDES YE	shull nought kutt in the outeside but	*on the inwarde partie all that fflesshe-mater that is more than y-nowe with a hoke and with a · Rasour*
xxxiii		doyng it away neuertheles	*wysoliche that vndre that eyƷe-lid where the here wexethe that ye kutte hym nought that*
xxxiv	WHAN	is don	
xxxv	HAUETHE	litill pilwes	*as in other cures of the ouer-turnynges of eyƷeliddes*
xxxvi	· ID EST · WE	haue saide	*aboue*
xxxvii	AND DOO	thoo litill pilwes within	*twies in a daye that erlyche and late*
xxxviii	AND WE	haue cured so many at the full	*in Tusken*
xxxix	AND ABOUTE BOLEYNE	we founden	*moo than aure elles · / ·*

Table 15. Structural complexity and reference chains in Themes and N-Rhemes in a narrative section in *H513*.

First, as regards **grammatical complexity and length of structures**, we observe that Themes contain much simpler structures than Rhemes (see Table 16). In *H513*:10r–10v, the Themes are realized by 19 NPs (11 pronouns and 8 unmodified nouns) and 2 PPs (marked Themes), while the N-Rhemes contain only 1 NP (*soche state*), but as many as 15 PPs[74] (1 with another embedded PP, 3 coordinated, 2 whose noun

---

[74] We have only counted PPs functioning as Adverbials, excluding those that are verbal or adjectival Complements.

is postmodified by a relative clause, 1 followed by a result clause correlating with *such*), 5 AdjPs (1 followed by a coordinated clause denoting "result" in somehow correlating with the intensifier *so*, 3 complemented by PPs), 1 AdvP and 3 Clauses (2 realized by transitive verbs with their Objects, 1 by two coordinated intransitive verbs). In *H513*:25r–25v, the Themes are realized by 19 NPs (15 pronouns and 4 nouns, only one of which is postmodified), 4 PPs (marked Themes, 2 containing given information, 2 for emphasis), 4 VPs (2 imperatives, unmarked Themes, and 2 introducing non-finite clauses), 6 AdvPs (5 used to sequence the protocol followed and 1 summing up the whole treament so far), while the N-Rhemes contain 14 NPs (6 postmodified by a PP or a clause, 4 coordinated), 18 PPs[75] (7 whose noun is postmodified by another PP or a clause), 2 AdjPs, 6 AdvP (3 followed by a result clause correlating with the intensifier *so*, 1 with metatextual anaphoric reference and 2 time adverbs). The striking difference between both extracts is the high number of NPs in the second one. This – we believe – is due precisely to the fact that the second extract is a narrative told by the writer, which means that the Themes will contain a very high number of first person pronouns, thus impeding the presence of other NPs in this position.

		NP	PP	AdjP	AdvP	Clause
H513:10r–v	Theme	19	2			
	N-Rheme	1	15	5	1	3
H513:25r–v	Theme	19	4		6	
	N-Rheme	14	18	2	6	5

Table 16. Grammatical complexity in *H513*:10r–10v.

Secondly, as regards **presumed reference and reference chains**, we observe that the number of chains and the number of items in each chain is greater in the Themes than in the N-Rhemes in the first extract, but not in the second extract. See Table 17 and Table 18.

---

75   We have only counted PPs functioning as Adverbials, excluding those that are verbal or adjectival Complements, and those within clauses.

H513:10r–10v deals with 25 ideational meanings.[76] The total number of reference chains[77] is 7, of which 1 is found only in the Theme and 1 only in the N-Rheme. The total number of long reference chains[78] is 4. We observe that the Theme has a small number of meanings in general (only 6 out of 25), that it is also the locus for the only unshared long chain in the text (pronominal references to the author) and that it participates in all long chains (4 out of 4: author, eyes, bad leeches and patients). Also, since the Theme usually presents given information, it is natural that most of the chains, short or long, should be initiated in the N-Rheme, not in the Theme (5 as against 2, out of 7). However, the two meanings first mentioned in the Theme (author, patient) are retrievable from earlier context. Finally, the N-Rheme contains the highest number of general meanings (21). It also contains the highest number of meanings participating in a chain (9), but this represents only 42%, while in the case of Thematic meanings the proportion is 100% (6 out of 6).

H513:25r–25v deals with 31 ideational meanings, of which only 14 meanings are found in the Theme, while the Rheme contains all of them.[79] The total number of reference chains[80] is 14, of which 1 is found only in the Theme ("reader") and 1 only in the N-Rheme ("excess

---

76 The meanings, which I have nominalized here, are the following: author, malady, eyes, obtalmy, cure, reader, bad diet, bad leeches, profession, sorrow, eye-whiteness, health, hollowness, eyelids, distemperance, vision, help, lack of nourishment, decay of the eye, troubled vision, crying, purgation, pill and brain.
77 Chains have at least three items. I do not consider that 2 references constitute a chain, but simply a repetition.
78 Since the highest number of reference items in a chain is 12, and the smallest for a sequence to be considered a chain is 3, we have decided to count as long those having at least 4 repetitions of the same meaning, which is the whole number below the mean: (12-3)/2=4.5; this is more reasonable than the next number above.
79 The meanings, which I have nominalized here, are the following: author, eyelids, patient, pill^1, pill^2 (these are different pills), wound, overturning, cure^1, cure^2 (again, these are different cures), cutting, disease, sponge, excess flesh, skills ("features"), reader, cicatrix, razor, carefulness, egg-white, oinment, healing, cicatrization, excess blood, itching, finger-shape, binding, spirit and blood, treatise on itching, hook, Tuscany, Bologna and other places.
80 Again, 3 reference items at least.

flesh"). The total number of long reference chains[81] is 5. Unlike the previous text, there are merely two chains whose loci are only the Theme or the N-Rheme and no long chains at all in a single segment. As expected, the Theme participates in 11 small chains (out of 14) and in 3 long chains (out of 5). A total of 3 chains are initiated in the Theme, 1 in the Rheme and 9 in the N-Rheme (out of 14), which is to be expected, since the N-Rheme is associated with new information that may be retaken thematically in subsequent clauses. Finally the N-Rheme contains the highest humber of meanings participating in chains (13). However, contrary to our expectations, the N-Rheme is also used in large number of small chains (11 out of 14), and of long chains (4 out of 5). This may, again, be attributable to the fact that it is a narrative text. In many clauses, the Theme is already occupied by the Subject (the first person pronoun referring to the author), thus preventing fronting of Rhematic information susceptible of eliminating chains from the N-Rheme.

	Total no. of meanings	Reference chains	Long reference chains	No. of meanings in a chain	Starting point of a chain
Total no.	25	7	4	–	–
Theme	6	1	1	6 (out of 6)	2
Rheme	10	0	0	4 (out of 10)	0
N-Rheme	21	1	0	9 (out of 21)	5

Table 17. Reference chains and meanings in *H513*:10r–10v.

---

81 In this text, the highest number of reference items in a chain is 17 and the smallest, as explained, is 3. Following the same procedure as for the previous text, long chains have a minimum of 7 reference items.

	Total no. of meanings	Reference chains	Long reference chains	No. of meanings in a chain	Starting point of a chain
Total no.	33	14	5	–	
Theme	14	1	0	11 (out of 14)	3
Rheme	11	0	0	9 (out of 11)	3
N-Rheme	33	1	0	14 (out of 33)	9
3 segments		6	2		
Th.+Rh.		1	1		
Rh.+N-Rh.		2	2		
Th.+N-Rh.		3	0		

Table 18. Reference chains and meanings in *H513*:25r–25v.

4. Conclusions

The analysis of the Thematic system in the two works has shown that this type of works, practical medical manuals, present neat patterns in all their sections, with internal differences according to the type of function a particular section or paragraph performs (classification, description/explanation, instruction or persuasion). The systematic placing of given and new information in Themes and Rhemes smoothly conveys the information, both theoretical and practical, to the reader. In all kind of sections, not only in descriptive passages, but also in surgical and medicinal exhortatory passages, this method of development is observed, despite the existence of other less predictable clause constituent arrangements.

The regular exploitation of Thematic patterns is found at many levels: whole text, sections, paragraphs, clause-complexes and sentences, and clauses. For this reason, we have made use of concepts such as macro-Theme/Rheme, hyper-Theme/Rheme, and Theme/Rheme. At whole text and major section level, there are noticeable differences between the works, *H513* making use of section titles and *H503* of short paragraphs or sentences, both acting as macro-Themes to the subsequent section. In *H503* an internal reiteration Thematic pattern links macro-Themes, independently of all intervening paragraphs. At paragraph level, in both works, we find an initial clause or sentence acting as hyper-Theme to the paragraph. Less systematically, we also find hyper-Rhemes. However, what is normally found at the end of paragraphs are persuasive authorial comments realized by clauses with marked Themes (claims of success, warning against bad leeches, mention of professional experience...). At clause level, both texts exploit the three basic types of Thematic progression patterns (reiteration, zig-zag and split-Rheme) for different purposes. The most common seems to be the zig-zag pattern, a powerful device to push forward not only arguments and explanations, but also instructions to the reader. The Themes recycling Rhematic material in this zig-zag pattern achieve three things mainly: they present the topic to be developed in the rest of the clause, they link causes and consequences in explanations of medical conditions, and they calque the chronological sequencing of medical protocols and recipe procedures. In the deployment of Rhematic material as Themes, the writer frequently uses dependent clauses and adverbials, but also nominalizations of process and action verbs, a method which will become standard practice in scientific English in later centuries.

Since Themes present summarized rewordings of given information, the grammatical structures found in them are less complex than those in Rhemes (and N-Rhemes), where lengthier structures are needed. Likewise, the number of different meanings in the Theme is smaller than in Rhemes. Reference chains of meanings tend to be more frequent and longer in Themes than in Rhemes, and they are usually initiated in Rhemes.

Two areas which deserve further investigation are the degree of dependence of the English texts upon the Latin original(s) as regards

Thematic structure, and a comparison with later medical treatises to ascertain when and in what type of technical and scientific works the change to modern scientific English style took place.

Antonio Miranda García

Setting MSS Hunter 503 and 513 Apart: A Quantitative Analysis[1]

1. Introduction

As a rule, authorship attribution studies attempt to discover the writer of an anonymous or disputed work from a list of putative candidates by analysing their stylistic features with a traditional or a non-traditional approach. Our purpose in this chapter is to demonstrate that the two main translations into Middle English of Benvenutus Grassus's ophthalmological work, Glasgow, Glasgow University Library, MSS Hunter 503 and MS Hunter 513 (henceforth *H503* and *H513*, respectively) can be distinguished quantitatively by employing some techniques of a non-traditional approach in authorship attribution. The authorial features detected in the texts through this methodology lead us to the inescapable conclusion that they must have been translated, compiled, or simply copied by two different people.

A more traditional linguistic analysis had already cast some suspicions against the possibility of a direct genetic relationship between both pieces. To give but an example: the words meaning 'eggs' were different in each treatise: the possibilities in *H503* were ⟨eggis⟩ and ⟨eggys⟩ (i.e. the strong plural of the Scandinavian borrowing *egg*), which is opposed to the weak plural forms ⟨ayren⟩, ⟨eyren⟩ and ⟨eyryn⟩ found in *H513*, which ultimately stem from OE *ǣgru*. This allowed us to assign a broad northern or East Midlands provenance to *H503* as

---

[1] The present research has been funded by the Spanish Ministry of Education (project FFI2008-02336). This grant is hereby gratefully acknowledged.

distinguished from *H513* which appears to be connected with other, more southern composition areas.

In this chapter we seek to prove that the two treatises can also be differentiated quantitatively, by counting and rating their word-types and tokens in the raw text, as well as their lemmas and word-classes in the resulting annotated corpus. Along with the count of the occurrences, close examination of the texts has unveiled moreover an important feature that may help explain the concurrent orthographical variations in the same page or folio and even in the same verse or line. The study, conceived to complement the synoptic, multilingual edition of Benvenutus Grassus' *Treatise on the Eyes*, fits in with a quantitative linguistics framework at least to a certain extent – since the words in the texts have been counted, weighed and rated. However, it can be considered a piece of research in computational linguistics as well inasmuch – since the results provided in the following pages derive after all from an annotated corpus that was handled with computer-based techniques.

We also aim to demonstrate that a one-to-one inter-textual correspondence can be established between the qualitative differences shaping the authorial fingerprint and the quantitative divergences resulting from item counting, in such a way that the latter are bound to confirm the former. Although no similar line of research has been found in the literature of authorship attribution (Love 2000), the possibilities offered by *H503* and *H513* are extremely attractive to the researcher: both texts are virtually contemporary, share the same language and topic, and have comparable text-lengths. However, due to the intrinsic condition of 'closed games' (Burrows 2002: 267) featuring this case-study, the conclusions drawn from the empirical results here should rather not be extrapolated to other cases, for they cannot confer a universal validity to the method.

2. Methodology

This work is based on the semi-diplomatic transcription of the Late Middle English treatises on the eyes as performed in this same volume by David Moreno Olalla (*H503*) and Teresa Marqués Aguado (*H513*) using hi-res photographs kindly provided by the University of Glasgow. The digitised images and their transcriptions can be consulted at <http://hunter.uma.es>. The texts which resulted from the transcriptions were annotated and each word/token was provided with a referential mark-up, which included title, author, date, the line(s), page or folio (recto or verso) where it occurs, along with a lemma and a Part-of-speech (POS) tag. The lemma encloses the word-types, which arise from morphological inflections, as well as the allomorphs which result from dialectal features or derive from a graphetic transcription.

The adoption of a lemma permits the retrieving of all related word-types as a single batch while avoiding that allomorphic variants are taken as different word-types, which would cause a distortion in the results. For the sake of homogeneity, the *eMED* entries were used whenever possible. Thus, the lemma {finger, n (1)} covers the variants ⟨fingers⟩, ⟨fynger⟩, ⟨fingurs⟩, ⟨fyngurs⟩, and the word-types ⟨browys⟩, ⟨brouwis⟩, ⟨browe3⟩, ⟨browes⟩, ⟨browis⟩ are grouped under a single {brŏue, n}. For convenience, a compound lemma is assigned to multi-word lexical units, be they phrases or chunks (*because of, as towchyng, for to, ere that, fro thens foreward, etc.*), compounds or Latinate glosses (*Benuomicius Grapheus, Cardus benedictus, erys vsti, virtus a deo data*, etc.). As for the POS tag, it includes the word-class, the subclass, and the accidence-related grammatical categories (tense/ degree, number, person, case, and gender).

The annotation is keyed into a MS Excel work-sheet, where each row stores the information as follows: the leftmost cells contain a sequential ID number, which keeps the original word order of the text, whereas the next cells hold the word itself, lemma, word-class, accidence, meaning(s), and the reference mark-up. Tagging is done by typing in the annotation for each word. Such time-consuming task is partially relieved by sorting all the homographs in succession, filling in the annotation for the first item in the list and replicating it for the homographs by dragging down the cursor. A context-sensitive manual disambiguation especially of homonymous function-words is, however, required afterwards. (See Moreno Olalla/Miranda García 2009 for a more detailed account.)

The next step is to turn the spreadsheet into a MySQL database which enables the information retrieval by means of simple queries (non-Boolean searches) or with complex ones (Boolean searches). A non-Boolean query can provide with a list and an index of words, lemmas, adjectives, etc., whereas a Boolean query can generate, for instance, a list or an index of the adjectives containing a given letter and/or beginning with such and such character. However, these queries cannot retrieve context-sensitive information. They would be unable to generate a list of, say "plural nouns containing a given character string which are preceded by a determiner, followed by a preposition, and occur in pages 13 through 15". To cope with this shortcoming, a specific-purpose Text Search Engine (called *TexSEn*) was devised that handles fully annotated texts and sifts quantitative and/or qualitative information from them (Miranda/Garrido forthcoming). This software, which manages all kinds of Boolean and non-Boolean text-sensitive queries and performs the tasks involving statistical treatment, concordance generation, and glossary-building, both word- and lemma-based, was used to retrieve all the data included in this contribution.

3. Lexical profile and vocabulary richness at word- and lemma-level

The studies of computational stylistics or stylometry have mostly relied on several parameters as variables for a linear discriminant function, such as word length (Mendenhall 1887; Brinegar 1963; Mosteller/ Wallace 1964, 1989; Hilton/Holmes 1993), the number of words in a sentence (Yule 1938; Mosteller/Wallace 1964; Michaelson/Morton/ Wake 1978; Frisher et al. 1996), syllables and stresses in a verse line (Cox/Brandwood 1959), punctuation symbols, or the distribution of some vowels, for example ⟨a⟩ and ⟨o⟩ to separate Shakespeare and Marlow (Merriam 1994), intertextual distance (Labbé 2007), proportions of nouns, adjectives, etc. (Mosteller/Wallace 1964, 1989; Yule 1944).

However, the word-unit has traditionally been the most recurrent item for its accessibility and ease of treatment (Burrows 2002, 2007). Its efficiency has not been surpassed by any other parameter of style below or above that level (Tallentire 1973), a fact which explains why lexical features have predominated over syntactic or semantic characteristics (Holmes 1998: 111). Common high-frequency function words have been frequently employed as discriminatory style markers in various experiments (Ellegård 1962; Mosteller/Wallace 1964; Burrows 2002; Miranda García/Calle Martin 2007), though also sporadic words have been used for the purpose (Burrows 2007). The advent of computers sensibly helped stylometry for the ever increasing availability of electronic texts and specific programmes able to retrieve the information required from them: even a common word-processor allows us to know the number of pages, words, characters, paragraphs or lines with a simple click.

As a preliminary study of the external evidence, we considered it convenient to compute the page/folio density (the average number of words written on a page or folio, in analogy with the measure 'folio' used to reckon the length of legal writings.[2] Actually, remarkable variations are found even when the number of lines per page/folio is kept unchanged. The standard density is established to range between 91 and 105 words in *H503* and between 416 and 450 words in *H513* (the average number of words per page/folio ± half the value of the standard deviation). As shown on Table 1, 63.7% of the pages in *H503* fit within the standard range (and a smaller percentage below standard)

---

2   The length ranges between 72 and 90 words in UK and Ireland, and around 100 words in U.S.

as opposed to only 50% of those in *H513* (and a smaller percentage over standard).

H503	Hits	%	*H513*	Hits	%
< 91	19	14.07	< 416	11	30.55
91–105	86	63.70	416–450	18	50.00
> 105	30	22.22	> 450	7	19.45

Table 1. Page/folio density in *H503* and *H513*.

Close examination of the MSS allows us to state two facts: (1) out-of-the-range pages are not consecutive but scattered across each treatise, and (2) the low density is not due to the use of ornamented letters or any sort of flourish, but rather to the number of abbreviations or Latin terms.

Next, the main study regards the lexical richness of the witnesses at word- and lemma-level, which requires the building-up of the word/lemma profile for each text. The word profile includes, among others, the count of the tokens (*N*), the word-types (*WT*) that constitute the vocabulary *V(N)*, the occurrences of the most common word (*MCW*), as well as the number of *hapax legomena* (*HL*) and *dislegomena* (*HD*) – that is, the words that occur just once or twice in the texts, respectively. It must be pointed out that the number of tokens in a mediaeval manuscript may slightly fluctuate depending on the decision of the person responsible for the transcription and/or the annotation, as he/she may decide to join separate chains of characters that could also be understood as a single word as in ⟨a nother⟩, ⟨bi cause⟩, ⟨ey lyddes⟩, ⟨an hey3⟩, etc., or, conversely, to split a chain representing two or three words as in ⟨nomore⟩ ('no more'), or in ⟨asonus⟩, ⟨asonus⟩, ⟨assonys⟩ ('as soon as'). Add to this the different counts produced by different text-analysis and/or word-processing programs (Hoover 2004: 479).

The vocabulary richness of a text has traditionally been assessed by implementing a series of statistics with the values in the profile. *N/V(N)* (the *Mean Word Frequency* or *MWF* for short) and its reciprocal *V(N)/N* (the *Type-Token Ratio* or *TTR* for short) are the most recurrently used expressions, but their results are not fully reliable when texts of unequal length are inadvertently compared (Tweedie/Baayen 1998: 324). This rate, which is dependent on N (the number of tokens or running words) becomes smaller as N increases, due to the fact that function words, which make up for roughly the half of N, are accounted just once. Many other statistics have been proposed as length-invariant (see Twedie/Baayen 1998 for a survey), Yule's *Characteristic Constant K*, and Zipf's distribution Z, which is widely accepted as the least N-dependent. As for K, this constant is assumed to measure the lexical repetition or repetition rate in terms of the elements in the frequency spectrum, that is, the number of word-types that occur once, twice, thrice, n-times, whereas Z is thought to assess the vocabulary richness of a text accurately as "an increase in Z leads to an increase in $V(N)$" (Tweedie/Baayen 1998: 331). The values for N, $V(N)$ and MCW are used for the calculation of the free parameter Z.

	H503	H513
$V(N)$	2580	2843
MCW	1131	1249
HL	1513	1709
HD	389	413
N	13306	15656
N^*	13201	—
N^{**}	13353	15936
TTR	0.19	0.18
MWF	5.20	5.51
K	168.44	178.91
Z	34283	33863

Table 2. Lexical values at word-level.[3]

---

3   N^*, which takes into account the words on page 13 (a replica of page 11), decreases with respect to N, whereas N^{**} increases as the tokens in the multi-word lexical units are counted individually. As these increases and decreases ($<10^{-2}$) are negligible, all the studies are based on the values for N.

As seen from Table 2, the values for *TTR* in *H503* and *H513* are 0.19 and 0.18, respectively, and those for *MWF* are 5.20 or 5.51, which means that there is a *WT* every 5.20 or 5.51 tokens. Judging from these data, the vocabulary of the first text is slightly richer than the second, an uncertain result for their different text-length: *H513* exceeds *H503* by 2455 words, which represents 15.68% of the tokens in the latter or 18.6% in the former. However, the same assessment is obtained with *K*, which is smaller in *H503* than in *H513*, as well as with *Z*, which is larger in *H503* than in *H513*. Given that the three constants show the same direction, it would not be too bold a statement to say that the vocabulary in *H503* text is richer than its counterpart in *H513*.

To minimize the effects of the *N*-dependency, the main study is replicated with a serial one by partitioning the *H503* pages into five sections or series (*S1–S5*) and the *H513* folios into six (*S1–S6*). This partition, however, does not bring about equal text-length series: the average text-length amounts to 2611 words, the longer exceeding the average by 195 words and the shorter being 161 words below the average, as shown in Table 3 below. Any text-length divergence may cause that the sections become ranked somewhat differently in terms of lexical richness depending on the statistics used: *TTR, MFW, K* or *Z*.

	H503					H513					
	S1	S2	S3	S4	S5	S1	S2	S3	S4	S5	S6
pp./ff.	1–27	28–54	55–83	84–110	111–137	1–6	7–12	13–18	19–24	25–30	31–36
V(N)	934	838	846	818	822	802	817	793	800	758	837
MCW	222	191	227	266	225	277	174	204	183	183	227
HL	618	542	563	521	544	526	528	528	567	488	563
HD	135	125	123	112	105	110	128	102	91	99	108
N	2806	2604	2655	2624	2617	2671	2592	2483	2450	2546	2676
TTR	0,33	0,32	0,32	0,31	0,31	0,30	0,31	0,32	0,33	0,30	0,31
MWF	3.00	3.11	3.14	3.21	3.18	3.33	3.17	3.13	3.06	3.36	3.20
K	164.9	154.0	170.7	204.9	183.6	246.0	156.2	177.7	171.5	181.8	202.1
Z	28421	20103	21892	21523	20004	18802	16993	19298	19746	14045	20159

Table 3. Lexical values at word-level (serial study).

If only Z is considered as a more reliable constant for the actual measure of vocabulary richness, it can be also stated that $H503$ is slightly richer than $H513$ on account of these facts: (1) Z for the series in the former is always larger than for those in the latter, if the sixth series is excluded; (2) the values for Z are kept within a range but in two outliers: Series One of $H503$ (28421) and Series Five in $H513$ (14045). The data somehow validate the conclusions drawn after the first study with the complete texts, though the tendencies are not so well-marked: in general, the larger the text-length difference, the greater the divergences to be found. When the values for K and Z are considered jointly, the assessment is liable to offer more reliability (Tweedie/Baayen 1998: 333, 350). The plotting of Fig. 1 allows us to distinguish between them with the exception of Series Six of $H513$ which overlaps the boundaries of $H503$.

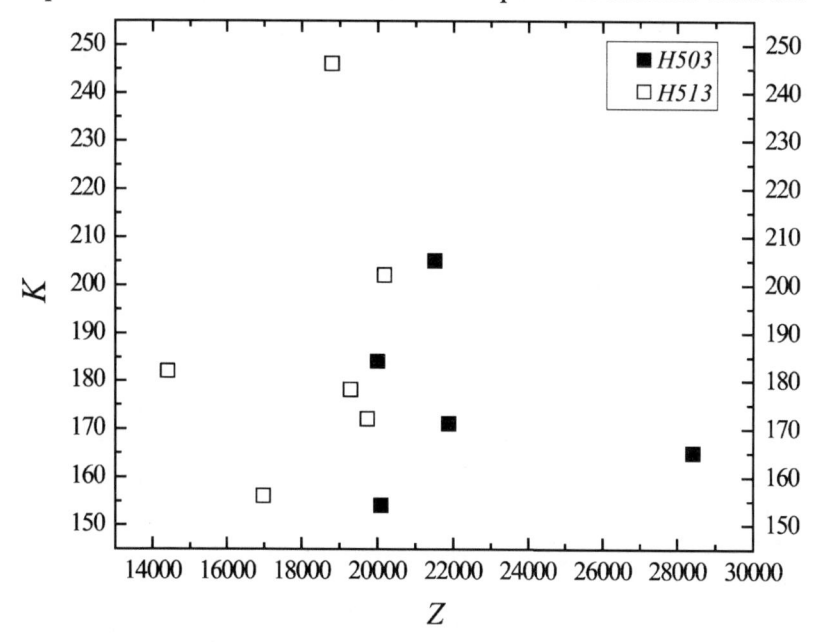

Fig. 1. Values for K and Z in the MSS series (words).

As the results are inconclusive, a new attempt must be made at lemma-level to cope with the great amount of allomorphs occurring in both treatises. The lemma count must be considered more accurate to assess the lexical richness of a text, inasmuch as the common divergences originated by Middle English allomorphs are alleviated through the disambiguation of homographs (Hoover 2001: 422; Burrows 2002: 268). The lemma profile as shown in Table 4 includes the accounting of tokens (N), the lemmas ($L(N)$) which constitute the vocabulary, the occurrences of the most common lemma (MCL), the number of lemmas considered as *hapax legomena* (HLL) and *dislegomena* (HDL), as well as the ratio between L and N (LTR) and its inverse function, that is the *Mean Lemma Frequency* (MLF).

	H503	H513
L(N)	1485	1545
MCL	1133	1318
HLL	643	672
HDL	217	229
N	13306	15656
LTR	0.11	0.09
MLF	8.96	10.13
K	184.37	193.12
Z	7004	6453

Table 4. Lexical values at lemma-level.

From the values for K and Z we can conclude again that the first treatise (*H503*) is also a bit richer in lemmas than the second (*H513*). For the sake of further validation of the data, a serial study is also carried out with the same partition criteria as in the study of words. This is shown in Table 5. The results obtained confirm the same trend: *H513* is less rich than *H503*, since greater values for Z are gotten from the latter (at least in four series) and the smallest value in Series Four exceeds those in Series Two and Five of the former. Likewise, when the values for K and Z are plotted, it is observed that the series of *H513* (on the left area) are detached from the series of *H503* (on the right area), with the exception of S4 (*H503*).

	H503					H513					
	S1	S2	S3	S4	S5	S1	S2	S3	S4	S5	S6
pp./ff.	1–27	28–54	55–83	84–110	111–137	1–6	7–12	13–18	19–24	25–30	31–36
$L(N)$	671	611	628	555	608	574	585	575	587	508	595
MCL	224	191	228	265	225	294	173	214	182	215	238
HLL	371	319	320	254	322	326	306	318	333	243	308
HDL	96	97	121	100	94	84	97	73	87	90	100
N	2806	2604	2655	2624	2617	2671	2592	2483	2450	2546	2676
LTR	0,24	0,23	0,23	0,21	0,23	0,21	0,22	0,23	0,24	0,2	0,22
MLF	4,18	4,26	4,22	4,28	4,3	4,65	4,43	4,31	4,17	5,01	4,50
K	184	168	187	220	197	272	164	192	180	199	213
Z	6815	5328	6233	4603	5699	5131	4334	5187	5255	3186	5143

Table 5. Lexical values at lemma-level (serial study).

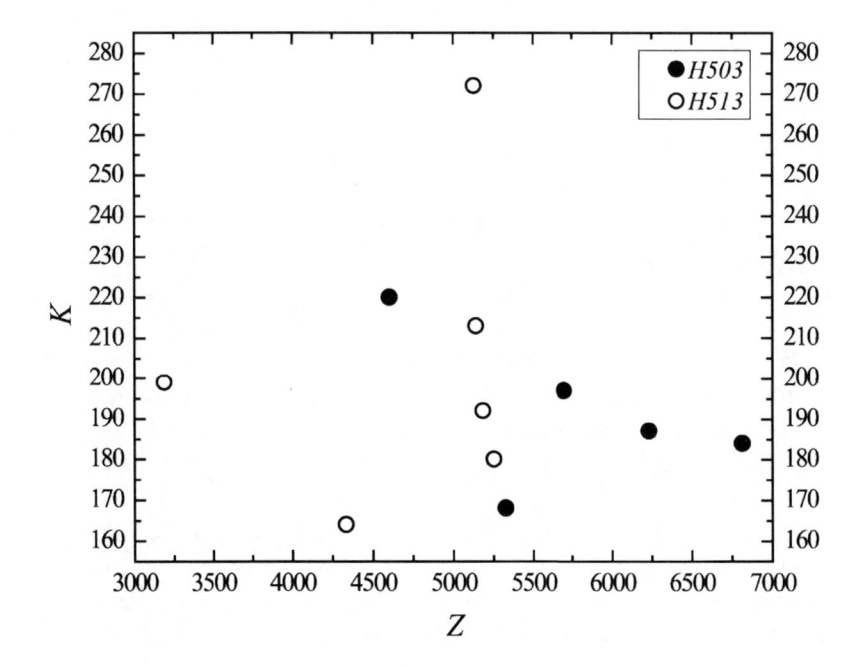

Fig. 2. Values for K and Z in the series (lemmas).

It it not surprising that the series with the greatest value for Z also exhibits the smallest for *TTR* or *LTR* (or else the largest for *MWF* or *MLF*), but this correspondence does not hold in the remaining series. Recall that *TTR* and *LTR* account for the average number of tokens necessary to find a new word-type or lemma (respectively, 5.16 or 8.96 in *H503*, and 5.51 and 10.13 in *H513*). *LTR*, while N-dependent as *TTR*, assesses the lexical or lemma variety of a text in the sense that the smaller the quotient, the larger the lexical variety. However, the ratio between *WT* and L (*WLR*), which appears to be N-independent, accounts for the orthographical variation of the words belonging to a given lemma, in the understanding that the ratio becomes higher with increasing variation due to Middle English inflections (grammatical accidents affect mostly nouns, adjectives, verbs, determiners, and pronouns) and/or common dialectal variants.

	N	*WT*	L	*TTR*	*LTR*	*WLR*
H503	13306	2580	1485	5.16	8.96	1.74
H513	15655	2843	1545	5.51	10.13	1.84

Table 6. N, *WT*, and L ratios.

In accordance with all the above remarks, it follows that *H503* is slightly richer from a lexical point of view than *H513*. Likewise, the former characterizes for showing a greater lexical variety and less orthographical variation. These conclusions agree with those drawn in previous studies, though a further evaluation is felt necessary after the analysis of the data in terms of word-classes. Moreover, the comparison of the lemmas in each treatise evinces that 885 are common to both, while 1260 are different from each other – of which 600 belong to *H503*, the remaining 660 to *H513*. Taking into account that only 10% of the lemmas are different in the referred texts, and recalling that their text-length differs in more than 15%, one could claim that *H503* clearly exceeds *H513* in terms of lemmas but for the fact that this result is also an N-dependent variable. On Table 7 the percentage of increase (Δ) of word-types and lemmas from one series to the next is calculated.[4] It is noticeable to observe that many a time the percentage becomes larger in *H513* than in *H503*, with the exception of lemmas in Series Five.

MSS/Series	S-1	Δ	S-2	Δ	S-3	Δ	S-4	Δ	S-5	Δ	S-6
H503 (pp.)	1-27	—	1-54	—	1-83	—	1-110	—	1-137	—	—
N	2806	92.80	5410	49.08	8065	32.54	10689	24.48	13306	—	—
WT	934	56.64	1463	30.14	1904	18.22	2251	14.62	2580	—	—
L	671	46.05	980	22.14	1197	11.86	1339	10.90	1485	—	—
H513 (ff.)	1-6	—	1-12	—	1-18	—	1-24	—	1-30	—	1-37
N	2671	97.04	5263	47.18	7746	31.63	10196	24.97	12742	22.87	15656
WT	802	67.08	1340	33.96	1795	19.44	2144	15.11	2468	15.19	2843
L	574	53.14	879	27.08	1117	14.86	1283	9.20	1401	10.28	1545

Table 7. Inter-series increase percentages.

4. Textual differences in terms of word-classes and grammatical categories

The second study, which relies on the annotated corpus of *H503* and *H513*, analyses the distribution of items in terms of word-classes and grammatical categories. The analysis is twofold inasmuch as both a general and a specific (or partial) treatment of the data are accomplished. Within the scope of the first approach Table 8 summarises the occurrences of each word-class, their percentage with respect to *N* as well as the punctuation marks *PM*, and the numeration marks *NM*, which are rated to the total number of items (*N*+*PM*+*NM*). The common normalization of the number of occurrences every thousand words is not provided as its calculation is trivial.

---

4   This increase is known as 'pace' by Tweedy/Baayen 1998: 323–352.

	H503				H513			
	Words	%	Lemmas	%	Words	%	Lemmas	%
Adjectives	721	5.42	222	14.95	710	4.54	181	12.19
Nouns	2967	22.30	662	44.58	3354	21.42	697	46.94
Verbs	2230	16.76	280	18.85	2580	16.48	315	21.21
Conjunctions	1458	10.96	31	2.09	1863	11.90	39	2.63
Adverbs	1009	7.58	157	10.57	1139	7.28	164	11.04
Prepositions	1736	13.05	40	2.69	2036	13.00	48	3.23
Interjections	2	0.01	2	0.13	1	0.01	1	0.07
Determiners	2065	15.52	46	3.10	2420	15.46	49	3.30
Pronouns	1118	8.40	45	3.03	1552	9.91	51	3.43
N or L	13306	—	1485	—	15655	—	1545	—
PM	2009	13.11	—	—	862	5.207	—	—
NM	—	—	—	—	36	0.217	—	—
N+PM+NM	15315	—	—	—	16553	—	—	—

Table 8. Distribution of words and lemmas in terms of word-classes.

The analysis of the results does not evince great percentual differences between *H503* and *H513* but for *PM*, which are more common in the first treatise (the result of such a difference being 8%). However, minor divergences (≥ 1%) point to individual features which may prove worthwhile for distinguishing between them: their difference is found to be greater for pronouns and conjunctions in *H513* and for adjectives and nouns in *H503* at word-level, and the same can be stated at lemma-level, setting nouns apart. To this exception other divergences must be added: the percentage of the remaining word-classes (adverbs, prepositions and determiners) is observed to be higher in *H513* than in *H503*, whereas the opposite phenomenon is found at word-level. The change of tendency detected requires close examination of all the data to find a plausible explanation, taking into consideration that nouns and verbs are the two word-classes more likely to display inflection marks. However, the results at lemma-level do not diverge when *N*, *V(N)* and *L(N)* are rated: *H503* turns out to be again richer from a lexical point of view, to contain larger lexical variety and to keep lesser orthographical variation.

	H503						H513					
	N	V(N)	L(N)	MWF	MLF	WLR	N	V(N)	L(N)	MWF	MLF	WLR
Adjectives	721	331	222	2.18	3.25	1.49	710	273	181	2.60	3.92	1.51
Nouns	2967	1165	662	2.55	4.48	1.76	3354	1242	697	2.70	4.81	1.78
Verbs	2230	673	280	3.31	7.96	2.40	2580	822	315	3.14	8.19	2.61
Conjunctions	1458	49	31	29.76	47.03	1.58	1863	72	39	25.88	47.77	1.85
Adverbs	1009	282	157	3.58	6.43	1.80	1139	291	164	3.91	6.95	1.77
Prepositions	1736	76	40	22.84	43.40	1.90	2036	99	48	20.57	42.42	2.06
Determiners	2065	106	46	19.48	44.89	2.30	2420	128	49	18.91	49.39	2.61
Pronouns	1118	97	45	11.53	24.84	2.16	1552	117	51	13.26	30.43	2.29
TOTAL	13306	2580	1485	5.16	8.96	1.74	15655	2843	1545	5.51	10.13	1.84

Table 9. *N, WT, L ratios* in terms of word-classes.

Therefore, the two treatises can be told apart on the grounds of their different word-class distribution. The results at word-level can plausibly be explained as follows: a greater use of adjectives in *H503* can be associated to a larger number of nouns which, in turn, favours a slight increase in verbs, and obviously a reduction in the use of pronouns; the opposite can be stated as regards the other treatise. A stylistic justification requires a further analysis to check whether the author/translator of the first treatise is more prone to nominalization than the second – who, at least to a certain extent, seems more prone to the use of pronouns. Likewise, it would be desirable to find out whether the first text is more descriptive on account of a larger use of adjectives, or whether the second text shows a greater cohesion due to the syndetic function conveyed by conjunctions; but such a research surpasses the scope of this work. Its accomplishment is, no doubt, worth attempting in a near future so as to confirm whether the hypotheses hold true.

The individual differences in terms of word-classes that characterize the first treatise from the second can also be accounted for by using the percentual distribution of *content words* (*CW*) and *function words* (*FW*) as a reliable feature in authorship attribution studies. Nouns, (qualifying) adjectives, verbs (auxiliary and modals excluded) and adverbs of manner are regarded as *CW*, whilst the remaining categories are taken as *FW*. The ratio between *CW* and *FW*, which ranges between 45% and 55% in most English texts irrespective of their style, genre or chronology, is the *lexical density* (*LD*) of a text (Miranda García/Calle Martín 2005). The *lexical density* confers upon the text a greater lexical or structural content: the larger the ratio, the more lexical content the text encloses and, conversely, the smaller the ratio, the more structural content the text displays. *Lexical density*, which is not *N*-dependent, is also found to be higher in *H503* than in *H513*, as shown in Table 10. A similar slight distinction is observed when the lexical density is calculated with the number of lemmas, though we must be aware that a new dependency can arise from the inherent feature of function lemmas, which constitute a *closed set*.

	\multicolumn{4}{c	}{H503}	\multicolumn{4}{c}{H513}
	Words	%	Lemmas	%	Words	%	Lemmas	%
CW	5772	43.22	1200	80.80	6441	41.14	1226	79.35
FW	7554	56.77	285	19.20	9214	58.86	319	20.64
LD	—	0.76	—	4.21	—	0.70	—	3.84

Table 10. Lexical density at word- and lemma-level.

Despite this, the different text-length of the treatises demands again a serial study in terms of word-class distribution to discover whether it is similar in each section and, otherwise, to analyse the likely divergent series which can shed light on the transmission process of the MSS. The partition criteria for the series and the computation methodology used in Table 11 remain unchanged, but only the percentages are shown for the sake of space in the page, along with the standard deviation (σ) that helps evaluate the existing divergences.

	\multicolumn{6}{c	}{H503}	\multicolumn{6}{c}{H513}
	S1	S2	S3	S4	S5	σ	S1	S2	S3	S4	S5	S5	σ
Adjectives	6.77	4.84	4.93	5.07	5.39	0.79	5.21	4.90	4.11	4.33	3.81	4.67	0.57
Nouns	20.92	22.50	23.88	21.57	22.70	1.13	22.17	20.56	22.03	21.67	19.64	22.61	1.08
Verbs	16.54	17.28	16.91	16.84	16.24	0.39	14.12	17.21	16.63	15.80	18.19	16.74	1.54
Conjunctions	11.44	11.10	10.47	11.05	10.70	0.37	10.94	11.84	10.43	12.90	13.12	12.18	1.18
Adverbs	7.88	7.76	6.78	7.51	7.99	0.48	6.07	7.72	7.09	7.55	7.97	7.14	0.75
Prepositions	13.22	13.52	12.62	12.88	12.99	0.34	15.17	13.77	13.09	12.16	11.63	12.18	1.39
Interjections	0.00	0.00	0.00	0.00	0.08	0.03	0.00	0.00	0.00	0.00	0.00	0.00	0.00
Determiners	14.50	15.28	16.23	16.43	15.21	0.79	17.64	13.93	16.83	14.98	15.48	14.31	1.48
Pronouns	8.73	7.72	8.17	8.65	8.71	0.44	8.69	10.07	9.79	10.61	10.17	10.16	0.72
N	87.33	87.03	85.51	88.59	86.00	1.20	93.10	94.70	95.39	94.52	95.18	94.69	0.90
PM	12.67	12.97	14.49	11.41	14.00	1.20	5.72	5.30	4.61	5.48	4.75	5.31	0.48
NM	—	—	—	—	—	—	1.19	—	—	—	0.07	—	0.57
N+PM+NM	100	100	100	100	100	—	100	100	100	100	100	100	—

Table 11. Serial distribution of the words in terms of word-classes.

The most noteworthy deviations which derive from σ can be summarised as follows:

- > 1 in nouns (*H503*), and in nouns, verbs, conjunctions, prepositions and determiners (*H513*)
- $\geq .75$ in adjectives and determiners (*H503*), and in adverbs (*H513*)
- $> .5$ in adjectives and pronouns (*H513*)
- $< .5$ in verbs, conjunctions, adverbs, prepositions, and pronouns (*H503*)

The results show a more steady distribution in terms of word-classes in the series constituting *H503* and similar trends are kept in the individual values for nouns, adjectives, conjunctions and pronouns. In other words, the serial study replicates the most significant data, which can be interpreted as a confirmation of the results obtained from the whole study. Some particular deviations can be explained when the text is carefully observed, as is the case of S1 in *H513*. The reason for these skews is found in the composition of the first folios listing the contents of the treatise. As expected, they fit into a noun phrase format where determiners, nouns, adjectives and prepositions predominate to the detriment of verbs, pronouns, adverbs, and conjunctions.

As indicated, a specific treatment of the grammatical categories is next accomplished focusing on some of the most divergent uses which help distinguish between the two treatises, namely, (1) the distribution of conjunctions denoting logical relations, (2) the use of tenses and modal verbs, (3) the paradigmatic frequency of personal pronouns, (4) simple and compound relative pronouns, and (5) the prefixed verbs.

(1) The communicative function "how to express logical relations" involves the notions of CAUSE and RESULT and, by extension, those of CONDITION and CONTRAST; depending on the relation marked, a great variety of sentences can be issued mostly by a using a conjunction. As already shown in Table 8, conjunctions are more common in *H513* than in *H503*, but this tendency is reversed if the conjunctions denoting cause-result are solely considered: 11.32% in the former witness as opposed to 12.51% in the latter. This may mean that the first author is more prone to signal this kind of scientific deductive discourse. In addition, the preference of a given modality instead of another also constitutes an authorial feature. Thus, the author of *H503* seems to prefer sentences containing a clause of cause or result (8.85% as compared to 5.90% in *H513*) rather than contrast clauses (3.57% as compared with 5.10% in *H513*).

	H503	%	H513	%
Cause	77	5.28	60	3.22
Contrast	52	3.57	95	5.10
Condition	1	0.07	6	0.32
Result	52	3.57	50	2.68

Table 13. Distribution of conjunctions denoting cause-effect relationship.

Setting MSS Hunter 503 and Hunter 513 Apart 161

(2) The use of tenses and modal verbs is also helpful to put the two texts apart as they differ noticeably in the use of the simple present tense and the imperative (41.48% and 16.82% in *H503* as opposed to 49.46% and 13.95% in *H513*, respectively). Concerning the lower percentage of imperatives in *H513*, it is plausible to argue that a balance can be roughly obtained by adding the occurrences of modal {shullen} which nearly double those in its counterpart. The distribution of modals is not homogeneous: {mōuen} occurs evenly and {cŏnnen} is practically non-existent in both treatises, whereas {willen} is more common and {mōten} practically of exclusive use in *H503*.

	H503	%	H513	%
Simple Present	925	41.48	1276	49.46
Simple Past	144	6.46	156	6.05
Imperative	375	16.82	360	13.95
Infinitive	289	12.95	304	11.78

Table 14. Distribution of tenses and mood.

(3) The paradigm of personal pronouns in each treatise contains individual features which are also interesting in authorship attribution studies. The figures are so illustrative that further explanations seem unnecessary.

	H503	%	H513	%		H503	%	H513	%
{ich}	92	12.67	19	1.78	{wē}	8	1.10	135	12.64
{thŏu}	8	1.10	29	2.72	{yē}	69	9.50	115	10.77
{hē}	115	15.84	97	9.08	{thei}	132	18.18	123	11.52
{shē}	—	—	5	0.47	hem	—	—	118	11.05
{hit}	302	41.60	427	39.98					

Table 15. Distribution of personal pronouns.

(4) Compound relative pronouns can also be helpful in distinguishing between the two treatises: the occurrences of the compound pronominal ⟨(the) whiche that⟩ and ⟨the which(e), the whych(e)⟩ are virtually exclusive to *H513*: there is only a handful of examples in *H503*.[5]

(5) Prefixed verbs are found to be more commonly used in *H513* than in *H503*.

The lemma-sorted KWIC-concordances of both treatises provide other features, mainly orthographical or graphemic, which also serve to separate the two works in quantitative terms, namely, the *-liche/-ly* dichotomy in the adverbs of manner, the alternating use of ⟨k⟩ and ⟨c⟩ for /k/ and the employment of ⟨y⟩ as a diacritic for vowel length.

(6) The Old English adverbs in *-līce* are found with both endings *-liche* and in *-ly* in *H513,* whereas *H503* displays only in the latter. Moreover, both endings can be irrespectively applied to one and the same stem in *H513*: ⟨erliche⟩, ⟨erly⟩, ⟨erlyche⟩, ⟨erlyiche⟩; ⟨oneliche⟩, ⟨only⟩, ⟨onyly⟩; ⟨parfiteliche⟩, ⟨parfitely⟩; ⟨sodaynliche⟩, ⟨sodenly⟩; ⟨softeliche⟩, ⟨softely⟩; ⟨whisely⟩, ⟨wisely⟩, ⟨wyseliche⟩, ⟨wyselyche⟩, ⟨wysoliche⟩.

(7) Unvoiced velar stops are represented by ⟨k⟩ or ⟨c⟩ in *H503* ⟨kut⟩, ⟨cut⟩, ⟨cutt⟩, ⟨cutte⟩, ⟨kutt⟩, ⟨kutte⟩, ⟨kutteþ⟩, ⟨kuttyng⟩, ⟨cerkyl⟩, but ⟨k⟩ is rarer in *H513* ⟨castethe⟩, ⟨castethe⟩, ⟨castithe⟩, ⟨cause⟩, ⟨circle⟩, ⟨sercle⟩, ⟨ache⟩; yet note ⟨kest⟩.

(8) Vowel length marked by means of ⟨y⟩ in ⟨boyth⟩, ⟨doyth⟩, ⟨cloyth⟩, ⟨goyth⟩, ⟨moyst⟩ is observed only in *H513*.

---

5   The examples are: *that haue þer humurs depedowne* **the whych** *causyth the ey to seme blak* (*H503* p. 8,5); *the poynt the corrupte water* **the whych** *ys the cateracte . and then* (*H503* p. 16,10); *that was betweyne þem . **The whych** doon . put no medycyne yn* (*H503* p. 52,10); *yn the stomake . Of* **the whych** *ys resoluyd a corrupte fumosytie þat* (*H503* p. 66,5); *after hys propre experyence ,* **the wych** *he had by long contynuance of* (*H503*, p. 1,5).

5. Conclusions

The two treatises have been studied from a quantitative perspective by a simple counting of tokens (words, symbols or marks of punctuation and numeration, etc.) as well as by their count of the items in terms of lemmas, word-classes, grammatical categories or accidence. Although some bias to the results could be argued due to human intervention in the processes of tagging and disambiguation, the possible distortion is deemed negligible, because the same criteria have been applied across the samples. In light of the previous analyses, it is not far-fetched to conclude that both treatises can be set apart by means of quantitative features, incidentally confirming also their different dialectal provenance established with a more traditional methodology (McIntosh/Samuels/Benskin 1986).

It has been demonstrated that the treatise *H503* is slightly richer from a lexical standpoint than *H513*, showing a greater orthographical variation and a larger lexical density. Moreover, the percentual differences found in the distribution of word-classes and/or grammatical categories (for example, the use of conjunctions to denote the cause-effect relationship, the tenses and moods more commonly attested, the paradigm of personal and relative pronouns, the spelling of the adverbs of manner, etc.) allows us to reach the same conclusion. To explain that the first treatise is richer than the second from a lexical point of view the hypothesis of a collaborative authorship is conjectured.

Although the main objective was thus reached, a side objective was to check whether the remarkable deviations found in the serial word-class distribution and/or the change of tendency in some analyses when switching from word to lemma level (the percentage of nouns and verbs in *H513* became greater than in *H503*) could be explained by the orthographical variation perceived across the two treatises. The first measure was to check that the raw data and the subsequent computations had not inadvertently become corrupt, but this operation proved useless for the coincidence of the results.

The next task was to work with the hypothesis of a collaborative authorship as the source for the orthographical variation in *H503*, as there is a debated and as yet unresolved question of "whether collaborative texts are always richer than texts from separate contributors" (Holmes and Forsyth 1995: 117). This approach required to locate a set of individual distinguishing features in certain passages (consecutive or alternating) as traits of authorial authorship. For this purpose, we scrutinized all the remarkable variants of each page of the witnesses and took them down into an Excel spreadsheet wherein the cells in the first row served to identify the page/folio number and the ones in the first column to hold the items being analysed for the existence of concurrent dialectal variants. Such items mostly involved the plural of nouns, 3rd person singular of presents, preterites, and past participles.

The detailed analysis of the observations has not yielded any satisfactory explanation of the phenomena as no complete allomorphic homogeneity was found in the columns. For instance, the morpheme *-es* was found to alternate freely with *-is/-ys* in the plural, *-eth* alternated with *-ith/-yth* as 3rd person inflection, and so did *-ed* with *-id/-yd* as preterite inflection. Had a systematic analogy of homologous variants been encountered in consecutive or alternating passages, we could claim the existence of one scribe who copied an exemplar compiled from sources translated from Latin by more than one people (each one using his own dialect) since the possibility for two hands had to be ruled out in view of the palaeographic examination. However, analogous phenomena such as ⟨*doyth*⟩, ⟨*boyth*⟩, ⟨*goyth*⟩, ⟨*cloyth*⟩, ⟨*moyst*⟩ did not occur on the same page or on adjacent pages/folios, while oppositely two variants concurred on the same page or even on the very same line (for example, ⟨*dyssoluyd*⟩ side by side with ⟨*dyssolued*⟩), which averted the possibility of drawing a reliable conclusion.

On the other hand, and as explained on footnote 7 of the foreword to the edition, the scribe of *H503* had a page of his exemplar duplicated: the text on page 11 is basically the same as that consigned on p. 13; but even there the spelling of some tokens differed from one version to the other, as seen from the following examples (the first excerpt is taken from page 11, the second from p. 13; it is important to indicate that the hand remains exaclty the same for both pages):

(1) **metis** . wherof a groos **fumosytee** resoluyd . ascendyth vp ynto the brayn . and from **thens**
metys . wherof a groos **fumosite** resoluyd ascendyth vp into the brayn and from **thence** .
(2) fallyth **downe** into the eyon . ¶ The **thyrde cateractte** curable ys also **whytysche**, but **it**
fallyth **down** into the eyon The **iijde Cateracte** curable ys also **whytylhe** . but **yt**
(3) turnyth into the **color** of ashes . and is **comunly gendrid** of the payn of the hede . as the
turnyth into the **colour** of ashes . and is **comonly gendryd** of the payn of the hede . as **of** the
(4) mygrym and such **other** . and **is causid** of gret **sorowe** . sumtyme . and of **grete** heuynes
mygrym and such **oyer** . and **ys caused** of gret **sorow** sumtyme . and of **gret** heuynes
(5) **cawsyng grette** wepyng . and sumtyme of **much** colde . and **much** watche and such **oþer** .
causyng gret wepyng . and sumtyme of **mech** colde and **mech** watche and such **oþer** . ¶
(6) And the **iiijth** spice of **cateracctis** curable . ys of **sytrynne color** . **and** it **ys comunly**
And the **forthe** spice of **Cateractys** curable is of **sytryne colour** . **And** it **is comunly**
(7) gendryd of exces **meete** and drynk **yndegest** . **and** also of gret **labour** . and sumtyme humurs
gendryd of exces **mete** and drynk **indigest** . **And** also of gret **labor** . and sumtyme humurs

This evidence somehow helps explain the concurrence of orthographical variants within the same text. It is not hard to describe the obvious features of each (in bold face) but it is not that easy to pinpoint them, one by one, and establish which of the two possibility is closer to the idiolect of the manuscript. A couple of examples of the two witnesses suffice to show the overlapping: (a) the nominal endings -*our* and -*or* alternate in *H503* (⟨*labo(u)r, colo(u)r⟩, barbo(u)r, humo(u)r*⟩ but only the -*our* ending is encountered in *H513*; (b) the allomorphs of the lemmas {much} and {such} are ⟨moch(e), seche, soch(e)⟩ in *H503*, ⟨much(e), mech, mych⟩ in *H513* and ⟨such(e)⟩ in both. Therefore, all these phenomena come to support the hypothesis of a collaborative authorship in the sense that the copyist may have used several exemplars at a time and he actually mixed them (sometimes a line, sometimes a sentence, some others a page). This behaviour cannot be easily explained unless motivated by any of the following hypothetical reasons: the need to complete a missing section, the convenience of finding an easier reading in the other model, or simply a mistake when switching from one to the other exemplar in a double proof-reading. Extravagant as they all may seem, no other valid theory holds for the non-systematic occurrence of alternative variants across the treatises.

DAVID MORENO OLALLA

Foreword to the Synoptic Edition[1]

1. General description

The text offered in the following pages is a synoptic edition of the ophthalmological work of Benvenutus Grassus (a treatise on the diseases and injuries of the eye variously called *Practica oculorum* and *De probatissima arte oculorum*) as it was recorded in six different manuscripts. The present edition provides the Latin text as given in Metz, Bibliothèques-Médiatèques de Metz / Département Patrimoine, MS 176, ff. 1r–16r [MS *M*] (which appears to be the fullest version available, see Eldredge 1993), together with the Provençal translation of Basel, Öffentliche Bibliothek der Universität, MS D.II.11, ff. 172r–177v [MS *B*], and the four Middle English versions identified so far: Glasgow, Glasgow University Library, Hunter MS 503 (V.8.6), pp. 1–137 [MS *H503*]; Glasgow, Glasgow University Library, Hunter MS 513 (V.8.16), ff. 2r–37r [MS *H513*]; London, British Library, Sloane MS 661, ff. 32r–46r [MS *S*]; and Oxford, Bodleian Library, Ashmole MS 1468, pp. 1–6 [MS *A*]. The present edition thus presents together for the first time at least one member from all the known textual families of this treatise, save the Old French translation.[2]

---

[1] The present research has been funded by the Spanish Ministry of Education (project FFI2008-02336). This grant is hereby gratefully acknowledged.

[2] The OF text, extant in a single manuscript (Paris, Bibliothèque Nationale de France, MS français 1327, ff. 38r–60v), was edited in 1901 by Pierre Pansier and Charles Laborde together with a reproduction of Henri Teulié's 1900 edition of the Provençal text. In the Introduction to this volume, they made a passing remark about the existence of a Hebrew version (Laborde/Pansier/Teulié 1901: 6) but did not provide a library shelfmark for this MS; I have found no reference to this Hebrew version outside their comment (it is not recorded in Steinschneider 1893's indexes, for instance). On the other hand, they were apparently ignorant of the substantial Middle English tradition.

Unfortunately, none of the known vernacular recensions furnishes a version of Benvenutus' treatise as complete as the Latin text provided by MS *M*. As a matter of fact, some of the non-Latin manuscripts are either acephalous (for instance, MS *A*) or atelous (such is the case of MSS *B* and *S*), while the two Hunterian versions, though complete, are probably translations from different abridgements of the original text. These two reasons serve to explain why long passages in MS *M* (whole sections in a few cases, as in §§4, 12–14, 32) are missing in the vernacular texts.

The English branch of the Benvenutus tradition is composed of two independent translations (Eldredge 1996: 30–37): Ashmole 1468 and Hunter 513 form one group (which Eldredge called *O*), and Hunter 503 and Sloane 661 form another (Eldredge's *O¹*). According to the proposed stemma, the Ashmole MS must have served as exemplar to Hunter 513, while Hunter 503 and Sloane 661 are two independent copies deriving from a common exemplar.[3]

The MSS in this edition have been edited collaboratively. Laurence M. Eldredge is responsible for the editing of the Metz MS, while Teresa Marqués Aguado prepared Hunter 513. David Moreno Olalla was in charge of the remaining four copies of Benvenutus' work used in the present edition (Ashmole 1468, Basel D.II.11, Hunter 503 and Sloane 661).

The transcriptions of the two Hunterian copies of the ME Benvenutus were made from fresh examination of the corresponding MSS *in situ*; they were later doublechecked using the high resolution images

---

[3] A glance to the ME texts makes the existence of two different families within the English tradition almost evident, but, while *H513* and *A* do seem to derive from a common lost exemplar, *H503* and *S* may not be at the same level in the stemma. These two MSS have a vertical, rather than a horizontal, relationship: they share common conjunctive errors, but no real separative ones. Moreover, the same hand, that of Joseph Fenton, wrote both *S* and part of the marginal comments in *H503*. It is extremely likely then that *H503* was the 'oulde Booke' that he mentioned at the beginning of *S* as the exemplar to his copy. See Pearson (2003: 239–242) for a biographical sketch of Joseph Fenton (*ca.*1565/1570–1634); MS *S* is mentioned in Pearson's article, but the direct link between *H503* and this MS was not recognised there either.

provided by the University of Glasgow.[4] The text of Sloane 661 is based on the black and white images provided by the British Library, while that of Ashmole 1468 and Metz 176 were taken from the microfilm. The Basel MS was transcribed from the facsimile that accompanies a translation of Benvenutus' treatise into Spanish (Udina y Martorell/Casas Homs 1967) and which appears to be a print of the microfilm.

Besides Benvenutus' treatise, the edition of the vernacular texts also includes a brief *apparatus criticus* that records the marginal annotations of the MSS (regardless of whether they were written by the main scribe of the text or by later readers) and such scribal alterations of the text as cancelations and erasures.[5] Marginal notes in the Metz MS, on the other hand, do nothing more than summarise the text, and thus have, with a single exception at section 58, been omitted.

The text of *M* has been edited with as little editorial interference as possible (only enough for clarity) following the philosophy that scribal errors which do not cause confusion should not be corrected. Where absolutely necessary, a reading from one or more other manuscripts has been inserted into the text in square brackets and a textual note added at the foot of the column. The edition of the Latin text additionally records the major variants from the following manuscripts: Naples, Biblioteca Nazionale MS VIII. G. 100, ff. 48r (51r)–67v (70v) (siglum *N* in the edition); Vatican, Biblioteca Apostolica, Palat. Lat. MS 1268, ff. 288r–314r (*VP2*) and Vatican, Biblioteca Apostolica, Regin. Lat. MS 373, ff. 29r–63v (*VR*). Readings from these manuscripts, which are inserted in square brackets, are supplied only for clarity and are not intended to represent all the manuscripts of the tradition. See on this subject Laurence Eldredge's contribution on this volume, and particularly pp. 24–27.

---

[4] Colour images of the two Hunterian Benvenutus, and of several other scientific ME MSS kept at the Special Collections section of Glasgow University Library, can be reached online at <http://hunter.uma.es>. Transcriptions of these treatises are also available there.

[5] The microfilm images of the Provençal MS may have been trimmed to make them fit into the page of the Spanish edition, and therefore there is a chance that part of the marginalia was lost.

2. Page arrangement

The transcriptions of the six different MSS have been distributed in columns on the page following two criteria: since the present volume is as a whole dedicated to the analysis of the English branch of the Benvenutus tradition, they have been set on the more central part of the page, while the Latin and the Provençal texts, which serve as a complement, accompany them in the outermost columns. Within the English translations, the Hunterian texts are again located in the more central place, while the rendering of the text in the Sloane and Ashmole copies stand in a secondary position at the bottom of the corresponding page. The reason behind this decision is that the two Glasgow MSS keep the more complete versions now available. Therefore, the reader will find – from left to right and from top to bottom – the text of Benvenutus' treatise as recorded in Metz 176, Hunter 503 and Sloane 661 on the left-hand pages, and those versions in Hunter 513, Basel D.II.11 and Ashmole 1468 on the right-hand ones.

It was decided from the start that the text of these manuscripts would be arranged in parallel columns, thus allowing the same matter to be read synopticly.[6] Eldredge's editorial division of the Latin text into eighty-two numbered sections, designed to facilitate reference, came in most handy for the purpose and thus served as a guide for the other versions. Presenting the text of the treatise in such a way is not without risks. While it makes comparison of data between the different witnesses a very easy task, it has also the drawback of leaving some pages virtually blank, since neither of the vernacular versions is a perfect rendering of the Metz text: all of them miss a number of sections – most conspicuously the Basel and the Ashmole versions, which are respectively atelous and acephalous.

To complicate matters further, Hunter 503 has sections 37 and 79 misplaced in comparison with the other witnesses. §37 was recorded

---

6 The same method had already been employed in Albertotti (1896) to present the versions of the Latin text contained in MSS Al, VR (left-hand side), N and VV. For the sigla, see Eldredge's contribution in this volume.

Foreword to the Edition 171

after §40 and therefore starts on *H503*:53.11 (note that §35 – the preceding section since §36 was not translated in Branch O^1 of the tradition – had ended at *H503*:49.16), while §79 appears after §81, starting on *H503*:135.9 (§78 had ended on *H503*:130.10). Needless to say, the text of Sloane 661, which is plausibly a sixteenth-century copy of this Hunterian text as stated above, could not but reproduce the same mistake as regards §37 (and, one can safely guess, also §79, had its scribe, J. Fenton, copied the whole exemplar – but for some reason he stopped after §58).

After some initial hesitations, synopsis finally got the upper hand over editorial integrity and the original arrangement of these two MSS was sacrificed by locating these chunks of text in the same place as the rest of versions. Such breaches have nevertheless been duly indicated in the text by adding a marginal reference to the folio/page and line, and a note in the *apparatus criticus*; a second reference similarly indicates the point where the MS arrangement of the text resumes.

There are a couple of additional flaws in *H503*. Page 12 of this MS was ruled in ink but remained blank, and the fragment on p. 13 merely repeats the words that had been already copied on p. 11.[7] Consequently they have been ignored for this edition, and our text jumps from p. 11 to 14. Moreover, this MS misses page 70, due to a mistake during the modern numbering of the folios: the paginator passed from p. 69 directly to p. 71. From this page onwards, odd pages are found on the left rather than on the right, which runs counter to the custom of most Western books.

---

[7] Differences between these two pages are minimal and consist mostly of alternative spellings such as the following (the first member represents the reading on p. 11): ⟨fumosytee⟩ : ⟨fumosite⟩ [1]; ⟨thens⟩ : ⟨thence⟩ [3]; ⟨thyrde cat*er*actte⟩ : ⟨iii[de] Cat*er*acte⟩ [4], etc. The only divergences of some substance are the mistake ⟨whytylhe⟩ [*H503*:13.5] instead of ⟨whytyshe⟩ [*H503*:11.5]; the inclusion of an extra word in ⟨as the⟩ [7] : ⟨as | of the⟩ [7–8] and the pair ⟨much⟩ : ⟨mech⟩ [11], which may have some dialectal interest. See also fn. 10 about the implications of the pair ⟨cat*er*accter⟩ [*H503*:11.13] : ⟨Cat*er*actys⟩ [*H503*:13.13].

3. Transcription philosophy

A sharp distinction must be made between the transcriptions policies of Latin and vernacular MSS. Latin was a very consistently codified language since the first century A.D. (Hale/Buck 1966: §52), and there is little variation in spelling that may help define spatial or temporal differences definitively. While there are some orthographic features that help differentiate Classical and Mediaeval Latin, for most mediaeval manuscripts they do not go much further than the use of ⟨e⟩ (or else, *e caudata* ⟨ę⟩) to represent the Classical Latin diphthongs ⟨ae⟩ and ⟨oe⟩ (cf. Classical L. *poenae* : Mediaeval L. *pene*) and ⟨c⟩ instead of ⟨t⟩ before consonantal ⟨i⟩ (cf. Classical L. *potio* : Mediaeval L. *pocio*) – a meagre harvest indeed, and too general to be of any real use to date a text with any precision.

On the other hand, the lack of national standards meant that spelling could vary greatly when dealing with Mediaeval Provençal and (most especially) Middle English, as demonstrated by *LALME*. The study of the way in which words are spelt in a MS is so revealing that it currently plays a role in locating the place of composition of a given Middle English text that is comparable to the analysis of morphemic variation only. Even the expansion of the abbreviations used in vernacular texts must be given a very deep thought: consider for instance the long-reaching implications that transcribing MS ⟨ſ⟩ as *-es*, *-is* or *-us* may have if we want to use that evidence to locate the text on the map, or ⟨⁹⟩ as either *-er-* or *-ar-*, if our intention is to date the text.[8]

Not only written variation, but also the very grammar of these languages must be taken into account before deciding which type of edition should be undertaken. To give an example: although there are of course exceptions, as a general rule the extensive use of grammatical cases in Latin makes the translation of a given sentence a relatively straightforward task, since the syntactic values of the components are well marked. This means, for example, that punctuation is normally

---

8   See Jordan 1974: §135 on the alternation *-es/-is/-us*, and §270 on the historical development of *-er*.

not a problem when one has to edit a Latin text, which serves to explain why national punctuation practices apply in most contemporary Latin editions. Although modernisation of the original punctuation in vernacular texts is also a common practice, there are voices against it, claiming that not only the presence or absence of a punctuation mark, but even the type of sign employed, can be relevant for the perfect understanding of the intended sense of a line. Modernisation of the original punctuation system of the MS could moreover be regarded as an attempt to force readers into editorial interpretations of the text.

This *caveat* is not restricted to punctuation only but must include also another feature that is rarely discussed in the introductions to modern editions: word separation. Again, within the Latin sphere this is an issue only with very obscure or mutilated texts: in normal practice, any editor would know unhesitatingly where to split the letter chain. The choice is less obvious for the editor of vernacular texts. Although most would probably agree in splitting MS ⟨aman⟩ into *a man*, there might be less *consensus doctorum* when it comes to what to do with MS ⟨anaddre⟩. Should this cluster be separated into *an addre* or rather into *a naddre*? The first policy would be in accordance with the contemporary standard spelling for the word (*an adder*); the second, with its etymology (OE *nǣddre*). And what shall we do with ⟨aneuete⟩? Both *an euete* ('an eft') and *a neuete* ('a newt') are accepted spellings in the *OED*![9]

These factors call quite naturally for a whole different editorial approach to the MS, depending on the language in which it is written. Whereas there seem to be only questions of detail on how to edit a Latin text, the editor of a vernacular MS must make a number of important decisions before ever laying his/her eyes on the volume – that is, unless the edition is expected to follow the guidelines set by a third party, usually a publishing house. All these decisions can probably be condensed into just two ideas that go hand in hand most of the time: the editor must define in advance the intended target of the volume (will it be read by specialists in the language, or is it oriented to a more general public?),

---

9   The same remarks are valid for the edition of Romance texts: it can be sometimes difficult to decide whether ⟨elmalaute⟩ in the Basel MS is to be separated as *e·l malaute* 'and the sick man' or simply as *el malaute* 'the sick man'.

and the personal and academic interests of the editor (is (s)he an expert in Literature, Linguistics, Palaeography...?).

The natural target for the present edition of Benvenutus' treatise is the specialist in Middle English; it coincides, therefore, with the fields of expertise of the several editors involved in the project. Accordingly, the editors' main driving force has been to present the diverse versions with as little interference as possible, and to leave the responsibility of interpreting the actual sense of the text to the final reader. Such a target must nonetheless include those scholars who are neither able to read Mediaeval scripts nor trained in the writing habits of the period, but are interested in the language or the contents of the treatise only. Making a complete palaeographical edition (let alone a full facsimile) would then have been awkward. This rationale explains, for example, that abbreviations in the MS have been expanded, but for the benefit of the specialist such expansions are marked in italics so that the scholar always have the chance to accept or reject the proposed transliteration. A full explanation of the transcription principles is given in the next section.

Since it caters for a different readership, this edition of Benvenutus' ophthalmical treatise may be thought of as a complement to the critical edition of the Middle English text that Laurence Eldredge published in 1996: his edition obviously had broader intentions and was designed to be accessible also to the non-specialist in Middle English. This can be seen from the editorial decision of using a base MS (Hunter 503, with additions from Hunter 513), the modernised punctuation and word division, the number of editorial interventions, the skipping of minor variants in the *apparatus criticus*, etc.

4. Editorial guidelines

To make the transcription as close to the MS as possible, the editors of the vernacular versions have indicated not only the folio/page but also the original lineation of the volume. The end of a line is marked by a

Foreword to the Edition 175

vertical line, that of a page by a double vertical line; numbers in the margin refer to the actual lines of the MSS; reference to a new folio/ page is similarly given in the margin between brackets. Rubrics are printed in boldface, but otherwise we have kept the texts as they appear in the MSS. Words are therefore spelt as they appear in the MSS. This means not only that word boundaries have not been normalized according to contemporary practices (thus, ⟨ou*e*reye lede⟩ [*H503*:92.15], ⟨a·naye⟩ [*H513*:25r.20] instead of *⟨ou*er* eye-lede⟩, *⟨an aye⟩), but also that such customs as using capital letterforms in the middle of a word (for example, ⟨nAme⟩ [*H513*:3v.25]) have also been maintained. The original capitalisation, punctuation and paragraphing of the MSS have thus been kept except for the Latin text, where they were modernised, as per the rationale expressed in the preceding section.

In all the vernacular MSS, capital ⟨J⟩ is the only letterform for both *I* and *J*, and therefore it can be safely transcribed on a per word basis (⟨Johannicius⟩ [*H503*:3.9] but ⟨Indie⟩ [*H503*:22.7]). The usage of ⟨U, V⟩ is on the other hand more complex: it is nowhere to be found in Branch *O* of the English tradition and the Provençal MS displays ⟨U⟩ only once (and it is a Lombardic letter: ⟨Uoletz⟩ [*B*:173ra.43]). The MSS of Branch *O¹* favour ⟨V⟩ both as a vowel and a consonant: ⟨Vuea⟩ [*H503*:3.16], ⟨Varius⟩ [*H503*:4.4]; ⟨Vngula⟩ [*S*:44r.19], but the scribe of Hunter 503 employed ⟨U⟩ at least once: ⟨Uitrius⟩ [*H503*:4.6]. To avoid confusion, then, the distinction between these two letterforms has been preserved. As for the Metz MS, its scribe used all four letterforms ⟨I, J, U, V⟩, although they do not necessarily have the same values as their contemporary counterparts.

As stated in the previous section, abbreviations have normally been expanded and marked in italics except in the case of the Metz MS, in the belief that there is little point in indicating that in a Latin text; see moreover the following section on conventional signs for the exceptions to this rule. Whenever possible, the expansion reproduces the most frequent spelling of the word when the scribe wrote it in full, irrespective of the standard spelling in Present-Day English (cf. for example ⟨w^ch⟩ standing for w*hitch* in *S*). Final tildes over ⟨n⟩, as in ⟨añ⟩, ⟨opynyoñ⟩, ⟨owñ⟩, etc. have been unexceptionally transcribed as *n*. The reader must be aware nonetheless that an alternative transcription -*e* may be more advisable at times, or else that such sign over the letterform may be otiose. A similar stroke that can be found in most MSS across final ⟨ll⟩, ⟨ch⟩ and ⟨gh⟩ (⟨well⟩ [*H503*:2.12], ⟨euerych⟩ [*H503*:15.6], ⟨þorugh⟩ [*H503*:107.4]) appears to have been used just to indicate the ligature and is thus considered otiose here, although in the orthographic system used by the scribe of *H513* it may arguably have stood for -*e* (see Marqués/Miranda/González 2008). Their position on this matter has been sacrificed for the sake of uniformity with the other witnesses. Some other minor modifications have been introduced that make the transcription of *H513* in the synoptic edition somewhat different from their 2008 version.

Letters or words added by the scribe above the line are bracketed in the text using the signs ⌊ ⌋. Of course this excludes standard suspension practices such as ⟨w^t⟩, ⟨þ^e⟩, where the raised letter is marked in italics (and the abbreviation expanded if necessary). Scribal cancelations, expunctuations, erasures and the like have been left out of the edition but have been recorded in the *apparatus criticus*. On the other hand, the errors that the scribes did not erase have been maintained, as in the following dittographies: ⟨after hys hys doctrine⟩ [*H503*:9.11], ⟨yn the | the begynnnyng⟩ [*H503*:47.12–13], ⟨of thys sekenes sekenes⟩ [*H503*:62.4], ⟨that that the eye⟩ [*H503*:119.14], ⟨herde me teche | herde me teche⟩ [*H503*:135.15–136.1]. The same policy applies to hypercorrections as well, cf. ⟨Take and hand|ful⟩ [*H503*:57.8–9].

The scribe of *H513* forgot to add the initial Lombardic letter ⟨O⟩ at the beginning of a new section sometimes. The instances are *H513*:8r.19, *H513*:26r.16 and *H513*:31v.18, corresponding to opening words of sections §§26, 58 and 69 of the edition. These have been corrected, putting the missing letterform into angular brackets < >.

Mistakes in brevigraphs have likewise been left uncorrected, as in ⟨hum*n*s⟩ [*H503*:5.15] instead of expected *hum*er*s 'humours'. The scribe of Hunter 503 frequently (but not always) employs the customary -*er*- abbreviation instead of the expected -*es*/-*is* one with the plural forms of 'cataract', 'egg' and 'ounce'; cf. ⟨Cat*er*acter⟩ [*H503*:17.6], ⟨egg*er*⟩ [*H503*:102.10] or ⟨vnc*er*⟩ [*H503*:33.5]. In all likelihood a mere scribal habit, this freak has been kept in the edition notwithstanding.[10] Another peculiar abbreviation is ⟨coniunctiã3⟩ [*H513*:16v.22], where ⟨3⟩ must stand for *m*, as the Latin text reads *coniunctiuam* here. Final ⟨3⟩ to indicate *m* is frequent in Latin MSS (see Cappelli 1990: xxxii–xxxiii), but not so in English ones (using the tilde was the rule there), probably because the sign might be confused with yogh and the tailed form of ⟨z⟩. Perhaps the preceding ⟨a⟩ had a tilde added over it precisely to make the value of the sign unambiguous.

5. Conventional signs

Apothecaries' abbreviations – including Troy weights – used in the vernacular treatises have been kept as they appear in the MSS, i.e. without expansion. While the signs for *ounce*, *dram* and *semis* look alike in all MSS, the abbreviation for *pound* differs from one codex to the other: thus, the scribe of *H503* preferred ⟨li⟩ joined with a horizontal stroke, while that of *H513* alternates that sign with a crossed ⟨l⟩; examples of both signs can be seen at f. 11r of the latter MS. For the readers' convenience, an overview of the Troy units is given as Table 1. This provides the usual meaning in Present-day English, together with their Metric System equivalents in grams; it must be noted nonetheless that the correspondences given here are built on the 1824 Imperial system, which

---

10   At first sight, the presence of ⟨r⟩ in the plural form of *egg* might seem defendable on etymological grounds since *ǣg* (the OE word for 'egg') belonged to the *es/os*-declension and had hence a nom./ac. pl. *ǣg-ru* (Campbell 1959: §635). But this is to be rejected, if only because ME *egg* is a Scandinavian borrowing originally from the *ja*-declension (Noreen 1892: §304). Besides, there is good internal evidence suggesting that the scribal choice of the alternative brevigraph is of no real consequence but simply a personal custom: as indicated in a preceding section, page 13 of *H503* is an imperfect duplicate of p. 11; on *H503*:11.13 the word 'cataracts' is spelt ⟨cate*r*accte*r*⟩, but ⟨Cate*r*actys⟩ on the twin line *H503*:13.13.

probably does not mirror perfectly the one used in England during the Middle Ages.[11]

gr	*granum*	grain			≈ 0.0648 g
Ɖ	*scrupulum*	scruple		= 20 grains	≈ 1.296 g
ʒ	*drachma*	dra(ch)m	= Ɖ.iij	= 60 grains	≈ 3.8881 g
℥	*uncia*	ounce	= ʒ.viij	= 480 grains	= 31.105 g
℔	*libra*	pound	= ℥.xij	= 5760 grains	= 373.26 g

Table 1. The Troy system units.

The number of units is expressed frequently after, rather than before, the abbreviation, a custom that remains even today in the case of currencies: £5 (where the pound sign still retains its usual mediaeval significance: *L* for Latin *libra*), and imitatively, also $5. But even so, the opposite is not uncommon, cf. ⟨iiij.ʒ⟩ [*B*:175rb.2] and similar examples in all the other MSS – except Hunter 513. The quantities are always expressed in Roman figures and sometimes separated from the corresponding unit by a *punctus*: ⟨ʒ.iiij⟩ [*H513*:11r.7] means therefore 'four ounces', and ⟨℔.iij⟩ [*H513*:36v.20] stands for 'three pounds'.

Fractions of these units were also in use. The symbol ⟨ß⟩ (transcribed *ss* in many editions) derives from Latin *semis* 'half' and indicates half a given weight; just like any other quantity, it normally appears after the unit: accordingly, ⟨ʒ.ß⟩ [*H513*:5r.18] is 'half a dram' (30 grains,

---

11   We should never lose sight of the fact that the original treatise was composed on the Continent, and the value of the units was sometimes divergent from one land to another. For example, a pound consisted on 16 ounces in France, and (just like most Western Romance regions, bar Southern Italy) a scruple was divided into 24 grains (1.55525 g); an ounce had therefore 576, instead of 480, grains. In the Kingdom of Naples and Sicily (which may have been homeland to Benvenutus) an ounce was divided into 10 drachms, and thus consisted of 600 grains (Jourdan 1840: 42–43). Within the English-speaking world, confusion among pharmacists were still common as late as the middle of the 20th century due to the coexistence of the Apothecaries' with the Avoirdupois system, made official in Great Britain in 1858 and as yet not completely abandoned. This is based on the division of a pound of 7000 grains into 16 ounces, in turn divided into 16 drams. The Metric system replaced the Apothecaries' in the US Pharmacopoeia only in the 1970s but, just like in the UK, avoirdupois units are still current for most everyday household purposes. On the ensuing conflicts see Stehle (1942).

approx. 1.944 g), ⟨ʒ.ß⟩ [*S*:37r.4] is 'half an ounce' (240 grains, 15.5525 g) and ⟨℔.ß⟩ [*H513*:11r.8] is 'half a pound' (2880 grains, 186.63 g). The scribe of Hunter 513 sometimes precedes this sign with an ampersand, as in ⟨ʒ.j. & ß rede | rose levis⟩ [*H513*:8v.13–14] 'an ounce and a half of red rose leaves'. Just like ⟨ß⟩ indicates half of a measure, the letter ⟨q⟩ (standing for *quarteron*) indicates a fourth part of a measure (< L. *quartus*), normally either an ounce's or a pound's. *H503* expresses the quantity in full in ⟨quarteron of an*n* vnce⟩ [*H503*:33.6], while the more businesslike scribe of Hunter 513 succinctly wrote ⟨ʒ q⟩ in the parallel passage [*H513*:9r.3].[12]

Similarly, and although strictly speaking it was not part of the Troy system, the *pennyweight* is another measure frequently encountered in English recipes. It is represented in MSS with the letter ⟨d⟩ (< L. *denarius*)[13] and officially defined as $^1/_{240}$ of a pound, or the twentieth part of an ounce (24 grains). But in many English recipes 'pennyweight' merely translated L. *scrupulum* (i.e. $^1/_{24}$ of an ounce; see Table 1 above), which goes to show how the French system was in full use in mediaeval England.[14]

The letters ⟨M⟩ and ⟨P⟩ are sometimes met in recipes too, mostly to measure dried herbs:[15] the first one, an abbreviation of L. *manipulus*, stands for 'handful' (as in ⟨rotis of fenell | rotis of p*er*sili wormode an*a* M j⟩ [*H513*:36v.19–20]), while the second measure, the abbreviated form for L. *pugillus* ('what can be held in the fist') is in fact a big pinch. Officially an eighth of a handful, a pugil will be more loosely defined in post-Mediaeval times as 'what two fingers and the thumb hold'

---

12   The *quarteron* should not be confused with the *quarte* [*H503*:83.6], which is a liquid measure of capacity corresponding to one-fourth of a gallon, i.e. about a litre, depending on the actual liquid to be measured; see Jourdan (1840: 52). Note that ⟨q⟩ stands for *quartus* 'fourth' in *H513*:14r.5.

13   Cf. *dwt*, its usual Pharmacists' abbreviation now, where *wt* simply stands for 'weight'.

14   For instance, see on the one hand 'an Englisse penny shall weye xvj cornys of whete taken owte of the myddyll of the ere. And xx maken an ounce' (Wright/Halliwell-Phillipps 1845: I/232) and, on the other, 'a scripule weyeþ a peny' (*MED*, *s.v.* scrūpul). Cf. moreover fn. 11 above.

15   See Crellin/Scott (1969: 57, fn. 34).

(see *OED*, s.v. pugil¹). This measure is never employed in Benvenutus' treatise.

Apart from Apothecaries' weights and measures, a few other abbreviations can be encountered in recipes as well that may strike some readers.

⟨R⟩ is the abbreviation of L. *recipe*, literally 'take (imper.)', whence the meaning 'recipe, prescription'. This sign customarily appears at the beginning of the formula, followed by a list of ingredients. The scribe of *H513* wrote the sign in red ink on the margins as a locating device. The sign, which still enjoys Pharmaceutical use, has been kept unexpanded in the edition.

The word *ana* (a transliteration of the Greek preposition ἀνά, which was sometimes employed with a distributive sense)[16] appears many times in medical treatises to indicate that the reader should measure the same quantity of each ingredient. *Ana* normally appears between the ingredients and the measure: ⟨Turbith, Aloes epatica ana ℥.j⟩ [*S*:34r.3] can then be translated as 'an ounce of turbith and another one of hepatic aloes'.

A sigma-shaped *s* between *puncti* (.σ.) is employed a couple of times in *H513* to abbreviate L. *scilicet* 'to wit, namely'; as with *recepta* above, this has also been kept unexpanded in the edition.

---

16   Cf. Liddell/Scott/Jones/McKenzie (1996: *s.v.* ἀνά, sense D): 'WITH NOM. of Numerals, etc., distributively'; see sense C.II.2 of the same entry as well.

Metz, Bibliothèques-Médiatèques de Metz / Département Patrimoine, MS 176, f. 1r

Biblio.-Médiathèques de Metz, MS 176, ff. 1r–16r

1ra **1. Incipit ars probatissima de | cura oculorum composita a Bene|uenuto Grapheo de Iherusalem.** | Auditores omnes audiant
5 aut | circumstantes qui cupiunt | audire nouam scienciam et ha|bere formam virtutem et addiscere Artem | Probatissimam de Cura Oculorum, a me | Beneuenuto
10 Grapheo compositam | secundum dicta antiquorum philosophorum | et meam experientiam, per longum exercitium | quod habui, eundo per diuer|sas partes mundi, medicando tam | in frigidis quam in calidis
15 regionibus | – adiuuante diuino auxilio; et semper | agendo in noticijs egritudinum oculorum et in | conualescentijs eorum secundum ac|cidencia cuiuslibet humoris – et iuua|tiuis et expertis medicinis.
20 Et omnes | circumstantias et probatissimas me|dicinas reducebam in scriptis, semper | no-

Glasgow, GUL, Hunter MS 503, pp. 1–135

A Grete phylosopher and | a [1] profunde phycycyane cle|pid. Be*n*nomicius Graphe|us, aft*er* the sentence of þe | of olde auctors of 5 phelozophie and of | phisyk. which he had radde. and after | hys p*ro*pre expe*r*yence. the wych he had by | long co*n*tynuance of his owne practik | yn dyu*er*se p*ar*ties of the worlde. boyth yn | hote 10 Regyons and colde. by influence | and help of goddys grace. compilyd & | made a boke of the sekenes of eyon. & | of her curys.

London, British Library, Sloane MS 661, ff. 32r–46r

[1] A great Philosopher & Profound Phisition cleped | Beneuenutus Graffeus, after the 32r sentence of the oulde | aucthors of Philosophye and of Physicke, w*hitch* he had redd & after his propper experience, the w*hitch* | he had by longe continuance of his owne 5 practize in | diuers p*ar*tes of the worlde, both in whoate regions, & in | coulde by influence and helpe of god his grace, | compiled and made a booke, of the diseases of the | eyes, and of there Cuers,

---

1 A] The Booke of Beneuenutus Grapheus ˻de Jerusalem˼ intituled, by him | Deus oculoru*m*, as I founde yt written in the English | tounge, in an oulde Booke *upper   margin* cleped] pag. 1 | Cap. 1. *outer   margin* 5 in¹] This Booke is | moste of yt pub|lished, by Burrou | in his Method | of Phisicke but | he [co *deleted*] stealeth | this, as he doth | all the rest of his Booke. wi*t*hout | acknowledging the Authores. | and yet hath | published yt verye fouls and lett owt | mutch *outer margin*

Glasgow, GUL, Hunter MS 513, ff. 2r–37r *Basel, Ö.B.U., MS D.II.11, ff. 172r–177v*

 Senhors auiatz me|descinas 172ra
proudas | et esperiencias delas |
curas dels uels e | de totas 5
malautias que po|don uenir als
uelhs faitas | per me ben uengut
desalern | las cals yeu ey pro-
uadas | sertanament afemnas es |
ad homes ioues euielhs:- | 10

Oxford, Bodleian Library, Ashmole MS 1468, pp. 1–6

Biblio.-Médiathèques de Metz, MS 176, ff. 1r–16r

tando et in mea memoria con-
ser|uando usquequo habui plenitu-
dinem | de omnibus egritudinibus
25   oculorum et cu|ris eorum, tam de
causis et accidentijs | superuenien-
tibus quam de curis necessarijs, |
pluribus colliriis et emplastris,
unctio|nibus et pillulis, purgatio-
nibus et | electuarijs, cauterijs et
30   abstinencijs a | contrarijs, [et]
regimine bonorum ciborum. Et |
imposui nomen proprium cuilibet
infir|mitati per se.

2. Hoc facto, omnia hec | congre-
gaui simul [ordinaui], et re|duxi in
35   scriptis in libro meo, et no|minaui
eum librum Artem Probatissi-
mam | Oculorum – et a me sic
nominatus est: | quia plena est
medicinis expertis | et probatis,
quia vidi quod necessarium erat |

30 et] M a   33 ordinaui] M ordinanti, N (f. 48[51]r) ordinati, VV (f. 166v), VP2 (f. 188r) ordinatiui

Glasgow, GUL, Hunter MS 503, pp. 1–135

And entitled thys boke. | and
clepid it. Deus oculo*rum*. Of the
whi|ch boke yn the fyrst Chapitre   15
he declarith | what an*n* eye ys. and
the makyng þ*er* of. || aft*er* oþ*er*   [2]
opynyon*n*. and also aft*er* his
own*n* | seying.

London, British Library, Sloane MS 661, ff. 32r–46r

[2] and intituled his booke | & called yt Deus oculoru*m*. In the first chapter | of the   10
w*h*itch booke he declares what an eye is, and | the makinge there of : after the opinion of
the Auntie*n*t | Phisitions, & allso after his owne sayinge

Glasgow, GUL, Hunter MS 513, ff. 2r–37r   *Basel, Ö.B.U., MS D.II.11, ff. 172r–177v*

Oxford, Bodleian Library, Ashmole MS 1468, pp. 1–6

Biblio.-Médiathèques de Metz, MS 176, ff. 1r–16r

humane nature, ideo quia auc-
40 tores | non ad plenum tracta-
uerunt de ista | sciencia sicut
fecerunt de alijs sciencijs | que
pertinent ad medicinam. Et
nullum | vidi tempore meo qui
recto tramite sciret | exercere – et
operari secundum artem inter
45 Christi|anos illam medicinam, que
magis | sit utilis nobis pro illo
1rb membro || quod illuminat totum
corpus, que scientia | erat preter-
missa et ibat ad manus | insipien-
tium, qui intromittebant se |
absque ratione et sine cognicione
5 artis, | et confundebant multos
homines | operantes ipsam cum
magno errore. |

3. Quid sit oculus? | Oculus est
callus concauus, ple|nus aque
10 clarissime, positus in fron|te
capitis ut ministret lumen toti |
corpori, adiuuante spiritu uisibili
cum | maiori lumine. Et est

Glasgow, GUL, Hunter MS 503, pp. 1–135

a eye is a rounde holow thyng. |
herde os the balle of the foote. or
as the | new scowrid basyn ful of
clere wate*r*. set | in the well of the   5
hede. to minystre lyght | to the
body. by influence of the vysyble |

London, British Library, Sloane MS 661, ff. 32r–46r

[3] an eye is | a rownde hollowe thynge harde as the baulle of the foote | or as the new   15
scowred bason full of cleere water | sett in the well of the head, to minister lighte to the |
Bodye by influence of the visible speritt sent from | the phantasticall celle, by a Sinow
clepid Neruus | opticus . with the helpe of great lighte ministred from | w*i*thout.   20

Glasgow, GUL, Hunter MS 513, ff. 2r–37r   Basel, Ö.B.U., MS D.II.11, ff. 172r–177v

2r **Of tonicle of the ey3en and the |**
humours and cataractus· |
Oculus anglice an ey3e is hard
holowe rounde full | of water and

---

1 the²] 1 *added in outer margin*

Oxford, Bodleian Library, Ashmole MS 1468, pp. 1–6

Biblio.-Médiathèques de Metz, MS 176, ff. 1r–16r

    instrumentum preci|osum, sic
ordinatum quod a parte nerui |
uisibilis extra concauitatem est
15 car|nosum, sed a parte palpe-
brarum est cla|rissimum. Et per
medium illius clari|tatis apparet
pupilla, per quam | spiritus
visibilis ueniens ad neruum con|ca-
uum habet exitum suum infra
20 aquas et | tunicas.
    4. Quid est callus concauus? |
Callus concauus est instrumentum
preciosum, | compositum cum
tunicis et humoribus, | et hoc
instrumentum siue membrum
pre|ciosum dicitur instrumentum
25 per similitudinem: | quia sicut
instrumentum liguti uel cythole |
est concauum, ad hoc ut sonus
diuersarum | cordarum repleat
totam concauitatem | instrumenti
ut simul in vnam vocem con|cor-
dent, ita oculus est concauus ut |
30 spiritus visibilis ueniens per

London, British Library, Sloane MS 661, ff. 32r–46r

Glasgow, GUL, Hunter MS 503, pp. 1–135

spyrit. sent from the fantastical
celle | by a synew clepid. Neruus
obticus, | with the helpe of a
gretter light mynys|tryde from 10
wyth oute.

Glasgow, GUL, Hunter MS 513, ff. 2r–37r   *Basel, Ö.B.U., MS D.II.11, ff. 172r–177v*

    y sette in the mydward of the |
5 frounte of the heued that it mynystre and yeue | lyght to the body thorowe helping of the visible spirite | and the outward lyght ¶ And the ey3e is said of the | senwe optico that is said holowe warefore opticus is | grewe and hit is saide holowe in latyn

Oxford, Bodleian Library, Ashmole MS 1468, pp. 1–6

Biblio.-Médiathèques de Metz, MS 176, ff. 1r–16r

    neruum | opticum repleat totam
concauitatem | oculi, donec
iungantur cum maiori | claritate
– et simul lumen corpori mi-
nis|trent. Et dicitur oculus ab
35 optico | neruo, vnde opticus
Grece, Latine | dicitur concauus.
    5. Quid est fons | capitis? Fons
capitis est antra|cillus ille in quo
siue ubi oculus | est positus. Et
40 fons dicitur ideo quia | cursus
lacrimales semper habent |
meatum per illum fontem, de
quo|cumque modo veniant per
tristiciam | cordis aut per frigidi-
tatem ipsius capitis. |

45 **6. De tunicis oculorum.** | Dicit
autem Iohannicius quod septem
sunt tunice oculorum, quarum
1va prima || vocatur retina, secunda
secundina, tertia | scliros, quarta
aranea, quinta | vuea, sexta cornea,
septima coniunctiua. | Si tunice

Glasgow, GUL, Hunter MS 503, pp. 1–135

and co*n*ueniently | ys the place
where the eye is. sett. clepid | the
well of the hed. for the habun-
dance | of wat*er*y hum*er*s & teris.
the whych ofte*nn* | yssu cu*m* out.
þ*er*. by cause su*m* tyme of sorow |
and heuynes of herte. su*m* tyme of   15
ioye. | & gladnes. and su*m* tyme
for habundance || of sup*er*fluytees   [3]
of hum*er*s causid of cold. |
    ¶ And for asmuche as eu*er*y
natu|rall ma*nn* hath such ij. wellis.
nature | hath sett i*n* eu*er*y hed ij
eyon. thus þan | bryefly shewid by   5
this auctor what | eu*er*y eye is.

London, British Library, Sloane MS 661, ff. 32r–46r

[5] And convenientlye is the place where the | eye is sett, called the well of the head,
ffor the ab|undance of watrye humors & teares w*hitch* often issue | from them. Some
tymes because of Sorrowe, and | hevynes of hearte, Some tymes of ioye & gladnes. | and   25
some tymes for abundance of superfluous humors caused of couldes.
[6] And for as mutch as everye Na|turall man hath 2 sutch wells, nature hath sett | in
everye mans head towe eyes. thus then breefe|lye is shewed by this Author what everye
eye is | consequentlye he sheweth how an eye is made. | ffirst he reherseth the opinion   30
of a great leche | clepid Johannitius and after he putteth hiw owne | opinion Johannitius
is his Isagoges sayeth that | an eye hath 7. tunicles or cootes 4. Colors, and .3. | humors   35

Glasgow, GUL, Hunter MS 513, ff. 2r–37r *Basel, Ö.B.U., MS D.II.11, ff. 172r–177v*

10 and Johannic*ius* | saith that ther ben seuene tonicles of the ei3en ¶ The | first he clepeth retentiua ¶ The secund se*cun*dina ¶ The | ·3ᵉ· Scliros ¶ The firthe aranea ¶ The·5· vuea ¶ The | ·6· cornea ¶ The ·7· coniunctiua ¶ These bene seuene |

Deuetz saber | que set son las tuni|cas dels uelhs segon | mayestre johan michi. la pri|meyra 15 es apelhada rethina | ¶ Ela segonda es apelhada | segondina ¶ Ela terssa. escli|ros ¶ Ela quarta. arania: | ¶ Ela quinta. vnea ¶ Ela

Oxford, Bodleian Library, Ashmole MS 1468, pp. 1–6

Biblio.-Médiathèques de Metz, MS 176, ff. 1r–16r

    oculorum sunt septem secundum |
5 Iohannicium, ergo cum prima tunica | frangitur tota substancia oculi [non] deuastatur. | Sed quia secundum nos non sunt nisi | due, et cum prima frangitur tota | substancia deuastatur et oculus
10 consumitur | cum suis humoribus; alia uero est per|forata, et propter foramen non potest | retinere humores oculorum quod non ex|eant postquam prima tunica erit frac|ta.

15 **7. Quid est tunica oculi?** | Tunica oculi est ille circulus cla|rus qui in multis apparet niger | ac varius, et per medium circuli | est foramen, de quo foramine ducitur | pupilla per quam spiritus uisibilis, |
20 veniendo per neruum con-

---

6 non] M *omitted*, VP2 (f. 288v), VR (f. 29v) non *added*

Glasgow, GUL, Hunter MS 503, pp. 1–135

consequently he shewyth | how an ey is made. ¶ First he reher|syth the opynyon of a gret leche clepid. | Johannicius, And after he puttyth hys | owne opinyonn. Johannici*us*   10 in his ysa|gogys seyth. that an ey hath vij. tuny|cles. or vij cootis. iiij. Colors. and iij | hum*ers*. The first tunicle or Cote ys cle|pid. Rectina. The secunde. Secundina. | The thirde. Scliros. The iiijth. Aranea. | 15 The vth. Vnea, The vjth. Cornea. The || vijth and the last.   [4] Co*n*iu*n*ctiua.

The first | coler is. Niger. that is blak. The ij^{de} is. | Subalbidus. whytyshe. the iij^{de}. is | Varius. that is dyu*er*se in color. The | iiijth is.   5 Blancus. yolow. ¶ The first | humo*ur* is callid. Uitrius. glassy or like | glas. The ij^{de} ys. Cristallin*us*.

---

6 he] e *added over the line* 3 is] va|rs *deleted*

London, British Library, Sloane MS 661, ff. 32r–46r

The first tunicle, or Coote, is called Re|tina the Second Secundina the thirde | Slyros the fourth Aranea the 5th vnea the .6. | Cornea, the 7th & last Coniunctiua.
[7] The first colo*r* | is Niger. that is blacke the 2. is Subalbidus, why|tish the thirde is   40 varius, that is diuers in colo*r* | the fourth is Glaucus, yealow. The first humo*r* | is called vitreus glassye or like glasse The .2. | is Christallinus like christall The .3. is Albu|genius like the white of an egg. Thus sayth || Johamitius But Beneuenut*us* . varieth from him in   32v Cootes | and in colors ffor as he sayeth an eye hath but | 2. tunicles or cootes as he hath proved by his Ana|thomye of Eyes, that is to saye by incytion or | cuttinge of a dead   5 bodye. The first coate he | calleth Saluatricem that is a Sauior for yt sa|ueth and kepeth the humors, The second tuni|cle or Coote is called Discoloratam. that is disco|lored or of

---

36 Retina] tina retin *deleted*

Glasgow, GUL, Hunter MS 513, ff. 2r–37r

    tonicles of the ey3e and yif the first
15 happeth to be bro|ke   or thorowe
any thinge ys perforate and for that
hole | may not holde the humors
of the ey3en ware þorwe | it
senwith that all the substaunce of
the ey3en is wasted | and the ey3e
withe his humors ys consumed

¶ The | tonicle of the ei3e ys that
20 clere sercle the which | to   many
it apperethe blak to other appereth
variaunce | and by the myddell of
the ei3e ther is an hole the | which
hole is said pupilla anglice. the
appell of the ey3e | bi the whiche
the visible spirite comyng by þe
holwe | nerffe hathe his oute
goyng and taketh lyght of a· ||

Oxford, Bodleian Library, Ashmole MS 1468, pp. 1–6

Basel, Ö.B.U., MS D.II.11, ff. 172r–177v

sex|ta.   cornea ¶ Ela septima   20
con|iutinia

¶ Editz que quatre | son las colors
dels uelhs:- la prumeyre. es negra ¶
Ela | segonda es quais blanca. | ¶
Ela terssa es uayra. Ela | quarta   25
es quais rossa ¶ E | yeu ben uengut
dic. que non | son mais doas
tunicas de | los uelhs que non an
ne|guna colhor que yeu o. ey |
esproath ben. et aysso es per | 30
amor dela humor. la qual | es

Biblio.-Médiathèques de Metz, MS 176, ff. 1r–16r

cauum, | habet exitum suum et recipit lumen | a maiori claritate. Et dicit Iohannicius | quod colores oculorum sunt quatuor: | niger,
25 subalbidus, varius, et glau|cus. Nos autem Beneuenutus di|cimus quod non sunt nisi due tuni|ce oculorum tantum, quia per maximum | exercitium et longa experimenta nostra | probauimus
30 et inuenimus per ana|thomiam nostram oculorum duas esse | tunicas tantum. Et primam vocamus | saluatricem, quia saluat et conseruat | totum oculum et retinet omnes hu|mores oculorum. Secundam vero vocamus | discolo-
35 ratam ideo quia non est color | in ea. Vnde dicimus quod nullus co|lor est in oculis sed accidit propter | situm humorem – scilicet propter claritatem | humoris cristallini, quia quando humor |
40 cristallinus est prope tunicas

Glasgow, GUL, Hunter MS 503, pp. 1–135

like cristal. | The iij^{de} is. Albigenius, like the white | of an egge. thus sayth Joha*n*nicius, | But. 10 Bennomicius. varieth fro*m* hym | in cotys and yn Colo*ur*s. For as he seyth. | an ey hath but ij tonycles or cotys. as he | hath p*r*oued by hys anothomie of eyon. | þat ys to sey by inocyon or kuttyng of a | dede body. ¶ The fyrst Cote he 15 callyth | Saluatrice*m*. that ys a sauyour. for it || sauyth and [5] kepyth the hum*er*s. ¶ The | *s*ecunde tonycle or cote he callyth. Discolora|tam, þat ys discolurde. or of no colo*ur*. | For as he sayth. In the ey of hym selfe. | ys 5 p*ro*purly no colo*ur*. but dyu*er*sytees of co|lurs þat apperen*n* yn the ey. for when | the cristallyne humor ys nyght the to|nycle

---

16 Saluatricem] The first cote | outwarde *added in outer margin in an Elizabethan hand*

London, British Library, Sloane MS 661, ff. 32r–46r

no color. ffor as he sayth in the eye | of him selfe is properlye no color, but diu*er*sityes 10
of colors that appeare in the Eye. ffor when | the Christoline humor is neare to the
tunicle | of the eye, then yt semeth of on color And | when yt is in the middest, then yt
semeth | of an other color. And when yt is depe w*ith* | in, then yt semeth of a third color 15
where of | he concludeth the the eye yt selfe is discolo|red and hath no color properlye.
And those | men that have the humors lowe sett and w*ith*in | there eyne seme blacke, 20
theye see best, for a tyme, | but when theye are about thirtye yeares oulde | or more then
there sighte begineth to decaye.| Theye allso that have the humo*r*s sett aboute | the
middest of the Eyes, theye com*m*onlye see well | younge and oulde, w*h*itch we call 25
graye, and these | manner of Eyne be subiecte to Ophthalmia & | Paniculus, and other

---

14 when] yt *deleted* **15** of¹] t *deleted*

De Probatissima Arte Oculorum 195

Glasgow, GUL, Hunter MS 513, ff. 2r–37r

2v   grete clerete ¶ And he seithe the
colours of the ey3en | ben foure
that ys to wete blake lowe white
varie | and yelwisshe ¶ Forsothe
Benemit*us* saye that ther | ben two
tonicles of the ei3en onyly
5   w*ith*outon mo / And | the first y
clepe Saluatricem for whi it saueth
all þ*e* | ey3e and it haldeth Ayen
all the humors of the ey|3en the ·2e·
tonicle y clepe discolorata*m*
an*glice*. vncoloured | tonicle · For
whi ther nys no colour in hit
wherfor y | saye that ther nys no
10   colour in the ey3en / And yiff | any
colour is sayne to w*ith*holden or to
comprehende | apperyng of colour
yiff hit fall for his place or for | the
clerete of the cristallyn humo*ar* for
whi whan | the cristallyn humo*ur*
ys nygh to the tonicles of the |
ey3en it comprehendith of one
15   colour and whan it | is in the
myddes than hit sheweth of

Oxford, Bodleian Library, Ashmole MS 1468, pp. 1–6

Basel, Ö.B.U., MS D.II.11, ff. 172r–177v

secca. e per amor de la hu|mor
cristallina. quar cant | la humor
cristallina secca es | pres delhas   35
tunicas es apar | duna colhor
equant sen deue | que intra preont
apar dau|tra color ¶ Don uos dic |
ques aquels ques an la hu|mor   40
preonda de dintre apa|ron los uelhs
negres eues|on mielhs que non fan
los | autres. et acap de trenta || ans   172rb
comenson apeioyrar ¶ Et | aquels
que an la humor al | mietz dels
uelhs aquels ues|on ben dela
pueriscia en tro- | ala uilesa ¶   5
Etenquestz uen | una enfermetat
als uelhs: | quen appelha hom ob
talmia | et aquelha cobre los uels |
als alquns enon pas atotz | ¶ Et   5
aquels ques anlas hu|mors pres
delas tunicas | eque son los uells
uayrs a|quels ueson ben en la

---

37 dautra] dau|ta *before correction,*
ra *expunged and* tra *added*   **2** talmia]
q *expunged*

Biblio.-Médiathèques de Metz, MS 176, ff. 1r–16r

oculi | videtur de vno colore, et quando est | in medio videtur de alio colore, | quando uero est in profunditate de alio | colore. Et sic
45 variatur vnus ab | alio secundum situm humorum. Quia si ocu|lus haberet colorem, omnis color vi|deretur esse de illo colore, sed
1vb quia || non habet colorem recipit omnem colo|rem. Vnde per simile si lingua haberet | saporem, omnis sapor videretur esse de il|lo sapore, sed quia non habet saporem, |
5 recipit omnem saporem. Et nonne quando co|lera dominatur in ore stomaci, omnia videntur | pacienti esse amara propter amaritudi|nem colere que est prope linguam? Vnde | illi qui habent humores in
10 profunditate | apparent oculi eorum nigri et melius vi|dent, sed postquam veniunt in spacio et | in etate xxx annorum deteriorantur. | Et illi qui habent humores in

Glasgow, GUL, Hunter MS 503, pp. 1–135

of the ey. than the ey semyth of oon*n* | colo*u*r. And whan*n* yt ys in the myddys. | þan it semyth of a 10 nother colour. and | when*n* yt ys depe wythyn. þan it semyth | of the iij^de colo*u*r. wherof he con- cludyth þ*at* | the ey of yt selfe ys discolurd and hath | no colurn pr*o*purly. ¶ Tho me*n* þat ha|ue the 15 hum*n*s lowe set and wythyn | her eyon*n* semen blake and þei see best || for a tyme. but when þei [6] cu*m* a bowt xxx^ti | wynt*er* or more. þan here syght begynnyth | to peyre. ¶ Thei also þat haue the hu|mers set a boute the middys of the eyon. | þei co*mmun*ly se wele 5 yong and olde. And | the Colo*u*r of the eyon ys meueable blak. | that we call grey. but often*n* yt ys seyn | þat i*n* þis man*er* of eyon. obtalmie. þat | is derknes of sy3t.

14 haue] no *deleted*

London, British Library, Sloane MS 661, ff. 32r–46r

diuers diseases, w*hitc*h shalbe | declared here after. for Eyes of this color | are more 30
subiecte to them, then of anye other | colo*r*. But theye that have the Humors situ|ate or
sett neare besyde the tunicles, have there | Eyes varied of diuers colors and inclyninge |
mutch to whitenes, and there sighte is not verye | good nether in youth nor age. ffor those 35
man*n*er | of Eyes are oftner vexed w*ith* fluxes humors & | teares then any others. ffor
when the visible || sperit descendinge by the hollow synowes, finde about the tunicle 33r
fresh abundance & plentye of corrupte | humors theye be the soner disgregate &
dissolved | from the Humors :

33 and] be *deleted*

Glasgow, GUL, Hunter MS 513, ff. 2r–37r

a·myddell co|lour ¶ And whan it is
low3 in the depthe thanne it |
shewith of a·nother colour· And so
o colour varieth | fro a nother after
his stede and place · For whi yiff |
the ey3e had any colour shuld be
20 seye of that colour | ¶ But for he
hath none colour therfor hit re-
seyueþ | colour as the tonge
lacketh sauour and it takethe |
therof sauour wherfor thoo that
hauen humo*ur*s | in the depir-
fundite ·i· in the depe y saye that
her | ey3en apperen blake that they
25 mowe the better seyn | after that
they comen to the age of · xxx$^{ti.}$
yeres þei | ben werse and tho that
hauen humo*ur*s in the medde ||
3r soche seyn well fro her youth tyll
here olde age and | her ey3en
apperen meuely blake ¶ But many
aposto|mys that me clepun obtol-
meys comon in soche ei3e | more
than in any othir ey3en ¶ And thoo

Basel, Ö.B.U., MS D.II.11, ff. 172r–177v

pueris|cia equant son uielhs non |
ueson ben ¶ E quant an als | en   10
los uelhs tropas tunicas e | tropas
lagremas et an los | palpelhs
uermels pus quels | autres enon
ueson trob ben |

Oxford, Bodleian Library, Ashmole MS 1468, pp. 1–6

Biblio.-Médiathèques de Metz, MS 176, ff. 1r–16r

    medietate | bene vident a puericia
15 usque in senectu|tem, et apparent
    oculi eorum mediocri|ter nigri, sed
    in multis de istis super|ueniunt
    obtalmie et panniculi quam in |
    alijs. Et illi qui habent humores
    iuxta | tunicas sunt varij et pendent
20 in al|bedinem, omnes non bene
    vident in | puericia neque in
    senectute sicut et | alij, quia magis
    superueniunt lacri|me et reuma in
    istis varijs quam in | alijs – et
    semper habent palpebras rubeas. |
25 Ideo dicimus quod idcirco non
    bene vident, | quia spiritus uisibilis
    veniendo per | per neruos conca-
    uos et inueniendo | humores iuxta
    tunicas, cicius disgre|gatur et
    refugit extra.

Glasgow, GUL, Hunter MS 503, pp. 1–135

And Panniclus. | that is smale   10
webbys. and oþer dyuerse |
dyseasis. whych shald be declaryd
here | after. thei grow rather þan
yn oþer maner | of eyenn colourid.
¶ But þei þat haue | humours
situat or set nyght be syde the
ton|nycles. haue eyen varied of   15
dyuers colours. | and hangynn
mych yn whitnesse. and || hir   [7]
syght is not right goode. neþer yn |
yowgth nor age. For yn þo maner
of eyon | haue bendyng humers of
teris more þan | yn oþer. For when
the uisible spirite des|cendyng   5
downn by the holow synews |
fynde a boute the tonycle fresche
habun|dance and plente of corupte
humors. | þei ben the sunner
disgregat and dyssol|ued from the
humers.

---

27 per²] VP2 (f.289v), VR (f. 30v) *omitted*

London, British Library, Sloane MS 661, ff. 32r–46r

Glasgow, GUL, Hunter MS 513, ff. 2r–37r   *Basel, Ö.B.U., MS D.II.11, ff. 172r–177v*

5   that ha|uen humours besiden the
tonicles ben diuerse and | they
hangen in the white ·i· in albugine
and suche | neyther they seen
nought in her youthe ne in | her
olde Age as in hem that hauen
moche of the | reume and teres
and such hauen rede eye leddes | ¶
10   Also y say they seen nought wele
these that ben | diuerse coloured ·i·
varij For whi the visible spirite |
comyng by the holowe norfes and
fyndyng the | humours by the
tonicles the sonner they departen
a|way and shenneth outward

Oxford, Bodleian Library, Ashmole MS 1468, pp. 1–6

Biblio.-Médiathèques de Metz, MS 176, ff. 1r–16r

30 **8.** Diximus | uobis de illis in quibus apparent oculi | varij et pendent in albedinem, qua de | causa multi illorum non bene vident. | Ammodo dicemus vobis de illis qui | habent oculos
35 mediocriter nigros, qua | de causa durat magis in eis visus quam | in aliquo istorum. Dicimus idcirco quia | humor cristallinus residens in me|dio et spiritus visibilis per neruos con|cauos facit
40 ibi residenciam, propter hu|morem varium et tunicas oculorum quod | retinent eum, et non potest ita cito disgre|gari.

9. Narrauimus vobis de illis | qui habent humores in medio oculorum | qua de causa durat magis
45 in eis | lumen quam in alijs.
2ra Expedire volumus ‖ vobis de illis qui habent humores in pro|funditate, et in quibus apparent | oculi eorum nigri et melius vident, | et

Glasgow, GUL, Hunter MS 503, pp. 1–135

¶ Also ys the | sight the feblere yn 10
them. þan yn þo | that haue þer
eyon meueablye blake. | In tho
pro*pur*ly þat haue grey eyon. the |
ly3t duryth bett*er* þen yn other. For
the | cristallyne beyng resydent yn
the mid|dys. makyth the visual 15
spiritys to ‖ abyde þere, wherby [8]
the glassy humore | and the
tonycle of the ey. ys kept yn | þat
it may not redely be disgregat
and | disp*er*bolyd.

¶ But yn þem that haue | þer 5
humurs depedowne the whych
can | byth the ey to seme blak as I
sayd be fore | bett*er* þan oþ*er*
seyn. for the depth of the c*ris*|tallyne humor fro the spirite of ly3t. |
co*m*myng from the synew obtik.
fyndyth | the large space. and 10

London, British Library, Sloane MS 661, ff. 32r–46r

[8] and allso the lighte is the febl*er* | in them. than in those that have there Eyes graye | 5
In those properlye that have there Eyes graye *the* sighte | dureth bettar then in others. ffor
the Christaline. | for the Christaline beinge resident in the middest of | Eye maketh the
visible spirit*tes* to abide there where | by the glassye humo*r* and the tunicle of the eye 10
is | kepte in that yt maye not readilye be disgregate | and disperced.

[9] But in those that have the Humo*rs* | depe into the Eyes the w*hitch* causeth the
ˌEyeˌ | to seme blacke, as I sayde before see farr bettar | then others doe: for the depˌtˌh 15
of the christalline | humor from the sperite of sighte com*m*inge from the | Opticke
synowe fyndeth the large space, and filleth | all the concavitye or hollownes of the Eye
before | yt passe from the glassye humo*r*. but as is sayde | it dureth not in manye to age, 20

13 Eye] Humo*urs* *deleted,* Eye *added over the deletion* **15** the] *del deleted*

Glasgow, GUL, Hunter MS 513, ff. 2r–37r

15   ¶ But tho that ha|uen her ey3en sumdell blake in hem the syght | lastethe longe tyme · For the cristallyn humo*ur* ys | restyng in the myddes and the visible sp*i*rite comy*n*g | by the holowe neruys and maketh ther residens for | the glacy humo*ur* ·i· viterum and the
20   tonicles of the | which weth- holden it and ther for it may nou3t | sone sparple abrode ne run*n*e a way

Basel, Ö.B.U., MS D.II.11, ff. 172r–177v

¶ Nowe shull | we seyn of hem that haue humours in the pro|fun- dite ·i· in the depthe and her ey3en apperen blake | and they seyn the more and that ther for ys good ||
3v   for the depthe of the cristallyn humo*ur* For the cristal|lyn humour fyndethe more space and refillethe

Oxford, Bodleian Library, Ashmole MS 1468, pp. 1–6

Biblio.-Médiathèques de Metz, MS 176, ff. 1r–16r

    in multis non durat usque in
5 se|nectutem. Dicimus ideo melius
    vident | propter profunditatem
    humoris cristallini, | quia spiritus
    uisibilis inuenit maius | spacium et
    replet totum spacium oculorum |
    et totam concauitatem, antequam
10 per|transeat humorem vitreum
    extra et | tunicas oculorum. Si
    uultis scire | qua de causa lumen
    oculorum in multis | istorum non
    durat usque in senectutem, | ista
    est causa: quia magis superfluunt |
15 et superueniunt cathari et fumo-
    si|tates in istis quam in alijs.
    10. Nar|ramus uobis de tunicis
    oculorum que | sunt septem
    secundum Iohannicium et secun-
    dum | nos due, et [explanauimus]
20 uobis quo|modo color et quare
    non est in ocu|lis quod accidit

---

19 explanauimus] M explanabimus, VP2 (f. 290r), VR (f. 31r) explanauimus

London, British Library, Sloane MS 661, ff. 32r–46r

for com*m*onlye in | these manne*r* of Eyes are oftne*r* trobled w*ith* Cata|ractes and fumosityes then any other.
[10] and thus | mutch for the Humors. |

Glasgow, GUL, Hunter MS 503, pp. 1–135

fulfillyth all the | concauyte of
holownesse of the ey. | ere yt
passe from the glassy humor. & |
the tonycle. but os ys sayd it
dureth | not in many to age. for
comu*n*ly in | thyes man*er* of eyen. 15
ar oftener gen||dred cateract*er* and [9]
fumo*us* sy3t*is* than yn | oþ*er*.

And as for the humors. thys auc|tor
and. accorde yn |

---

3 and] *a blank follows where the name of the* auctoritas *would be written. The name appears in the outer margin in tiny letters:* Joha*n*nici*us*.

Glasgow, GUL, Hunter MS 513, ff. 2r–37r

    all | that holwenes of the ey3en
But why her syght | endurethe
nought in hem or in many of these
5 in to | her olde age that ys for
many fumositeys and many |
catarrecte habunden in suche more
than in any oþer |

Basel, Ö.B.U., MS D.II.11, ff. 172r–177v

    ¶ And nowe speke we of the
humours of the ey3en | and of her
Anothomye ther for y saye that
ther | ben thre humours of the
whiche the first is said | albu-
10 gine*us* for it is lyche the white of
the naye of | a henne ¶ The
secunde is cleped humour cristal-
lyn | for it is liche to the cristall ¶

Aras uos | uuelh dire delas 15
hum|ors dels uelhs. edic uos | per
serth que son tres ¶ Ela pri|meyra
es coma album du|ou ¶ Ela 20
segonda es coma | cristalhs ¶ Ela
terssa es co|ma colhor deueyre

Oxford, Bodleian Library, Ashmole MS 1468, pp. 1–6

Biblio.-Médiathèques de Metz, MS 176, ff. 1r–16r

      propter situm humorum, et quomo-
      do | variatur vnus ab alio, et qua
      de | causa videt vnus melius quam
      alius. | Ammodo procedamus et
25   dicamus de | humoribus ocu-
      lorum. Dicimus ergo | quod tres
      sunt humores oculorum: primus |
      dicitur albugineus, secundus
      cristallinus, | tercius uitreus.
      Albugineus dicitur | quia similis
30   est albugini oui, cristal|linus quia
      assimilatur cristallo, vitreus | quia
      assimilatur vitro.
      11. Nunc volumus | vos docere
      qualiter oculus est compositus | in
      capite cum humoribus suis,
      secundum | anathomiam nostram
35   probatissimam quam | fecimus et
      ita inuenimus. Est enim | oculus
      quedam concauitas in summita|te
      nerui obtici, et concauitas illa est |
      plena aqua glauca uel glaucosa, |
      et est diuersa aqua illa in tribus |
40   manieribus, scilicet: in specie et

London, British Library, Sloane MS 661, ff. 32r–46r

Glasgow, GUL, Hunter MS 503, pp. 1–135

De Probatissima Arte Oculorum 205

Glasgow, GUL, Hunter MS 513, ff. 2r–37r
The thirde humour | humour
vitreus humour glasy for it is liche
white | glasse

Basel, Ö.B.U., MS D.II.11, ff. 172r–177v

¶ wherfore it is to vndyrstonde that
15 ther ys | a·maner holwenes in the
ouer p*ar*tie of optici nerffe | and
that holwenes is full of water
yelwisshe and | Departed in thre
partis and in thre diuisiouns in |
kynde in name in figure and in
felynge ¶ wherfor | the first spice
in kynde of felynge ys liche the
20 white | of a·naye ¶ And the
second as it were a fresshe gu*m*|me

¶ Als uels | uos dic ques vn. nerui
for|cat que ua al seruelh. et a|quel   25
nerui es cauatz. et a en | si aquelha
con cauitat hum|or. quar es plena
duhumor | que es partida entres
maney|ras. quar launa maneyra |
resembla album duou ¶ Ela | 30
segonda maneyra es coma | goma
fresca. laterssa coma lart | deporc |

Oxford, Bodleian Library, Ashmole MS 1468, pp. 1–6

Biblio.-Médiathèques de Metz, MS 176, ff. 1r–16r

```
           in nomine et in | figura et in tactu.
           Vnde prima | species est in tactu
           similis albugini oui, | secunda
           autem sicut aqua congelata, |
           tercia uero habet tactum sicut
    45     gumma | recens. Et omnes sunt
           in vna substancia | et non sunt
    2rb    separati in vna figura || et habent
           diuisionem in tactu et sic de |
           nomine. Vnde primus [humor] est
           ille quem | Iohannicius vocat
           albugineum, | secundus quem
    5      vocat cristallinum, tercius | quem
           vocat vitreum. Et omnes | iste
           ordinaciones sunt secundum
           ordi|nacionem Dei, composite in
           instrumento | capitis cum vij
           tunicis coopertis | a parte palpe-
           brarum secundum Ioannicium. Et
    10     secundum | anathomiam proba-
           tissimam, quam | probauimus et
```

---

2 humor] M color, VP2 (f. 290r), VR (f. 31r) humor

London, British Library, Sloane MS 661, ff. 32r–46r

Glasgow, GUL, Hunter MS 513, ff. 2r–37r

¶ The third hathe in felynge as it were swy|nes larde whan it is soden ¶ And alle ben in sub-sta|unce and ben nought departed and ben in one fi|gure Saue thei haue a·Distinccion in the felyng |
25 and   in nAme where for the first is that Johannici*us* | albuginem the secunde cristallyne the third vitreus |

Basel, Ö.B.U., MS D.II.11, ff. 172r–177v

Oxford, Bodleian Library, Ashmole MS 1468, pp. 1–6

Biblio.-Médiathèques de Metz, MS 176, ff. 1r–16r   *Glasgow, GUL, Hunter MS 503, pp. 1–135*

inuenimus, quod hoc est | instrumentum quod est coopertum a parte | palpebrarum de duabus tunicis. | Et illam tunicam quam
15   Iohannicius | coniunctiuam vocat, inuenimus totam | integram – que oculum amplificabat | mediocriter siue per medium, et nos | vocamus ipsam saluatricem, et habet | tactum sicut pellis callosa et est |
20   tenuis subtilissima ad modum | spolij cepe quando commeditis de eis | crudis, et inuenitis sub cortice | intrinseca a parte cepe illum panni|culum folij.
25   **12.** Est alia tunica quam | nos vocamus discoloratam, et inue|nimus quod occupat omnes tres humo|res circumcirca, et erat nigra per | medietatem. Illa nullum colorem | habebat sed apparebat
30   lucida sicut | cornu lucidum, et ab illa parte erat | perforata – et illud foramen erat | rotundum et

London, British Library, Sloane MS 661, ff. 32r–46r

Glasgow, GUL, Hunter MS 513, ff. 2r–37r   **Basel, Ö.B.U., MS D.II.11, ff. 172r–177v**

Oxford, Bodleian Library, Ashmole MS 1468, pp. 1–6

Biblio.-Médiathèques de Metz, MS 176, ff. 1r–16r

erat ita magnum | ad modum vnius
grani milij. Simile | erat separata a
35   tunica predicta salua|trice, quam
Iohannicius vocat coniunc|tiuam,
quod poterat stare inter | vnam et
aliam extra foramen, medium |
grani frumenti. Et dicimus quod |
aliquando inuenimus eleuare
40   catharac|tam a separacione quam
facimus de | ea, aut cum credimus
ipsam mittere | inferius sicut
facimus de alijs | catharactis. Et
ipsa exit de | concauitate per illud
45   foramen et | permanet inter vnam
tunicam et aliam, | ita quod
2va apparet extra oculum quasi || aqua
congelata putrefacta. Vnde
dici|mus quod per illud foramen
exit | spiritus visibilis et recipit
lumen a | maiori lumine.
5   **13.** Et inuenimus similiter | aliud
foramen a parte cerebri in sum|mi-

London, British Library, Sloane MS 661, ff. 32r–46r

Glasgow, GUL, Hunter MS 513, ff. 2r–37r *Basel, Ö.B.U., MS D.II.11, ff. 172r–177v*

Oxford, Bodleian Library, Ashmole MS 1468, pp. 1–6

Biblio.-Médiathèques de Metz, MS 176, ff. 1r–16r

    tate nerui concaui, [sed] tamen |
ab illa parte intrinseca, ubi
tenetur | oculus a neruo, erat
tunica dis|colorata perforata, sicut
10 est a parte | palpebrarum. Et
tunica predicta erat | cooperta ex
omni latere de callo, et super |
illum callum inuenimus carnosi-
ta|tem viscosam. Tamen a parte
palpebrarum | inuenimus pellicu-
15 lam circundan|tem tunicas claras
per quas in|trat spiritus uisibilis,
per foramen | in intrinseca parte,
et resultat intus | infra humores, et
recipit lumen | per aliud foramen
20 quod dicitur | pupilla ad maiorem
claritatem. |

14. Diximus uobis de humoribus |
oculorum et nomina eorum, et
patefeci|mus qualiter compositus
est oculus | in capite, et quo modo

---

6 sed] M se, VP2 (f. 290v), VR (f. 31v) sed

Glasgow, GUL, Hunter MS 503, pp. 1–135

London, British Library, Sloane MS 661, ff. 32r–46r

Glasgow, GUL, Hunter MS 513, ff. 2r–37r

Basel, Ö.B.U., MS D.II.11, ff. 172r–177v

Oxford, Bodleian Library, Ashmole MS 1468, pp. 1–6

4r Of the complexions of humoures and of the sub‖staunce of whom they ben nourshed //
Therfore y | saye that the complexiou*n* of the first albuginosi hu|mour is colde and moyste ¶ The ·2ᵉ· for sothe is colde | and drie ·i·

Biblio.-Médiathèques de Metz, MS 176, ff. 1r–16r

25 est concauus et | plenus de omnibus humoribus, | et vij tunicis compositus secundum | Iohannicium et secundum nos de duabus | tunicis tantum. Ammodo dicamus de | complexionibus et substantia
30 vnde nutriuntur. | Dicimus ergo complexionem primi | humoris, scilicet albuginei, et dicimus | quod est frigidus et humidus, cristal|linus frigidus et siccus, vitreus | similiter frigidus et siccus
35 – sed tamen minus | habet de frigiditate quam alij, quia tempera|tur frigiditas sua per calorem san|guinis qui est in palpebris, ideo | quia magis ei uicinatur quam alij. | Et dicimus quod
40 humor uitreus | et cristallinus nutriuntur a gum|mositate neruorum, et albugineus | a gummositate cerebri.

Glasgow, GUL, Hunter MS 503, pp. 1–135

London, British Library, Sloane MS 661, ff. 32r–46r

Glasgow, GUL, Hunter MS 513, ff. 2r–37r   *Basel, Ö.B.U., MS D.II.11, ff. 172r–177v*

    crystallyn ¶ The thirde is colde and
5   drie | ·i· vitreus but netheles it
hathe lesse of coldenes | than of
drinesse for his coldenesse is
temperate in to | hete of blode the
whiche is in the ey3e leddes þe |
whiche is more ny3 than any othir
humo*ur* / And | sithen that
humo*ur* vitreus and cristallynus
10 ben | nourshed of the gu*m*mosite
of the neruis and the | humour
albugenosus is nourshed of the
visco|site of the brayne

Oxford, Bodleian Library, Ashmole MS 1468, pp. 1–6

216   *De Probatissima Arte Oculorum*

Biblio.-Médiathèques de Metz, MS 176, ff. 1r–16r

      15. Ammodo | procedemus de infirmitatibus | superuenientibus et
45 earum curis necessarijs, | et primo de catharactis. | Dicimus ergo quod vij sunt species ||
2vb catharactarum quarum 4 sunt curabiles | et iij incurabiles. Vnde explanare uobis | volumus primo de illis que sunt cura|biles, quia per
5   certum cognoscitur incer|tum, et non econuerso. Prima ergo spe|cies est illa que est alba | sicut calx purissima; secunda est alba | tamen uertitur in colore celestino; tercia | est alba tamen assimilatur
10 cine|ricio colori; quarta uero apparet quasi | citrina, sed de ista specie scilicet citrina | pauce et pauce inueniuntur. Dicto | de speciebus catharactarum curabilium | quot sunt et de coloribus

——————————————

6 est¹] dicimus uobis *expunged*
9 tamen] uertitur *expunged*

Glasgow, GUL, Hunter MS 503, pp. 1–135

Now after he hath tau3t what | an   5
eye is. and how it ys | mayd. and
of the colour | and of the humors
of eyon. he conse|quently by-
gynneth to trete of the infir|mytees
of an ey. and after of the curys. |
And fyrst he begynnyth to trete of   10
ca|teracter. And after hys hys
doctrine a ca|teracte is nou3t ellys.
but a corupt | water. or a water
congyeld lyke a crude | gendred of
humers of the ey. dystempred | be   15
twyx the tonycle. and set be fore
the || ly3t of the ere. and the   [10]
crystallyne | humor. And of this
maner of cateracter | þer be vij.
maner of dyuers spices. wher|of
.iiij. be curable. and .iij vncura|ble.   5
And fyrst he tretyth of the iiij |

——————————————

11 cateracte] cataracte *added in outer margin in an Elizabethan hand*
2 humor] 7 manner | of Cataractis *added in outer margin in an Italic hand*

London, British Library, Sloane MS 661, ff. 32r–46r

[15] Now that he hath taughte, what and Eye is & howe | yt is made, and of the Colors.   25
and of the Humors | He consequentlye begynneth to intreate of the infir|myties of the
Eyes. And after of there Cuers And | first he begineth to intreate of the Cataracte: and |
after his doctrine a Cataracte is noughte ells, but | a corrupte water, or a water congeled   30
lyke crudde| ingendred in the humors of the eye. distempred be|twixte the tunicles, and
sett before the lyghte of the | Eye and the Christalline humor. And there be .7. | kindes of
Cataractes where of 4. be curable & | 3. vncurable: and first he intreateth of the fowre || 35
that be curable, He sayeth that the first of the | Cataractes that be curable, is like brighte   33v

——————————————

24 howe] Cap .2. *outer margin*   28 and] A Cataracte & | what it is. *outer margin*   33 7] 7. kindes of | Cataractes. | 4. Curable. | 3. vncurable. *outer margin*   34 of¹] 4. *deleted*   35 fowre] that be. *lower margin*   1 that¹] The first Cu|rable, Cata|racte. *outer margin*

De Probatissima Arte Oculorum 217

Glasgow, GUL, Hunter MS 513, ff. 2r–37r

¶ Of the ·7· spicis and kyndes | of catarractis ·i· of westis that ben in the ey3en | //
The first spice is curable the
15 whiche is white | as clerist chalke ¶ The secunde is white and | is liche to the whitnes of firmament ¶ The ·3^{e·} | is white and is liche a·skyn ·i· cuuers colours ¶ And | thre other kyndes of catarractis that suen ben vn|curable · Forsothe wo speken of the first kynde the |
20 whiche is liche clerest chalke and that fallethe in | the ey3e ofte thorough smytyng in the ey3e howe |so euer it be smyten weth outforth weth stone or | with staffe or weth rodde ¶ The seconde kynd of | catarractes that is liche to the
4v firmament white || we sayen that hit comethe fro the stomake and fal|lethe in to the brayne sendethe it to the ey3en ¶ The | third that is white liche the colour of Asshyn*n*

Oxford, Bodleian Library, Ashmole MS 1468, pp. 1–6

Basel, Ö.B.U., MS D.II.11, ff. 172r–177v

Aras uos uelh dire de | las 35
enfermetatz dels | uels edelas curas ¶ E | prumeyra ment delas car|actas que son en. vij. ma|neyras eson quatre que se || podon curar 172va
¶ Etres que non | ¶ Elaprumeyra es quepot | curar es coma caus pura et | aquesta uen entorn lo uelh. |
os ambaston o. am uergua | os 5
am lopoinh. o. am peyra | o am uent. os am semblans | causas. ¶
Ela segonda es | coma color celestina euen | delestomach per 10
manjar ma|las uiandas. ela fumo-sitat | monta en latesta. ¶ Ela ter|ssa espessia es blanca. coma sen|res. et aquesta enfermetat | uen 15
als uelhs per tropa dolor | detesta. coma es emigranea. o. | per tropa freior detesta. o per | trop plorar. o per trop uelhar | oper angozia ¶
Ela quar|ta es pessia es sitrina. es 20

18 per] *a expunged*

Biblio.-Médiathèques de Metz, MS 176, ff. 1r–16r

15 earum. Nunc | volumus uos docere de accidentibus et | curis earum secundum virtutem et Artem Nostram | Probatissimam Oculorum. Dicimus ergo | quod prima species est illa que est alba sicut | calx purissima. Accidit
20 propter percussionem | accidentem in oculo quoquomodo oculus | sit percussus exterius – aut cum virga, aut | cum baculo, aut cum stipite, aut cum lapide |, aut cum arangio quando homines | ludunt aliquando in plateis, et similia istis. |
25 Secunda autem species que est alba et as|simulatur colori celestino, dicimus uobis | quod procedit a stomaco et accidit occasione | malorum ciborum, ex quibus resoluitur | fumositas grossa; et
30 illa fumositas | ascendit ad caput et intrat cerebrum, | et cerebrum mittit ad oculos. Tertia | species, que est alba et que conuertitur | in

Glasgow, GUL, Hunter MS 503, pp. 1–135

curable. He seyth þat the fyrst of þe | curable cateractys ys lyke ryght briȝt | whyte chalke or alabastre vele polys|hyd. and is causyd of a stroke yn the | ey. 10
wyth a styk. or wyth a stone or any | oþer outwarde vyolence. ¶ The secunde | cateractte curable ys sumwhat white. | and lykenyd much to a celestyal color. | and this procedyth from the stomake. | and is comunly causyd of 15
wykkyd || metis. wherof a groos [11]
fumosytee resol|uyd. ascendyth vp yn to the brayn. & | from thens fallyth downe into the eyon. | ¶ The thyrde cateractte curable ys al|so whytyshe. but it turnyth into 5
the | color of ashes. and is comunly gendrid | of the payn of the hede. as the mygrym | and

---

12 cateractte] 2. *added in outer margin in a late hand* **4** also] 3. *added in outer margin in a late hand*

London, British Library, Sloane MS 661, ff. 32r–46r

white | chaulke. or Alabaster finelye polished. and is cau|sed of a stroke in the Eye. with a stycke, or with a | stone or any other outwarde violence. The second | curable Cataracte is some what white, and likened | mutch to a celestyall color and this procedeth from | the Stomacke, and is commonlye caused, of naughtye | meates where of a grosse vapor resolved ascen|dyth vpp into the braine, and from thence fawleth | downe into the Eyes. The thirde curable | cataracte is allso whitish, but yt torneth into the | the Color of asshes, and is commonlye engen|dred of the paine of the heade, as the megrim & | sutch like. and is caused of great sorrowe some | tyme, and of great heavines causinge great | weepinge, and some tyme of mutch coulde & | mutch watchinge and sutch like The 5 10 15

---

5 or²] The seconde | kinde of Cu|rable Cata|racte. *outer margin* **11** downe] The thirde | kinde of Cura|ble Cataracte. *outer margin* **13** asshes] and *deleted*

Glasgow, GUL, Hunter MS 513, ff. 2r–37r

comþᵉ | of moche wo as of emy-
gr*a*nis and sum tyme for moch |
5   coldenes of wepyng and of teres
letyng and wa|kyng and such other
moo ¶ The 4 kynd of catarract*es* |
is that that is in colour citrine and
hit comethe of | moche drynkyng
and of ouer moch etyng and of
gre|te trauell in many folke it
10 comethe thorowe ma|lancoly
humour ·/· |

Basel, Ö.B.U., MS D.II.11, ff. 172r–177v

a|questa uen per grant moue|ment
de moth manjar. eper | gran
trebalh euen per humor | eper
malencolia

Oxford, Bodleian Library, Ashmole MS 1468, pp. 1–6

Biblio.-Médiathèques de Metz, MS 176, ff. 1r–16r

    cinericio colore, accidit ex multo
    do|lore capitis, sicut est dolor
35 emigra|neus. Et aliquando accidit
    propter nimiam | frigiditatem, et
    propter nimiam angustiam et |
    planctum lacrimarum, et uigilias
    et | similia illis. Quarta species,
    que est | quasi pertinens in citrino
40 colore, dicimus | quod accidit ex
    multo potu et multa com|mescione
    et per magnum laborem, et |
    dicimus quod generatur in multis
    ex humore | melancolico.
    16. Diximus vobis causas et
    accidentia | catharactarum cura-
45 bilium. Ammodo do|cebimus
    uobis curam earum. Et ita dicimus
    quod omnes iste species quatuor ||
3ra curabiles nunquam possunt curari
    nisi | prius compleantur et bene
    confirmentur, | et postquam sunt
    complete et confirmate | hec sunt
5 signa: quia ab illa hora | inantea
    paciens nichil uidet nisi | clari-

Glasgow, GUL, Hunter MS 503, pp. 1–135

such other. and is causid of gret
so|rowe. su*m* tyme. and of grete
heuynes | cawsyng grette wepyng.   10
and sum|tyme of much colde. and
much wache | and such oþ*er*. ¶
And the iiij*th* spice of | cat*er*acct*er*
curable. ys of sytrynne color. | and
it ys comu*n*ly gendryd of exces |
meete and drynk yndegest. and   15
also | of gret labour. and su*m* tyme
humurs || malencoly.   [14]

¶ Thyes iiij spices ben*n* | curable.
but neu*er* tyl þei ben growu*n* | and
confermed w*ith* his signe. And

---

11 wache] t *added between* a *and* c *over the line in a late hand* || watchinge. *added in the outer margin in an Elizabethan hand* **12** of] 4 *added in outer margin in an Elizabethan hand* **16** humurs] After this | page you | follow to the | 14. page *added in outer margin in an Italic hand*

London, British Library, Sloane MS 661, ff. 32r–46r

fourth | sorte of Curable Cataractes is of Citrine colo*r* | and yt com*m*onlye caused of   20
excesse in meates & | drinck*es* vndigested and allso of great labour | and some tymes of
melancholye humors. |
[16] These fowre kindes of Cataractes be curable | but neu*er* till theye be growen and
confirmed | And the signes to knowe when yt is confirmed | are these, when the patient   25
seeth noughte but | the brightenes of the sonne by daye or the moone | by nighte or a
lanthorne w*ith* a candell, lighte, | An many lewde letches not knowinge the cau|ses nor   30
properties of these manner of Cataract*es* | thincke to Cuer them, w*ith* purgations,
Powders, | and plaisters but theye be deceaved, for these manner of diseases maye not be

---

19 sorte] The 4*th* kinde | of Curable | Cataract*es*. *outer margin* **25** And] The signes of | Curable Cata|ractes. *outer margin*

**Of the Cure of the· 4· kindes of
Cate|ractus curabill & of
worching with nedill |**
The Cure of these foure kyndes of
catarrac*tes* | forsaid is for to witte
15 first at begynnyng | that all these
kyndes of catarrac*tes* curable that |
they maye neu*ere* be well y holpen
but they be com|plete and con-

---

11 Of] 2 *added in outer margin*

Oxford, Bodleian Library, Ashmole MS 1468, pp. 1–6

¶ Aras uos | uuelh dire delas 25
autras cur|as da questas enfer-
metatz | edic uos ques aquestas
espes|cias non sen podon ben
curar | en tro que sian ben com-
plidas | eben fermadas ¶ Et 30
aque|st es losenhalh en que
cone|yssiras cant ceran ben
com|plidas que lomalaute no | pot
lo lum del solelh si non | enlauia. 35
olo lum dela can|delha si non de

Biblio.-Médiathèques de Metz, MS 176, ff. 1r–16r

 tatem solis in die et lumen lu|cerne
in nocte. Multi stolidi me|dici
ignorantes causas credunt ipsos |
curare cum purgationibus et
10 pulue|ribus, sed falluntur quia iste
catha|racte nunquam possunt curari
neque cum | medicinis laxatiuis
neque cum pul|ueribus neque cum
electuarijs neque cum | collirijs,
ideo quia sunt subtus omnes |
15 tunicas oculorum. Et sunt gene-
rate de | humoribus oculorum,
scilicet: de humore albu|gineo,
quia occasione supradictorum
accidentium, | humor albugineus
dissoluitur in parte | et putrescit.
20 Et illa putrefactio est quasi | aqua
coagulata et ponitur ante | lucem
inter tunicas et humorem cris|talli-
num. Vnde Sarraceni et Arabes |
vocant ipsam ilmesarac, id est in
latino | aqua celestina. Alij antiqui
25 philosophi vo|cabant ipsam
putrefactam in oculis. | Nos autem

Glasgow, GUL, Hunter MS 503, pp. 1–135

the | tokyn of hyr conplexion or
confermy*n*g | is. when the 5
pacyent seyth ry3th now|ght. but yf
it be bry3tnes of the su*n*ne | by
day. or the mone by ny3t or a
lan|te*r*ne. And many lewde leches
not know|yng the causes nor
prop*ur*tes of thyes ma|ne*r* of 10
Cat*er*acties weyn*n* to cure þem
w*i*th | purgac*i*ons. powders. and
plastrys. | but thei be disceyuyd.
for thyes mane*r* | of diseasys may
not be curid oonly by | medycyns
neyther ynward nor out|warde. nor 15
pr*i*ncypally. but by thys | craft that
ys callyd. Ars acuaria. || that ys to [15]
saye the craft of nedyl. In whych |

16 craft] Ars Acua|ria *added in outer
margin in an Italic hand*
1 craft…nedyl] first cure of ey *added
in upper margin in a late hand*
whych] The Cuer | of Cararac|tes. by
the | Needle *added in outer margin in
an Italic hand*

London, British Library, Sloane MS 661, ff. 32r–46r

cured onlye | by medicines nether inwarde nor outwarde: | But by this crafte that is 35
called Ars Acua|ria that is to saye, to cuer by the Needle, In | whitch crafte who so will
procede artificiallye || muste begin thus. ffirste he muste purge his braine | w*i*th pills 34r
called Pillulæ Hierolimitanæ w*hi*tch are | thus made. Take Turbith, Aloes epatica ana
ʒ j. | Macis, Cubibæ, Masticis, Anethi, ana ʒ j. Beate | them all into fine powder, and 5
make them vpp | into a masse w*i*th the Juyce of roses. And with | the pills let the patient
be first purged. And | the nexte daye followinge about nyne of *the* clocke | while he is
fastinge sett him oue*r*thwart a forme ry|dinge wyse. and sitt yo*w* allso on the forme | 10
w*i*th him face to face. and cause the patient | to houlde his whole Eye close. w*i*th his

34 outwarde] Ars Acua|ria *outer margin* 37 artificiallye] muste *lower margin* 3 j] Pillulæ
Hiero|solimitanæ. *outer margin* 9 rydinge] wysse *deleted*

Glasgow, GUL, Hunter MS 513, ff. 2r–37r

  firmed and whan they ben well
  com|plete and redy to be cured ¶
  these ben the signes For |why fro
  that houre before they seen nought
20 but | the clerete of the sonne in
  the way the lyght of | the day or
  elles symplych thei seen right
  nought | ¶ wher for many leches
  that ben folys and vnkun|yng of
  this Crafte and that knowen naught
  þis | cause wonen for to helpe in
25 hem w*ith* purgacions | w*ith*
  pouders wethe oynementes or
5r wethe coleries || and they ben
  begilyd for why thoo cataract*es*
  ben undyr | the tonicles of the
  ey3en and ben engendred of
  humo*urs* | of the ey3en ·i· of the
  humour albuginoys · For why |
  thorugh accacion of the forsaid
5 causes the humour | albuginoys
  ys dissoluid in p*ar*tye and hit rotith
  and | that roted is as it were water
  congelid and crudded | and it is

Oxford, Bodleian Library, Ashmole MS 1468, pp. 1–6

Basel, Ö.B.U., MS D.II.11, ff. 172r–177v

nuytz o dese|ra ¶ Don uos fau
saber q*ue* | motz megges son que
uo|lon curar. aquestas enfer|metatz. 40
am polueras. o. am | ayguas. o. am
colliris. o am | medecinas laxati-
uas eson | ne maluadament en-
gan|natz. car totas aquestas en|fer-
metas || son engendas de so|tas las 172vb
tunicas e son engenra|das. de las
humors secas ede | la humor que
sembla. album | duou. quar 5
aquelha humor | se disol
esepoyriga coma ayga | poyrida
econgelhad ene met | se entre las
tunicas. ela hu|mor cristallina ¶ Et
yeu | ben uengut uos diray las | 10
curas que sedeuon far. las | quals
yeu per sert uos dir q*ue* | ey
esprouadas lonc temps | per
lagracia dedieu. ¶ Pru|meyra ment 15
uos purguaretz | lo seruelh. am
uostras pillu|las las quals uos auem
fay|tas et annom ierosolimitan|as. ¶
Ɍecep. ʒ.i. turbit. aloes | espaci-

Biblio.-Médiathèques de Metz, MS 176, ff. 1r–16r

  et prouidi magistri Saler|nitani
  vocamus ipsam catharactam, | ideo
  quia aqua illa putrefacta ponitur |
  ante lucem, id est ante pupillam
30 inter | tunicas et lumen oculorum.
  Ergo non | possunt curari cum
  pulueribus neque cum | alijs
  medicinis, que dari possunt
  intrin|sece et extrinsece, nisi
  secundum magiste|rium nostrum et
35 Artem Probatissimam | Oculorum
  a nobis Beneuenuto Gra|pheo
  compositam. Et hec est cura: |
  Primo oportet in hac cura purgare |
  cerebrum pacientis cum pillulis |
  nostris Iherosolomitanis a nobis
40 com|positis, ad quas Recipe ʒ 1
  turbit, a|loe epatici ʒ ß, macis,
  cubebe, mas|ticis, croci ana ʒ 1 et
  conficiatur cum succo | rosarum.
  Et in sequenti die post pur|ga-
  cionem in hora tercie, ieiuno
3rb stomaco, fa||ciatis sedere pacien-
  tem in vno scamp|no ut equitet, et

Glasgow, GUL, Hunter MS 503, pp. 1–135

craft who so wyll procede arty-
fycyally. he | must begyn thus.
Fyrst he must porge his | brayn
wyth pelett*is* callyd. Pillule
ihero|solimitane. wherof thus is 5
the maky*n*g. | Take turbite. aloes.
epatica. of eu*er*ych | a nownce.
Macys quibyb. Mastic*is*. and. |
dylle. of eche of þem a dram. and
beete | þem into pouder. And
confecte þem w*ith* | the Jows of 10
rose. And make þ*er*of pelat*is*. |
And when he hath youen the
pacyent | purgac*i*on. on the day
next foloyng a|bowt ix. of the clok
whyle he is fastyng. | do hym sitte
ou*er*thwhart rydyng wyse. | and 15
sytte þou also on the stoke yn
lyk|wyse face to face. And do the
pacyent || to holde the hole eye [16]
cloos w*ith* hys oon hand | And

―――――――――――――
6 euerych] Pill. Jhero|solimitane
added in outer margin in an Italic hand

London, British Library, Sloane MS 661, ff. 32r–46r

owne hand | and charge him that he sytt steadfastlye, and | not to stirr, and then blesse
the, and begin thy | worke in the name of Jesus Christ, and w*ith* | thye lefte hand (if yt 15
be for his lefte eye) lyfte | vpp his eye lydd, and w*ith* the other hand, put | in the Needle,
made for that purpose, into that | syde ˻of the eye˼ nexte to the eare. and ˻thurle˼ yt
thorough | the tunicle called Saluatrice. and allwaise stirr | yo*ur* fingars too and froo till 20
yow touth w*ith* the | poynt of the Nedle the corrupte | water the w*hitch* is the Cataracte,
and then begin | to remove downewarde from aboue (w*ith* the pointe | of the nedle) the 25
sayde corrupte water from | before the sighte, and dryve yt downe levell | and there kepe
yt still w*ith* the poynt of the | Nedle as longe as yow maye saye .3. or 4. tymes | ou*er*

―――――――――――――
14 thy] thyn *MS*, n *deleted* **17** vpp] t *deleted* **18** purpose] o *deleted* **19** thurle] thrust *deleted*,
thurle *added over the deletion* **22** the³] tunicle called *deleted*

De Probatissima Arte Oculorum 225

Glasgow, GUL, Hunter MS 513, ff. 2r–37r

    putten afore the lyght and afore the ey3e ap|pill bitwene the tonicle and the cristallyne humour | the which the Sarazyns and the Arabies
10 clepen | hit amesarca that is in latyn aqua· putrefacta in | englisshe water y roted in the ey3e ¶ Of the whi|che it sheweth openly that they mowen nought be | holpon withe poudres neither w*ith* other medecyns | y putte in the ey3e sithen the mater· and all the
15 humo*ur*s | of the ey3en w*ith*yn the tonicles ben conteyned ¶ This | is the Cure first to pourge the brayne withe oure | pillull of Jerusalem ¶ ℞ turbith aloes epatik an*a* ·℥·ij· | mac*es* cucube aneti mastic*es* an*a* ·℥·ß make hem w*ith* the | Juse of rose ¶ In the secunde
20 day folowyng after þ*at* | purgacion

---

17 ·℥·ij·] pelles | of tour|bethe *in outer margin in a late hand*

Oxford, Bodleian Library, Ashmole MS 1468, pp. 1–6

Basel, Ö.B.U., MS D.II.11, ff. 172r–177v

cum. ℥.ß mastec. cubebas | 20
safran. ℥. ecofis lon. am suc | de rosas efassa purgar loser|uelh. e que fassa fum de las de|uant ditas causas. erescepia | per lonas 25
lofum. et en lautre | iorn segent tu faras lo pacient | sezer desobre .i. banc. ecaulgue | sobre lobanc. elomayestre sega | deuant el. efassa lui tener los | uelhs clauses 30
et amlauna | man leue lapalpelha del uelh | desobre et am lautra man ten|ga vna agulha dargent etrau|que am lagulha lo uelh dela | part blanqua deues laurelha | 35
efaraso torssen lagulha. equa*n*t | seras pres delapupilla tu res|clauras luelh am lagulha. e | metras lacaracta rasclan de | sota la 40
pupilla o de sobre | ecant tuauras pauzada laca|racta en son loc non layces la|gulha tost mais temlan

---

40 la] pullu *expunged*

226 — De Probatissima Arte Oculorum

Biblio.-Médiathèques de Metz, MS 176, ff. 1r–16r

  tu sedeas simile | cum ipso pacien-
te facie ad faciem. | Et teneat
5 paciens oculum sanum | clausum
et incipe curare alium | in nomine
Ihesu Christi. Et cum vna manu |
subleua palpebram superiorem et
cum | alia manu teneas acum
argen|team, et ponas illam acum a
10 parte | lacrimalis minoris et
perfora ocu|lum cum acu, tor-
quendo et distor|quendo cum
digitis tuis donec | tangas cum
puncto acus aquam | illam putre-
15 factam, quam Sarraceni | et
Arabes vocant ilmesarac et | inter
nos dicitur catharacta. Et inci-
pia|mus desuper cum puncto acus,
et re|moueas ipsam a loco ubi
manet, | id est ante pupillam, et
20 facias ipsam des|cendere inferius,
et sustineas ipsam | ibi cum puncto
acus per tantum | spacium tem-
poris quod 4 uel 5 pater noster |
possunt dici. Postea remoueas

Glasgow, GUL, Hunter MS 503, pp. 1–135

charge hym that he syt stydfastly |
styl and styre not. And þen blysse
the. | and begyn thy craft in the
name of ih*esu* | cryste. and w*ith* 5
thy lyfthand lyft vp hys | oon ey
lyd. and w*ith* þin oþ*er* hande put |
yn thy nedyl made þer fore on
the | forþ*er*syde from the nose.
and softly thyr | the tonycle.
Saluatrice, And alwey | wryth thy 10
fyngers too and fro tyll | þou
touche wyth the poynt the co|rupte
water the whych ys the cat*er*|acte.
and then begyn to remeue
down|ward from a boue wyth the
poynte | the sayd corrupte wat*er* 15
fro be forne | the sy3th. And dryue
yt down beneth || and þ*ere* kepe [17]
yt styl w*ith* the poynt of the |
nedyl as long as þou mayst sey.
iij. | or .iiij. tymes. Pater noster.

---

16 beneth] and þ*ere* kepe *added in lower margin*

London, British Library, Sloane MS 661, ff. 32r–46r

yo*ur* pater noster. then remove easelye yo*ur* | nedle from yt, And if yt happ to ryse vpp 30
a|gaine bringe yt downe againe to the corner of | the eye nexte to the eare. But here yow
must | take great hede that after yow have once tow|ched the Cataracte, thowe shiftest no
more thy | fingars too and froo, till yt be placed, as is || sayde before. And then softlye 35 |
drawe out thy | nedle as yow put yt in. Allwaise thyrllinge | thy fingars too and froo, till 34v
thy Nedle be all | out. and then make a plaister of cotton or of | fyne tow, w*ith* the white 5
of an egg and laye | on the sore eye. and let him lye vppon his | backe in his bedd for the
space of .9. dayes. | after charge him that he stirr not his eye all | that tyme, and thrice in
the daye & thrice in | the nyghte remove the plaist*er*. 10

---

35 is] sayde before *lower margin*

De Probatissima Arte Oculorum 227

Glasgow, GUL, Hunter MS 513, ff. 2r–37r

    make the pacient to sitte on astole
and | thou shalt sitte w*ith* the
pacient face to face · and lete |
hym holde his one ey3e shitte and
thou shalt begyn|ne and blesse
a·crosse wise on the maladie in the
na|me of ihesu criste and w*ith* that
25 one hande holde a | siluere*n*
nedyll and put that nedyll in the
5v lasse || *pa*rtie lacrimal ·i· there as
the teres come*nn* oute and
perys|she the ey3e w*ith* that nedill
twynyng toward and | froward
w*ith* thi fyngers till thou touch w*ith*
the poynte | of that nedill that
water so roted ·i· putrefyed the |
5 whiche is cleped a·cataracte and
thou shalt begynne | fro the
vnderward withe the poynte of the
nedill | and remoue fro that place
where it dwellethe and | w*ith* that
nedyll make hit to discende and
goo doun and | susteyne it so in so
long tyme till thou mayste saye

Oxford, Bodleian Library, Ashmole MS 1468, pp. 1–6

Basel, Ö.B.U., MS D.II.11, ff. 172r–177v

per | espasi. de catre pater
nostres || disens ¶ Epueis osta 173ra
lagulha el | nom dieu en aquelha
maneyra | torsen que tulay mesist.
epueis | tu faras aisso amlos detz
en tor|sen edeues tusaber ques am 5
la | poncha dela dicha agulha tu
de|ues ostar aquelha ayga poyri|da
ecant auras fayt aysso a|ias de
coton mulhath am cla|raduou 10
etulomet de sobre lu|elh del
malaute. efay lon iaser | enuers en
son leyt en tro aia | passatz. ix.
dias egarda quelh | nos mude ¶
Ecascun dia tu | mudaras locoton 15
doas uega|das en lo iorn. et alanuit
fin | al terme de. ix. iors en lo
loc.: |

Biblio.-Médiathèques de Metz, MS 176, ff. 1r–16r

 acum plane desuper – et si accidat
25 quod re|uertatur sursum, reducas
 ipsam | ad partem minoris lacrima-
 lis, id est | uersus aurem. Sed nota:
 postquam | posueris acum in
 oculo, non debes | ipsam extor-
30 quere nisi prius collo|cetur
 catharacta a parte sicut su|perius
 dictum est. Postea plane et |
 suauiter extrahas acum sicut | intus
 misisti, torquendo et ex|torquendo
35 cum digitis tuis. Et | extracta acu,
 facies tenere oculum | pacientis
 clausum. Item habeas | bombacem,
 et intingas in clara oui, | et ponas
 super oculum pacientis, | et facias
40 ipsum iacere in lecto su|pinum
 usque ad 9 dies, oculis clau|sis ita
 quod non moueatur. Et clara | oui
 semper superponatur, ter in die
 cum | bombace et similiter in
 nocte, usque | ad predictum
 terminum.

Glasgow, GUL, Hunter MS 503, pp. 1–135

Than | remeue esely the nedyl
therfro. And it | hape to ryse vp   5
ayen. bryng it down*n* | a geyne to
the corner of the ey to the
ere|warde. But here be ware þat
after ty|me the nedyl hath towchyd
the Cat*er*act*er*. | þou schalt no
more wrythe thy fyng*ers* | to &   10
fro. tyl þat it be set yn hys place. |
as it ys seyd be fore. And þan
softlye | drawe out thy nedyl as
þou put it yn. | ¶ Alway thyrllyng
thy fingurs to | and fro. tyl yt be all
owte. And a non | make a plaster   15
of coton*n* or of flaxe herd*is* || w*ith* [18]
the whyte of an egg. And ley it on
the | the sore eye. And do hym lye
down in hys | bed wydeopon ix
days. After charge hym | that he
ster not hys eye all that tyme. & |
thryys yn the day. and tryys yn   5
the | nyght remeue the playster.

London, British Library, Sloane MS 661, ff. 32r–46r

Glasgow, GUL, Hunter MS 513, ff. 2r–37r

10   foure | or fyue pater nosters and
than take vp thy nedill | euyn and
yif it falle that it come ayen than |
turne it ayen vpward to the lasse
tery p*ar*tie toward | the ere ¶ And
knowe thou well that thy nedyll |
shall haue an hafte that it maye
15   w*ith* thy fyngers | turne aboute ¶
And Also whan thou haste putte |
that nedyll in the ey3e thou shalt
not drawe her | oute till the
cataracte be all y gadered as it is
said | aboue ¶ And than thou shalt
drawe thi nedyll play|nelych as
thou puttest yn wyndyng ayene
20   wyndy*n*g | the nedill w*ith* the
fyngers ¶ And the nedyll y
drawe*n* | oute make the pacient to
holde his ey3e y shitte | ¶ And
after loke thou haue cotu*n* y putte
and y watte | in the glayre of A
neye and ley it on the sore ey3e |
and make hym to lygge in his
25   bedde vp right till | ix dayes the

Basel, Ö.B.U., MS D.II.11, ff. 172r–177v

Oxford, Bodleian Library, Ashmole MS 1468, pp. 1–6

Biblio.-Médiathèques de Metz, MS 176, ff. 1r–16r *Glasgow, GUL, Hunter MS 503, pp. 1–135*

45 **17.** Et sit locus | ubi ipse iacet	And he to | to lye yn a derke
3va obscurus, et come||dat in illis	house. ¶ And for hys | dyet the ix
diebus oua sorbilia | cum pane; si	days. lete hym ete rere egg*is* |
est iuuenis bibat | aquam, et si est	wyth breed. And yf he be yong &
senex bibat vinum | bene limpha-	strong. | lete hym drynk water. 10
5 tum. Multi autem | precipiunt et	And yf he be | yn age. lete hym
uolunt ut comedat | carnes	drynk wyne medlyd | wat*er*.
recentes et gallinas. | Nos uero	Som*m* byd hym ete fresch flesche |
istud prohibemus, quia | multum	and he*n*nys. but we for bedde yt.
nutriunt – et posset ha|bundare per	for þei | be noryschyng of mych
10 multum nutrimentum | sanguis in	blode. ¶ Ther | myght be gendryd 15
oculis, et hoc esset | contrarium	yn the eyon that || my3te be [19]
nostris curis. Finito | numero ix	cont*ra*ry to oure cure. ¶ when | the
dierum faciat sibi signum | sancte	ix days ar past. make on the eye |
crucis, surgat a lecto, et | abluat se	
15 cum aqua frigida. Et | deinde	**8** dyet] Diate *added in outer margin*
paulatim conuersetur in factis |	*in a late hand* **1** my3te] mighte
suis.	*added in upper margin in an Elizabethan hand*

London, British Library, Sloane MS 661, ff. 32r–46r

[17] and let him lye \| in a darke place And for his dyett the .ix. dayes \| let him take reare egg*es* w*ith* bread. and if he \| be younge and stronge, let him drincke water & \| if he be in age, let him drincke wyne. medled w*ith* \| water Some councell him to eate fresh flesh &   15 hennes. but we forbid yt, for theye doe brede \| mutch bloode. and mighte breed offence to the eyes \| to hinder our Cuer. when the nyne dayes be \| past make on the eye the signe of the crosse \| and let him ryse vpp, and wash well his face \| & his Eyes w*ith* fayre coulde   20 water and after \| that faull to sutch busines as he hath to doe. \|

16 theye] l *deleted* **18** to] The Seconde \| dressinge *outer margin*

Glasgow, GUL, Hunter MS 513, ff. 2r–37r

    ey3en bethe shitte so that he be
naught | meued and the glayre
6r shall be renewed thries on || the
day and so often sithes on the
nyght to the forsaid | terme of ix
dayes /
and the place where the pacient |
shall ley moste be derke withe oute
any wynde and | make hym to ete
in thoo dayes rere ayren netheles |
5 yef he be yonge he shall dryngke
water ¶ yef he | olde wyne weth
water many comaunde to eten |
capons and hennes but we forbede
it for theinour|shyng moche and
that byhappethe that thorugh |
moche nourshing blode habunth in
10 the ey3e and is | contrarious to
oure cures ¶ But whan the sum*m*e
of | tho ix· Dayes been passed
make ther a·signe of the | crosse
and leten hym arise fro his bedde a
make hym | wasshe hym selfe
w*ith* colde water ¶ And afterward |

Basel, Ö.B.U., MS D.II.11, ff. 172r–177v

ondormira sia ben escur el |
malaute manie debos hueus | en   20
la braza cueitz o en layga o | e sian
molhs emanie pauc bl|anc ¶ E sies
ioues beua ay|ga. et sies uielhs
beua del vin | ben temprat. garda
que non | manie de deguna carn   25
car noi|ririan trop et engenraria
tro|pa. sanc et seria contrasis al|a
cura ¶ E quant aura co*m*|plit los
sobre ditz. ix. iorns le|ue se el   30
nom dieu elaue se la|ue sen lacara
ab ayga fregga e | pauc epauc
fassa sas fasendas |

Oxford, Bodleian Library, Ashmole MS 1468, pp. 1–6

Biblio.-Médiathèques de Metz, MS 176, ff. 1r–16r

18. Et tali modo curantur | omnes catharacte curabiles, scilicet | calcina, celestina, cinericia, et citri|na. Et si quis aliter curaret, nisi | secundum magisterium nostrum et Artem | Probatissimam Oculorum, ignoraret | causam et curam. Et hanc curam | vocamus nos acuare, ideo quia | fit cum acu argentea uel de | auro puro uel de ferro. De ferro | autem prohibeo quia tria possunt | inde contingere pericula: primo quia | durum est, et ex duricia sua | dissoluit ubicumque tangit. Secundo | quia si catharacta est dura, ac | de separacione quam tu facis ante | lucem posset puncta acus frangi |

Glasgow, GUL, Hunter MS 503, pp. 1–135

a tokyne of the crosse. and let hym | ryse vp. and wasche wele hys face & | hys eyon*n*. wyth fayr colde water. and | after that doo hys occupac*i*on that he | hath to doon.

and yn thys wyse be cu|ryd all the Cat*er*act*is* curable. ¶ And | who that wyll cure hem oþ*er* wyse shall | dysceyue þemselfe ignorant of the true | craft of curyng. And thys crafte a fore|sayde ys callyd the nedyll crafte. for | it ys excercysed & don*n* w*ith* the nedyll. | But alway be ware that the nedyll | be of golde or of syluer. or of clene || spanesh laten. and yn no wyse of | yren*n* nor of stele. And þat ys for the | hardnesse þat dyssoluyth suche as | yt towchyth. ¶ Another

5

10

15

[20]

14 nedyll] NB. *added in outer margin in an Italic hand*

London, British Library, Sloane MS 661, ff. 32r–46r

[18] And in thi wise be cured all curable Cataract*es* | and who so will cuer them otherwise shall de|ceave him selfe, beinge ignorant of the trew | crafte of Curinge, And this craft aforesayd | is called the Nedle crafte ffor yt pratized | and done w*ith* the Nedle. But beware that | the Nedle be made of goulde, or sylu*er* or of | cleane spanish lattin, and in no wyse of | Iron or Steele. for that by the hardnes yt | dissolveth what yt towcheth. An other cause | is that if the Cataracte be harde in the dra|winge downe there of the poynt mighte breake | for Iron & steele are verye brittle, and the poynt | of the Nedle abydinge in the Eye, mighte cause || a consumption of the Eye, through abundance of | teares and greatnes of paine.

25

30

35

35r

28 and] The Needle to | be of Goulde | or Silu*er* or | of Spanish latin *outer margin* 36 Eye[1]] l *deleted* cause] a consumptio*n lower margin*

Glasgow, GUL, Hunter MS 513, ff. 2r–37r
he shall be kepte a lytell and a litell
in his doyng // |

Basel, Ö.B.U., MS D.II.11, ff. 172r–177v

15   And in this maner shull be cured
     all the cataract*es* cura|ble that is to
     weten th*e* chalke white cataract*es*
     the | welken white asshen white
     and the citrine cataract*es* | ¶ And
     who euer curethe in any other
     maner he can | nought here causes
     of his Cure / And this cure we |
20   clepen the cure w*ith* the nedyll
     and su*m*me clepen hit | the
     magelyng · For it is Done w*ith* a
     nedill of siluer | or of golde ¶
     withe a·nedill of yren y forbede
     for | thre noyes may ther of befalle
     First for the nedill | of yren is
     harder than golde or siluer and
25   thorugh | his hardenes he dis-
     solueth where euer he touchethe |

¶ Et en aquesta maneyra se | curon
totas las caractas cu|rablas las   35
quals son de color | caulsina
celestina cinere es | citrina. et en
autra no sen de|uon curar ¶ E de
ues saber | que tu non deues
meggar am|bagulha deferr   40
nidelaton car | trop son duras.
Mais arge*n*t | es humils o aur |

Oxford, Bodleian Library, Ashmole MS 1468, pp. 1–6

Biblio.-Médiathèques de Metz, MS 176, ff. 1r–16r

  et remanere in oculo. Et si puncta |
  acus remaneat in oculo, ab illa |
35 occasione tota substantia oculi
  con|sumeretur propter dolorem
  oculorum semper | lacrimando.
  Tertio quia | magis dolet et
  ponderat et sen|tit per suam
  duriciem quam si esset de |
40 argento uel auro. Habetis |
  contraria de ferro que possunt
  contin|gere inde in opere nostro.

19. Nunc di|cemus vobis de auro et
  argen|to. Dicimus quod ambo sunt
45 bona | propter puritatem et
3vb molliciem eorum, sed || tamen
  aurum magis clarificat propter |
  dominium suum, quia frigidum et
  humidum | est in occulto suo. |

Glasgow, GUL, Hunter MS 503, pp. 1–135

cause ys. | for yf the Cateracter be 5
harde yn draw|yng down*n* therof.
the poynt my3te | ly3tely breke.
for yron & stele arne | frayle and
brytyll. and so the poynt | abydyng
yn the eye my3te cause of |
consumpc*ionn* of the eye thorugth 10
ha|bundance of terys and gretnese
of | payne.

---

12 payne] The first | kinde of |
Cataracte *added in outer margin in
an Elizabethan hand*

London, British Library, Sloane MS 661, ff. 32r–46r

Glasgow, GUL, Hunter MS 513, ff. 2r–37r *Basel, Ö.B.U., MS D.II.11, ff. 172r–177v*

¶ The 2^{e.} yif the cataracte be of
6v harde departy*n*g || a yenst the
lyght or the sight of the ey3en
myght | the poynte of the nedill
breken And so leve stille in | the
ey3e and so thorugh soche a
chaunce the sub|staunce of the ey3e
5 myght be loste thorugh mysche|fes
of hym wepyng ¶ The third forsoth
the nedill | of yren more greuethe
and more wey3th and the | pacient
felithe his hardenes more than it
were | of siluer or of golde
¶ But of siluer or of golde boþe |
ben full good for her clennes and
10 her softenes But | golde moste
clarifiethe for his dominiu*m* for it
is | moste in his *p*ropriete

Oxford, Bodleian Library, Ashmole MS 1468, pp. 1–6

Biblio.-Médiathèques de Metz, MS 176, ff. 1r–16r

20. Audiuistis a nobis causas
species et | accidencia et curas
catharactarum | curabilium.
Ammodo dicemus et doce|bimus
uos diuisionem que est inter |
vnam et aliam de restauracione
luminis, | in quibus earum post
restauracionem | melius videant.
Verbi gratia: illa que | est alba
sicut calx et accidit propter |
percussionem, ut superius dictum
est, faci|lius curatur – et tamen non
bene vident, | ideo quia propter
percussionem quam susti|nuit in
oculis, humores oculorum, sci-
licet: | cristallinus, albugineus, et
vitreus, | dissoluuntur in parte,
sicut dissoluuntur | in alijs partibus
corporis humores quando | aliquis
est percussus gladio uel ba|culo et
alijs similibus. Modo habetis |
speciem, causam, diuisionem de
restauracione | luminis de prima
catharacta.

Glasgow, GUL, Hunter MS 503, pp. 1–135

¶ Thys spyce of Cat*eract*is is | as
the aucter seyth easely & sone
cu|red. but yit þei þat ben cured
seen*n* | not ryght wele forasmuch
as the || humor yn the eye ys yn
p*ar*ty dysgregat | & dyssoluyd by
the stroke. and be bru|ser therof.
whych stroke was cause of | the
Cat*er*acter.

13 cured[1]] NB. *added in outer margin in an Italic hand* 3 of] NB. *added in outer margin in an Italic hand*

London, British Library, Sloane MS 661, ff. 32r–46r

[20] This kinde of | Cataracte is as my Autho*r* sayeth easelye and | soune cured. But those that be cured doe not | see perfectlye well, because the humo*r* in the | Eye is in p*ar*te dysgregate and trobled by the | stroke in brusinge there of: w*hitc*h stroke was cause | of the Cataracte.

Glasgow, GUL, Hunter MS 513, ff. 2r–37r   *Basel, Ö.B.U., MS D.II.11, ff. 172r–177v*

    Of restoring of | lightes &   U o l e t z   a u z i r   l a d i f e r e n | c i a
    dyu*er*se worching in this 4 | daquestas caractas || curablas. Jeu   173rb
    cataract*es* | uos dicques a|quelhas que es
    Of diuerse restoryng of lyght after   decolor calsina | pus stost se cura.
15 dyu*er*se | kyndes of cataractes for   Mays elha fa | peior uista car uen
    why they be nou3t | euen ne   al uelh per colp |
    parfitely y seyn as thus verbi
    gra|cia ¶ Of the first kynd of
    cataract*es* that is white | as it were
    Chalke the whiche ys be cause of
    smy|tyng and lyghtly ys cured ¶
20 But he seythe nou3t | well for
    why thorugh stroke the humours
    of the | ey3en albuginosus cristal-
    linus and vitreus ys | dissolued in
    p*ar*tie and that is that the sight of
    hem | is nought possible to be
    restored p*ar*fitely ne to tur|ne to the
    first kynde of helthe

---

12 lightes] 3 *added in outer margin*

Oxford, Bodleian Library, Ashmole MS 1468, pp. 1–6

Biblio.-Médiathèques de Metz, MS 176, ff. 1r–16r

21. Dicto | de prima specie catharactarum, nunc do|cebimus vos de secunda. Dicimus uere | de secunda specie catharactarum, que est alba | et conuertitur in celestino colore, si est | bene curata cum acu sicut | superius dictum est, dicimus quod ad sanitatem pristi|nam luminis reuertitur. Et si vultis | scire qua de causa accidit eis, di|cimus quod propter puritatem humorum et ha|bundanciam spiritus visibilis exeuntem | in oculis; vnde firmiter credatis quod illi | qui paciuntur de secunda specie melius vi|debunt quam de omnibus alijs speciebus. |

Glasgow, GUL, Hunter MS 503, pp. 1–135

¶ The secunde spyce of | Cateracter curable yf it be welle cured w*ith* | the nedyl as it is seyd be fore the ly3te | turneth ayen*n* to hys fyrst bryghnes. | for by purenes of the humurs whych | be not dyssolued. And also for habun|dance of the vysible spyrit yn the eye. | And therfore tho þat be cured of thyes | man*er* of Cat*er*acter. seen bett*er* þan oþ*er*.

4 of] The second *added in outer margin in an Italic hand* 10 eye] Those that | be cured | of this Ca|taracte : See | bettar after | then those | that be cu|red of the | other Cata|racte Caused of a strooke | or outward blowe *added in outer margin in an Italic hand*

London, British Library, Sloane MS 661, ff. 32r–46r

[21] The second kinde of curable | Cataracte if yt be well cured w*ith* the Nedle | as is beforesayde, the sighte retorneth againe to | his first brightenes, because the humors be not | dissolved, or trobled, and allso for the abundance | of the visible sperit there remayninge. And | therefore those that be cured of these manne*r* | of Cataract*es*, have there sighte bettar then the | other.

8 curable] The seconde | kinde of Cura|ble Cataracte. *outer margin*

Glasgow, GUL, Hunter MS 513, ff. 2r–37r
¶ Of the ij^{de} spice ‖

Basel, Ö.B.U., MS D.II.11, ff. 172r–177v
¶ E l a u tra   celestina siben es   5
cura|da pus perfeytament home
ne | uetz edaquesta uen per grant |
abundantia edumors secca. |

Oxford, Bodleian Library, Ashmole MS 1468, pp. 1–6

240   *De Probatissima Arte Oculorum*

Biblio.-Médiathèques de Metz, MS 176, ff. 1r–16r

22. Dicto de secunda specie, dicere uolumus | vobis de tercia que est alba et pen|det in colore cinericio. Dicimus ergo | quod postquam erit
40 curata sicut superius | diximus et recuperatum erit lumen, non | diu permanebit in eodem statu, | nisi iuuetur cum alijs medicinis, | scilicet cum isto diaolibano nostro Ihero|solomitano, frequencius
4ra sumendo: || ℞ olibani ʒ ij, gariofili, nucis musca|te, nucis indice, croci ana ʒ ß, boni cas|torei ʒ 1, hec omnia puluerizentur | et cribellentur et cum bono melle
5 de|spumato conficiantur et fac inde electu|arium, de quo recipiat paciens ie|iuno stomaco ad quantitatem bone castanee, | in sero etiam similiter quando intrabit lectum. | Et custodiat se a cibarijs
10 contrarijs, | et semper utatur cibarijs digestibi|libus et calidis et humidis et bonum | sanguinem

Glasgow, GUL, Hunter MS 503, pp. 1–135

¶ | The thyrde spyce of Cat*er*acter curable. aft*er* | that yt ys cured w*ith* the nedyl. and the | syght   15
recou*er*ed. yf it dure not long yn || that astate. lesse þan it be holpen   [22]
w*ith* oþ*er* | medycynes. as w*ith* oure electuarie that | we calle, Diolibanu*m* salernitanu*m*, | And wyth good dyet as yt schal be tolde | after. The makyng of oure.   5
Dioliba|num, ys thys. Take olibanu*m*. ij. vncys | Clouys. Notemygys. notys of Indie. sa|feron of eche lyke that ys of ycche a dram. | and an halfe. of good castor*er*. a dram. | Bete all   10
thyes to powder. and sars þem | and confete hem to gedder wyth claryfy|ed hony. and make electuarye. And of | thys lete the

---

13 The] 3. *added in inner margin in an Elizabethan hand* 5 Diolibanum] Diaolibanu*m* | Salernita|num *added in outer margin in an Italic hand*

London, British Library, Sloane MS 661, ff. 32r–46r

[22] The thirde kinde of Curable Cataracte | after that yt is cured w*ith* the Nedle, and *the* seighte | recovered, if yt endure not longe in *that* estate | then let yt be holpen w*ith* other medicines, as | w*ith* our Electuarie that we call Diolibanu*m* Sa|lernitanum. and w*ith* good   20
dyet, as yt shalbe taught | hereafter. The makinge of our diaolibanu*m* | is after this manne*r*. Take Olibanu*m* ij ownc*es* | Cloves, Nutmegge Nutt*es* of India saffron ana ʒ j ß | of good Castoreu*m* ʒ j. Beat all these to powder, & | serse them, and confecte them   25
together w*ith* cla|rified honye. & make of them an Electuarje. | And of this let the patient receave in the mor|ninge fastinge. the quantitye of a good chesnutt | or walnut & as Even   30
to bedwarde, as mutch And | let him for his dyett vse meates of good digestio*n* | hoate

---

16 Cataracte] The thirde kinde | of curable | Cataracte *outer*   *margin* 20 Salernitanum] Diolibanu*m* | Salernita|num *outer margin* 23 ownc*es*] ℞ *outer margin*

Glasgow, GUL, Hunter MS 513, ff. 2r–37r

Oxford, Bodleian Library, Ashmole MS 1468, pp. 1–6

Basel, Ö.B.U., MS D.II.11, ff. 172r–177v

¶ Elaterssa cura ques colhor
sine|risia non pot curar luelh
alp*ri*|mer estament tornar. si non |
sa iuda daquest colliri. olec|tuari
loqual anom ierosoli|mitan eque
non ma*n*ie souen | Pren ℨ.ii. de
ieroffle denotz mu|scada. ede noz
dindia ede safra | aitant delaun
com del autre | .ß. ℨ edebon
castor | .i. ℨ. totas aquesta causas
fay | ben poluereiar passar per .i.
cre|bellador subtilh. et am debon |
melh escumath detot encemps |
tufaras .i. lectuari. elo passie*n*t |
prenda daquelh letuari ama|neyra
duna castanha. loma|tin cant leuara.
equant se col|quara. gardessen de
cauzas co*n*|trariosas efay lon usar
de uian|das de bona degestion
caudas | es humidas edaquelhas
que | engeron bon sanc. garda
ten | sempre mays de causas

18 ℨ] e polueriza o *expunged*

Biblio.-Médiathèques de Metz, MS 176, ff. 1r–16r

generantibus. Et custodi|at se
semper a frigidis et siccis. Caueat |
sibi a carnibus vaccinis, caprinis, |
15 et hircinis, ab anguillis frigidis, a
ce|pis crudis, quia multum offen-
dunt | et ledunt eos. Et de hoc
sumus experti, | quia multi uene-
runt in cura nostra | qui non
habebant catharactas completas, |
20 et nos dabamus eis ad come-
dendum | cepas crudas, ob hoc ut
cicius com|plerentur et magis
firmarentur. | In hyeme uero
semper bibat vinum | calidum in
quo ponatur saluia et ruta, et
25 cus|todiant se a coitu plus quam
possint, | et nunquam intrent
balneum uel | stupam. Et si uelint
intrare et se balne|are, preparent
sibi vnam in domo sua | cum aqua
30 decoctionis camomille et | aliarum
herbarum odoriferarum et teneant |
faciem suam extra tinam ut

Glasgow, GUL, Hunter MS 503, pp. 1–135

pacyent resceyue yn the | mornyng
fastyng. the quantite of a | good   15
chasteyn. or of a walnot. And || at   [23]
eue to bedward asmuch. ¶ And |
for hys dyet þat ye vsyn dygestyble
me|tys hote and moyst. whych
engender | good blode. And let
hym be ware of con|trarius metys.   5
and for cowes fleshe | ghetys
fleshe. and eelys. and such oþer. |
and specyally of rawe onyons. for
they | be specyally contrarius. as I
haue p*re*uyd | be exp*er*yence. For
many haue come too | me w*ith*   10
Cat*er*actys not fully confermede. |
I made hem q*uo*d he to ete rawe
onyons | to conferme w*ith* the
Cat*er*act*is*. and they | were sone
spede. wherfore rawe onyons | be
noyows to the sy3te. And yn

---

6 oþer] On*n*yons *added in outer margin in an Italic hand* 9 too] NB. *added in outer margin in an Italic hand*

London, British Library, Sloane MS 661, ff. 32r–46r

and moyste. w*hitch* ingender good blood And | let him beware of contrarye meates, and
⌊eschew⌋ | Cowes flesh, and Goates flesh, and Eeles, & | sutch like, & especiallye rawe   35
Onyons for | theye be verye hurtfull as I have proved || by experience ffor many have   35v
come to me with | Cataract*es* not fullye confermed, And I made | them to take rawe
onyons, to hasten the confir|minge of the Cataract*es*. and yt mutch hasten yt | And   5
therefore I saye rawe Onyons be hurtfull | to the sighte, and in winter let *the* patient |
drincke hoate wynes in w*hitch* let be put Sage | and rewe. let astaine from the Companye
of | women, nor let him not come into any bath or | stove. But if he will bathe, let him   10

---

33 eschew] for | co *deleted,* eschew *added over the line* 36 proved] by experience *lower margin* 1 by] NB. *outer margin* 6 let] put *deleted*

Glasgow, GUL, Hunter MS 513, ff. 2r–37r

Basel, Ö.B.U., MS D.II.11, ff. 172r–177v

freggas | escecas. ede carn debuou
edeboc | ede cabra. ede anguilhas
ede | als eboletz e cebas cruzas   35
esem|pre. mais pren ebeu uin caut |
enque aia saluia eruda egar|desen
de femna pus que poyra | egarde
sen de baynh si non en | vna   40
cornuda es dedins met | erbas
caudas. so es. camamil|la et erbas
flayrans ben enon | tengua locap
dedins lobainh | que lo fum
delayga lin faria || mal en los   173va
uelhs aras uos a|uem dich de la
terssa. |

Oxford, Bodleian Library, Ashmole MS 1468, pp. 1–6

Biblio.-Médiathèques de Metz, MS 176, ff. 1r–16r
fumosi|tas recedat extra tinam et ne
noce|at oculis suis.

Glasgow, GUL, Hunter MS 503, pp. 1–135
wynt*er* | lett nat the pacyent
drynk hoote wynes. || yn whych
be put sawge & rewe. And ab|stene
he from co*m*menyng of women. |
nor let nat hym com in no bath nor
stew. | and yff he wyll algatt*is* bath
hym. lete | hym enter to a stewe
or fat wyth the | wat*er* of the
decocc*i*on of Camamyl or oþ*er* |
swete smellyng herbys. but lett
hym | kepe hys hede w*ith*out the
wessyl þat | the fume cu*m* not yn
to hys eyon. for | þat were
noyo*us*. The forsayd electu|arye of
Diolibanu*m* salernitanu*m*. ys | also
good as he seyth to a voyde terys
& | to dystroye þem. And so yt ys
also for | almaner peyne of the
mygryme that ys | caused of
flume.

15
[24]

5

10

15

10 electuarye] pag: 22 *added in outer margin in an Italic hand*

London, British Library, Sloane MS 661, ff. 32r–46r
bath in | a decoction of Chamomile or swete smel|linge herbes, but let him kepe his head
w*ith*out | the vessell that the fume come not into his | eyes, for that is hurtfull to them
The | foresayde Diolibanu*m* Salernitanu*m* is allso good | to avoyd teares, and so distroye   15
ʟ   them ˩, and so it is | allso for all manner of payne, of the megrim | that is caused of
Rhume.

11 Chamomile] of *add,*   *deleted* swete] sem *add,*   *deleted* **15** foresayde] Againste teares | & waterye | Eyes. *outer margin*

Glasgow, GUL, Hunter MS 513, ff. 2r–37r   *Basel, Ö.B.U., MS D.II.11, ff. 172r–177v*

Oxford, Bodleian Library, Ashmole MS 1468, pp. 1–6

Biblio.-Médiathèques de Metz, MS 176, ff. 1r–16r

    23. Audiuistis de | tertia specie
catharactarum curabilium | et
contraria que sibi contingere
35 possunt | et regimina bonorum
ciborum. Et docui|mus uos bonum
electuarium pro ista | infirmitate et
pro alijs infirmi|tatibus oculorum
que superueniunt | de humoribus
40 frigidis, et non tantum ualet |in
istis sed eciam valet ad con-
strin|gendum lacrimas et ad
omnem dolorem | emigraneum qui
uenit de reumate. | Docuimus vos
4rb de tercia specie catha||ractarum
curabilium, ammodo volumus |
vos docere de quarta. Quarta |
species que est quasi citrina
dicimus quod | est durissima inter
5 omnes alias et | rotunda, et
quando capis ipsam cum acu | non
debes ipsam ponere nec reducere |
inferius quia non staret propter
ro|tunditatem et duriciam suam,
sed | pone ipsam a parte lacrimalis

Glasgow, GUL, Hunter MS 503, pp. 1–135

¶ The iiij[th] spyce of || Cateracter [25]
curable. þat ys of colour Citry|ne.
ys herder þan any of the oþer.
And | also yt ys rownder.
wherfore yt may | not be leyd
ryghtdowne yn the ey. for | yt 5
wylnot abyde þere. for the
rownd|nesse and hardnes þereof.
And þere|fore ys must be leyd yn
the corner of | the ey to the ere
warde. and þere be kepte | with
the nedyll a good whyle as yt ys |
beforeseyd. ¶ But hyer fynyally I | 10
wyl ȝe knowe. ȝe þat wyll be |
practyfe yn the acurye crafte. þat
noon | of þies. iiij curable cater-
act*is*. yt ne|dyth to doon from clene
metys absty|nence. as I haue 15
preuyd by experyence || saue [26]
oonly yn the thyrde spyce. whe|re
neuerthelesse yt behouyth alwey |

---

10 I] NB. *added in outer margin in an Elizabethan hand* **11** wyll] knowe *deleted*

London, British Library, Sloane MS 661, ff. 32r–46r

[23] The fourth | kinde of curable Cataracte is of a citrine | color, yt is harder then any 20
of the Other | and allso yt is rownde. wherefore yt maye | not be cowched ryghte downe
in the eye, for | yt will not abide there. by reason of the | roundnes and hardnes there of,
and therefore | yt muste be cowched in the corner of the Eye | toward the eare, and there 25
be kepte with | the Nedle a good while as is before sayde. | But here to conclude. I let
yow to vnderstand | that doe purpose to practize the Acuarye Crafte | that none of these 30
4[or]. curable Cataract*es*, but | are to be done after abstinence from meat*es* And | after,
allwhise to administer sutch thing*es* as maye | comfort and norish the visible spiritt.

---

19 kinde] The fowrth kinde | of curable Ca|taracte *outer margin Hand B*

Glasgow, GUL, Hunter MS 513, ff. 2r–37r

7r   it yn and afterward whan thou drawest oute the ne|dill turne thi honde fro the p*ar*tye of the nose and | therafter drawe it oute smothely twynyng and re|twynyng with thi fynger as thou haste in the
5   cure | of agulyng afore ¶ where for we saye you þ*at* all þoo | that haue hade of soche infirmites of ey3en withe | soche manan*er* cataractis curable for her cinericiam | asshynnes it nedethe nought hem to haue abstine|nce of metis for we be exp*er*te of it for it
10 noyethe | hem nought ¶ Also it be houethe for to haue nour|sshyng and confortatiuis that her nervis were | comfortid by the whiche the visible spirite myght | be ioyed and kept in y3en

Basel, Ö.B.U., MS D.II.11, ff. 172r–177v

Aras uos uoli dire enom | dedieu dela quarta ques | acolor citrina.   5
et yeu uos | dic ques es redonda epus du|ra quelas autras equant tu | lan tocaras am la agulha delar|gent tu lan deues metre desota | ben so   10
es dela part delnas de|ues lo blanc dela part delaure|lha torsen am los detz | lagulha. ayssi com uos aydit | desobre es aquestz non cal trop | gardar de uiandas car nos   15
si | auem motas vegadas provat | empero si lin couen alcunas | uegadas de cauzas conforta|tiuas perforssa |

12 am] lagulha *expunged*

Oxford, Bodleian Library, Ashmole MS 1468, pp. 1–6

Biblio.-Médiathèques de Metz, MS 176, ff. 1r–16r

10   minoris | et fige bene ipsam ibi.
     Et postea cum | extraxeris acum
     uertas manum tuam | a parte nasi,
     postea extrahes acum | plene
     torquendo et retorquendo | cum
15   digitis tuis, sicut habes in | cura
     acuandi. Vnde recordamur | vobis
     karissimi quod omnes illi qui
     fuerunt | passi de omnibus
     speciebus catharac|tarum cura-
     bilium, preter cinericiam, | non
     oportet eis facere fieri abstinen-
20   ciam a cibis, | quia experti sumus
     de hoc, quia non | nocet eis; sed
     tamen oportet eis dari | conforta-
     tiua et nutritiua, ut nerui | confor-
     tentur per quos spiritus visibi|lis
     semper resultat in oculos. |

Glasgow, GUL, Hunter MS 503, pp. 1–135

to haue confortatiuus & neutry-
ty|uus of the vysible spiryt yn the |
eyon.   5

London, British Library, Sloane MS 661, ff. 32r–46r

De Probatissima Arte Oculorum 249

Glasgow, GUL, Hunter MS 513, ff. 2r–37r   **Basel, Ö.B.U., MS D.II.11, ff. 172r–177v**

Oxford, Bodleian Library, Ashmole MS 1468, pp. 1–6

Biblio.-Médiathèques de Metz, MS 176, ff. 1r–16r

24. Iam expleuimus uobis tracta-
tum | catharactarum curabilium et
docu|imus uobis causam accidentia
et curam | de omnibus secundum
experientiam nostram | et Artem
Nostram Probatissimam Ocu-
lorum. | Deinde reuertamur ad
illas tres | species que sunt
incurabiles, vnde di|cimus de
prima specie incurabili. | Prima
species incurabilis est illa quam |
medici Salernitani uocant guttam |
serenam, et hoc est signum
cognoscen|di eam: quia pupilla est
nigra et | clara ac si non haberet
illam maculam, | et inter concaui-
tatem oculorum apparet | in colore
sereno, et oculi semper mo|uentur
cum palpebris suis quasi | tre-
mendo ac si essent pleni argen|to
viuo. Et nos iam vidimus mul|tos
qui fuerunt cum illa infirmitate. |
Vnde dicimus quod accidit eis ex
utero mater|no pro aliqua corrup-

Glasgow, GUL, Hunter MS 503, pp. 1–135

¶ The iij cterac*ter* vncura|ble be
thyes. The fyrst. lechys of | salerne
call. Guttam serenam. And | thys
ys the sygne of knowyng, | The
pyupyl of the ey. þat ys place | yn
the myddys of the eye. where ys |
the resydence of the sy3te. ys
blake | and clere astowe yt hade
no spotte. | & the ey ys meuyng
alwey w*ith* the lyd|dys tremelyng
astow þei were ful | of quyk
syluer. And thys Cateract || ys
causyd of a corrupc*i*on of the
moders | wombe. And þerfore. tho
comu*n*ly that | haue thys Cat*er*acte
byth blynde borne. | Off whom
quod he I haue assayd w*ith* |
dyu*er*se medycyns to cure many.
but | yt wolde neu*er* be. I cowd

5 vncurable] The 3. vncu|rable
Cata|ract*es* added in outer margin in
an Italic hand 7 salerne] pag: 72
added in outer margin in an Italic
hand

London, British Library, Sloane MS 661, ff. 32r–46r

[24] The | three Cataract*es* vncurable be these. The first | the letches of Salerno call
Guttam Sere|nam. And this is the signe to knowe yt. The | Pupill of the Eye is blacke and
cleare as || though yt had no spott, and the Eye is movinge | all waye w*ith* the lydd*es*
tremblinge as though | theye wer fullof Quicsilu*er*, and this Cataracte | is caused of some
corruption the mothers | woumbe. and therefore those commonlye that have | this
Cataracte be borne blynd. Of whom | (quoth the Auth*or*) I have assayed with diuers |
medicines to have cured manye. but yt would | neu*er* be. I could neu*er* here that any
sutch | wer cured. But note that I perceaved of | diuersityes of these kinde of Cataract*es*
ffor | some of them mighte see the brightenes of the | sonne, and went by the waye with

34 three] The .3. vncu|rable Cata|ract*es*. Gutta Sere|na. *outer margin* 37 as] though *lower margin*

Glasgow, GUL, Hunter MS 513, ff. 2r–37r

    Of ·3· maner cata|rataractus vn curable & how þey schal be knowe |
15 Of the thre maner of kyndes that be vncurab|le of cataractis of the whiche maystirs of sale|ren clepen guttum cerenam an*glice* a·shere goute | ¶ And these ben the signes of her knowyng · For why | the ey3e appull ys blak and clere as
20 though he had | no spotte bitwene the holwenesse of the ey3en appereþ | in a·shire sorowe and the ey3en mouen alway w*ith* þe | ei3e liddes as they were quakyng and as thei were | full of quyk syluer Of the whiche when they see | the clernes of the sunne or of the day
25 or the sta|ture of any thinge and ther leuythe in som*m*e of soche | ey3en atantelette of lyght tyll her

---

13 cataratactus] 4 *added in outer margin*

Oxford, Bodleian Library, Ashmole MS 1468, pp. 1–6

Basel, Ö.B.U., MS D.II.11, ff. 172r–177v

Aras uos uuelh dire de | las 20
caractas que no sen | podon curar
¶ Et yeu ey | uos dieh que sontres.
la pru|meyra es blanqua. elos
meg|ges desalern. la apelhon go|ta 25
serena ¶ Et aquestz son los |
senhals enque las pot hom
co|noycer ¶ Car lapupilla es clara |
enegra. ededins en la concaui|tat 30
dels uelhs apar de color se|ren. Si
non a enlapupilla degu|na taca elos
uels semouon. | tot iorn quais
tremolon. elas | palpelhas coma si
eran plenas | dargent viu ¶ Enos 35
auem ne | uist trops daquelha
malau|tia et auem curatz assatz
per | la grassia dedieu
egasanhatz | debos floris |
Es aquesta malautia si | uen en lo 40
uentre delam|ayre per alcuna
humor | corompuda que es dintre
per | so aytals homs nayson sen||sa 173vb
lum ¶ Enos auem prouath | guerir
curar aquels emais nos |

Biblio.-Médiathèques de Metz, MS 176, ff. 1r–16r

4va cione que dominatur || ibi, et ideo
nascuntur sine lumine. Et | nos
probauimus multos illorum |
curare cum varijs et diuersis
me|dicinis, et nullum potuimus
5 curare. | Vnde sciatis karissimi
quod nunquam vidimus | nec
audiuimus aliquem ante nos | qui
posset eos juuare. Tamen aliqui
is|torum vident quasi claritatem
diei | et vadunt per viam oculis
10 apertis | ac si viderent, et multi
de illis sunt | qui vident staturam
hominis uel alicuius | alterius rei,
et in quibusdam istorum per|manet
illud tantillum luminis usque in |
finem vite sue. Et aliqui de istis
15 ta|libus sunt in quibus non durat |
uel nichil vident ac si non habe-
rent | oculos. Vnde karissimi ita
uere diximus | vobis quod si
omnes isti qui paciuntur | talem
infirmitatem que dicitur gutta |
20 serena – tam diximus de illis qui

Glasgow, GUL, Hunter MS 503, pp. 1–135

neu*er* heer þat | ony such was
cured. But nat for | þan I prœuyd
wele þat of thies ma|n*er* Cat*er*actys
were dyu*er*sytee. For sum | of 10
them myȝte see the bryȝtnes of |
the son*n* and went be the way
wyth | opon ey. as thow þei had
p*er*fyȝtly | seyn. And sum myȝte
see the statu|re of a man and of a
best. or of a | nother thyng. and 15
not els. And || sum had thys lytle [28]
p*ar*te of lyȝte to her | lyues ende.
and of sum yt vanyshyd | a vaye.
and þei hade nomore syȝte |
astowe þei neu*er* had none.
wherfor | I wyll that ye knowe all 5
thyes ma|ner of Cat*er*act*er* ben
vncurable lesse þan | god cure
þem. For the neruys obtyk | be so
opylate that ys such man*er* of
sy|newes ben so stoppyd &
mortifyed þ*at* | no medycyn may 10
helpe yt. And þ*er*|for thyes
cat*er*actys we clepyn. Gut|tam

London, British Library, Sloane MS 661, ff. 32r–46r

open Eyes. | as thought theye had seene p*er*fectlye. And some | and some mighte see the 15
stature, of a man, and | of a beast, and coulde disserne nothinge eles: | and some have had
this kinde of sighte to there | lyves ende. and in some yt hath vanished awaye. | Therefore
I woulde have yo*w* to knowe that all | these mann*er* of Chataract*es*, be vncurable ex|cepte 20
god doe cuer them. ffor the opticke sy|nowes be so stopped, that no medicine can | helpe
yt. And these kynde of Cataract*es* we | call Guttam Serenam. ffor it is caused of | a 25
corruption com*m*inge from the braine in the | mann*er* of a dropp of water. w*h*itch
corrupteth. | and dissolveth all the humors of the eye | that from theare forwarde, the
hollow synowes | be so stopped and ou*er*layed, that the visible Spi|rytt maye no more 30
passe downe by them.

De Probatissima Arte Oculorum 253

Glasgow, GUL, Hunter MS 513, ff. 2r–37r

7v dethe day ¶ And ‖ some ther be
suche that vtterlyche that seen
right | nought right as the hadden
none ey3en ¶ wher|for wetethe well
that they that seen somdell | and
tho that seen right nought for this
5 kynde | of cataract*es* w*ith* no
maner of medecyne ne wethe | no
crafte may be mended ¶ Ryght as
we haue | as sayed and prouid
w*ith* many dyu*er*se medicynes |
and w*ith* none we myght nought
spede ne helpe | ¶ wherefore yif
me yeue all the golde of the
10 worl|de and all the leches thorugh
trauailled ther none | of hem w*ith*
no medecyn may helpe But oure
lorde | Jh*es*u crist thorow his
vertue ¶ And that is why | they
ben so vncurable It is for nerui
optici ·i· the | holowe neruis ben so
15 fer stopped and so for mortifi|ed
that no helpe may hem saue ne
helpe ¶ And | we clepen thes

Oxford, Bodleian Library, Ashmole MS 1468, pp. 1–6

Basel, Ö.B.U., MS D.II.11, ff. 172r–177v

nonpodem negun curar e si
aqu*e*ls | donauan tot laur delmon
non | poyrian curar ¶ Eson alcus 5
q*ue* | ueson laclaretat del iorn
pauc | euan am los uelhs ubertz |
coma si uesian ¶ E son alcus - |
que ueson la ombra delhome o |
dautra causa. eson alcus que | 10
noueson nient coma si non a|uian
huelhs ¶ Efam uos sa|ber que auem
daquestz non - | ual medecina car
iamays | no sen poyran curar car 15
los ner|uis son secatz. dels uelhs.
car | una humor uen delceuelh
dego|tan coma gota dayga efa
cecar | los neruis dels uels |

---

6 pauc] euen *expunged* **14** iamays] n *expunged*

Biblio.-Médiathèques de Metz, MS 176, ff. 1r–16r

vident | aliquantulum, sicut
superius diximus, | quam de illis
qui visum ex toto ami|serunt
– vnde credatis quod si quilibet |
25 istorum haberet totum aurum de
mundo | et totum vellet dare, et si
omnes | homines de mundo essent
medici, | non possent eis ullum
juuamen|tum dare, nisi Deus et
Dominus noster | Ihesus Christus
30 faceret illud cum sua | diuina
virtute. Ideo quia nerui | coticij uel
obtici sunt ita opilati | et mortifi-
cati quod nullum auxilium |
pertinens ad medicinam posset
eos | juuare. Et vocamus eam
35 catha|ractam serenam ideo quia
generatur | a quadam corrosione
descendente | a cerebro ad modum
gutte aque, | et descendit sic
repente quod omnes | humores
40 oculorum corrumpit et | dissoluit
a loco suo, tali modo quod ab | illa

Glasgow, GUL, Hunter MS 503, pp. 1–135

serenam. For yt ys gendyrde | of a
corrupc*i*on co*m*myng downe
from | the brayn yn the man*er* of a
drope of | water. whych 15
corruptyth & dyssol||uyth all the [29]
humurs of the ey. that fro | thens
foreward. the concaue or the
ho|low synewys be so stoppyd &
ou*er*layd. | that the vysyble spiryte
may nomore | passe down*n* by 5
them.

London, British Library, Sloane MS 661, ff. 32r–46r

Glasgow, GUL, Hunter MS 513, ff. 2r–37r *Basel, Ö.B.U., MS D.II.11, ff. 172r–177v*

    cataracte serenam ·i· shere or
bright | ¶ For it is engendred of a
corupcio*n* destroyng | and
desendyng fro the brayne in the
maner of a· | Droppe of water and
20 it comthe doun sodenly that | it
rotithe and croumpith all the
humours of the | ey3en and losethe
hem and dissoluethe and than | fro
that tyme that it is so fallen nerui
optici | anon ben stopped

Oxford, Bodleian Library, Ashmole MS 1468, pp. 1–6

256 — De Probatissima Arte Oculorum

Biblio.-Médiathèques de Metz, MS 176, ff. 1r–16r

  hora inantea nerui concaui |
  opilantur sicut superius diximus. |
  25. Narrauimus uobis de prima |
  specie catharactarum incura-
45 bilium | et diximus causam
4vb accidencia et signa. || Nunc
  narrare et dicere uolumus uobis |
  de secunda specie incurabili.
  Secunda species | incurabilis est
  illa que apparet intus | oculis quasi
5 viridis in colore sicut lip|pitudo
  que est in aquis in multis | locis.
  Vnde sciatis quod ista species
  catha|ractarum incurabilis est | et
  non paulatim venit, sed | subito
10 descendit et ita repente quod | ab
  illa hora inantea paciens nichil |
  uidet ac si non haberet oculos.
  Vnde | dicimus quod ista species
  est deterior omnibus alijs. |
  Audiuistis signa, nunc explanare |
  uolumus vobis causam et acci-

---

7 est] illa que apparet *expunged*

Glasgow, GUL, Hunter MS 503, pp. 1–135

¶ The secunde | man*er* of
Cat*er*actys vncurable ys the |
whych apperyth w*ith* yn the ey of
grene | color. lyke water stondyng
yn wa|try placys not much meuyd.
nor re|newed. And thys Cat*er*acte   10
ys the worst | of all o*þ*er. And ys
gendred & causyde | of oue*r*mych
coldnes of the brayn. of | gret
betyng yn the hede. fer fastyng |
and such other. ¶ The thyrde
vn|curable Cat*er*acte. ys when the   15
pupyl || ys dylated and sprede a   [30]
broode so fer. | that no cerkyl may
be seyn w*ith* yn the | tonycle any
of thyes iij labourth yn | veynne. |

---

5 secunde] *2 added in outer margin in an Elizabethan hand*
14 vncurable] *3 added in outer margin in an Elizabethan hand*

London, British Library, Sloane MS 661, ff. 32r–46r

[25] The | second manne*r* of Cataracte vncurable, is that | w*hitch* appeareth wi*thi*n the eye of greene | colo*r*, like water standinge in watrye places | not mutch movid. and this Cataracte is the | worst of all others, and is caused of oue*r*|mutch couldnes of the Braine.   35 and vehem*ent* |repellinge in the heat and sutch like. The || thirde kinde of vncurable   36v Cataracte is when *the* | Pupill is dilated & spred abroode so farr | that no circle maye be seene wi*thi*n the tuni|cle And who so laboreth to cuer any of these .|3. Cataract*es* doth   5 losse his labor. |

---

30 The] The seconde | vncurable Cataracte *outer margin* **37** The] thirde *lower margin* **1** thirde] The thirde | vncurable | Cataracte. *outer margin*

Glasgow, GUL, Hunter MS 513, ff. 2r–37r   Basel, Ö.B.U., MS D.II.11, ff. 172r–177v

¶ The secunde kynde of vncura|ble
cataractis ys that the which
25 appereth in ey3e all | grene
colour in to the likenes of the
8r grenes that || is in the water that is
stondyng in many lakes // | ¶
wherfor knowell that this maner of
cataractes | comethe in to the
ey3en litell and lytell but it
co|methe sodenly so fro that houre
5 forward he seithe | no more this
maner of cataractis is worse þan |
all the othir that ben vncurable for
it comethe | of ouermoch coldenes
of the brayne and of ouer|moche
sorwe full wepyng and ouermoche
ang|wysshe and wakyng and for
10 drede of betinggus | and for
moche fastynge ¶ The thirde maner
of | vncurable cataractes ys that
the whiche whan all | the appell of
ei3e apperethe y made abrode or

Aras   uos uuel dire lase|gonda   20
maneyra ques es | quais uertz enon
sepoth | curar. euen soptament
coma | lautra elos uels son clars e
non | potdon ueser coma sinon   25
auian | uelhs ¶ Et aquesta es pus
ma|la delas autras et aquesta uen |
per per tropa freior delseruelh
eper | trop plorar dels uelhs eper
trop | uelhar eper trops deiunis.   30
eper | enflament deltest |
¶ Aras uos uuelh dire laterssa |
maneyra quees quant la pupi|lla
apar alargada es apar blan|ca   35
onegra esquesta non sepot | curar
am neguna medecina del | mont |

Oxford, Bodleian Library, Ashmole MS 1468, pp. 1–6

Biblio.-Médiathèques de Metz, MS 176, ff. 1r–16r

15   dencia qua | de causa ista species incurabilis proue |nit in oculis. Dicimus quod accidit per nimiam | frigiditatem cerebri et planctum lacrimarum, | et per nimiam angustiam et uigili|as, per magnum
20   timorem et uerbe|raciones capitis, per multa ieiunia, | et similia. Expleuimus de secunda specie, | deinde explanare volumus vobis | de tercia. Tercia species incurabilis est | illa in qua tota pupilla apparet
25   dila|tata, tali modo quod non videtur ibi | circulus tunice oculorum sed totaliter | lux apparet alba uel nigra. Postquam | ita est dilatata firmiter credatis quod | nullum juuamen quod pertinet ad
30   me|dicinam posset eos juuare – et si quis | vult ipsos juuare inuanum laborat. |

Glasgow, GUL, Hunter MS 503, pp. 1–135

London, British Library, Sloane MS 661, ff. 32r–46r

Glasgow, GUL, Hunter MS 513, ff. 2r–37r   *Basel, Ö.B.U., MS D.II.11, ff. 172r–177v*

    spred|de abrode thorugh such
　　maner that the the circle | of the
　　ey3e is nought seyn þer ne none of
15　the to|nicles But all the naterall
　　lyght after that it | is so spredde
　　abrode that none helpe maye
　　helpe | hem that longethe to the
　　medecyne and who so | trowethe
　　to helpen in vayne he trauaylethe
　　for it | shall neuer be done ·/·

Oxford, Bodleian Library, Ashmole MS 1468, pp. 1–6

Biblio.-Médiathèques de Metz, MS 176, ff. 1r–16r

26. Audiuistis karissimi quot sunt species ca|tharactarum et inter vnam et aliam | diuersitates et causas et accidencia earum. |
35 Modo incipiamus in nomine Domini | nostri Ihesu Christi de alijs infirmitatibus | diuersis et uarijs superuenientibus in | oculis occasione 4 humorum, scilicet: sanguinis, | flegmatis, colere, et
40 melancolie – et primo docebi|mus vos de sanguine. Et dicimus | quod propter multitudinem sanguinis ascen|dit aliquando in oculis quedam rubedo | et ardor, et illa rubedo et ardor postea | reuertitur
45 in pruritum, et palpebras | tali modo depilat quod non remanet ibi
5ra || pilus. Et si infirmitas ista steterit | per annum ut non curetur, facit palpe|bras reuersare. Vnde dicimus quod antequam | paciens perueniat ad illum statum |
5 adiuuetis ipsum cum isto

Glasgow, GUL, Hunter MS 503, pp. 1–135

Now after the doctryne & | 5
knowlege of Cat*eracter* and | the nombre of them*m*. and | whych be curable. and whych nat. | And the cures of the curable. and the | knowlege of the causes of vn- 10
cura|ble. ¶ Now I wyll q*uod* he speke of o*þer* | sekenes causyd & occasyonyd of the | iiij hum*ers*. as blode. flewme. color. | & malyn- colye. ¶ But first of the | sekenes 15
causyd of blode. for oftentymes ||
for multitude of blode *þer* [31]
growyth a red|nes yn the ey. w*ith* a grete brynnyng. | and after yt tornyth into grete ycche, | And thys dysease makyth the here of | the ey lyddys to fall a wey. And 5
of | many yt semyth non here. And yf | thys sekenes be nat curyd in a yere. | yt wyll make the eye lyddys to turne | vp. & make the pacyent bleryed. wher|for ere yt cu*m* to the 10
poynt yt may be | curyd q*uod* he

London, British Library, Sloane MS 661, ff. 32r–46r

[26] Now after the doctrine and knowledge of Ca|taract*es*, and the number of them, and w*hi*tch be | curable and w*hi*tch are not, and the cuers of | the curable, and the knowledge of the causes | of the vncurable Cataract*es*. Nowe I will | speake of the diseases of the 10
Eyes caused | of the fowre humors as of blood, fflegme | Choller and melancholye. But first of those | diseases caused of Blood. for oftentymes tho|rough the multitude of blood, 15
there groweth a | reddnes in the Eyes, w*ith* a great borninge, and | after yt torneth into a great ytchinge And this | disease maketh the heare of the Eye lydd*es* to fall | a waye. And if this syckenes be not curedd | in a yeare, yt will make the eye lydd*es* to torne | vpp. and 20
make the patient bleare eyed, where|fore or ever yt come to that poynt yt maye be | cured

---

6 after] Cap°. 3. *outer margin* 13 Choller] Of diseases | of the Eyes | caused of | Bloode. *outer margin*

De Probatissima Arte Oculorum 261

Glasgow, GUL, Hunter MS 513, ff. 2r–37r

20 <O>f maladi*es* comyng | to þ*e*
ey3en of 4 humours & first of
blode & the | Curyng |
Of maladies of ey3e comyng of the
foure humo*urs* | and first of hem
that comen of blode And | we saye
you that for the mochelte of
8v blode || sum*m*e tyme comethe
a·maner of redenes w*ith* bryn|nyng
and turnethe in to yeyche and it
driethe | the ey3e liddes in suche
maner that ther leuyþ | none heres
¶ And yif this in firmite stonde
5 any | whyle and is nought holpen
it maketh the ey3e |liddes to ouer
turne ¶ where for when suche |
ben founde ye shullen helpe hem
w*ith* oure coleri | of ierusalem ¶ ℞
tutie of Alexandre ·ʒ iij w*ith* | ℔
·ij· of good white wyne and in

Basel, Ö.B.U., MS D.II.11, ff. 172r–177v

¶ Aras uos uulh dire enom de |
dieu delas autres em fermetatz |
delhs uelhs diuersas que uenon | 40
oper tropa sanc oper car alcunas |
uegadas lo sanc monta als uels |
euen gran ardor eson mot uer|mels
etaquelha ardor enerme || lesa 174ra
corenlas palpelhas entalma|neyra
que alcunas uegadas noy | layssan
pelheth ¶ Esiaquesta en|fermetat
non es tost curada fa|ra las 5
palpelhas reuersegadas | per so
aiudaretz lor en aquesta | maneyra.
fay colliri ierosolimi|tan ¶ Recep
detutia alexandrina | ʒ .i. am doas
liuras de bon uin | blanc. episa o
ben coma sal emes|cla ben emeth 10
tot en .i. ola noua | emescla. ʒ .i.
derosas seccas efay | o tot bolhir
alfoc suau entro que | sia lo vin
co*n*sumath alamietat | epueis colha
o tot per .i. drap d*e* | lin egarda 15

---

19 comyng] 5 *added in outer margin*
8 of] ℞ *added in outer margin*

---

6 aquesta] m *expunged*

Oxford, Bodleian Library, Ashmole MS 1468, pp. 1–6

Biblio.-Médiathèques de Metz, MS 176, ff. 1r–16r

  collirio | Iherosolomitano: ℞ tutye
alexandrine ʒ 1 et | puluerizetur et
distemperetur ad modum | salse
cum duabus libri boni vini al|bi, et
10 ponatur in olla noua; et adiun|gatur
ʒ 1 rosarum siccarum, et cum
predicto | vino bulliant ad lentum
ignem | donec vinum reuertatur ad
medie|tatem. Postea coletur per
pannum line|um et seruetur in
15 ampulla uitrea. | Et de illo bis in
die in oculis mittatur, | scilicet
mane et sero. Et sic omnes
pacientes | liberabuntur per vnam
ebdomadam, et | postquam
composuimus hoc collirium |
infinitos homines cum ipso
20 libera|uimus adiuuante Deo. Et
recor|damur uobis quod antequam
medicetis | eos, faciatis eos
minuere de vena | que est in medio
frontis si sint juue|nes, et si sint
25 senes purgetis eos cere|brum cum
pillulis nostris que sunt contra |

Glasgow, GUL, Hunter MS 503, pp. 1–135

with my Colery. that ys cle|pyd.
Colerium iherosolimitanum. that |
ys mayd yn thyse wyse. Take
tutie | of alexandrye ann vnce and
be yt to | smale powder. and 15
temper yt with ij. ℔ || of whyte [32]
wyne þat ys a quarte. And | put yt
yn a new erthyn pote. And | put
þerto ann uncer of dry roses.
And | boyle yt wyth a sokyng fyre
tyl the | wyne be half wasted. 5
Then clense | yt throught a lynnyn
cloyth. And | kepe yt yn a vyall of
glas. and mornn | and yeuen put yt
yn to hys eyon. | And yf yt be
takyn be tymes. the pa|cyent 10
schalbe curyd with yn a weke. or |
ij. at moost. And wyth thys quod
he | I haue holpyn manny.
Neuerthelesse | or the practyser
begyn. lete hym make | the

---

12 that] nota | Colerium |
Jerosolimi|tanum. *added in outer
margin in an Italic hand*

London, British Library, Sloane MS 661, ff. 32r–46r

with Collerium Jerosolimitanum. that is | made after this sorte. Take Tutie of Alex.| j 25
ownce and beate yt into verye fine powder. | and temper yt with ij ℔ of white wine, and |
put yt into a new earthen pott, and put there|to j ownce of dryed roses: and boyle yt with |
a soafte fyer till halfe the wine be consumed | then straine yt through a fayre lyninge 30
cloth | and kepe it in a violl of glasse, and put of | yt into the patientes eyes both
morninge and | eveninge. and if yt be applyed at the begin|ninge, the will be cured with a
weke or towe | at the moste Neuerthelesse before he doe | applye yt, let the patient (if he 35
be younge) || be let blood on the mediane vaine, and if he be | oulde purge his braine 37r
with Pills made againste | the Itch. After this sorte Take Aloes Hepaticke | redd Saunders,

---

24 made] Collerium Je|rosolimitanum *outer margin* **31** kepe] lepe *before correction*
36 younge] be let *lower margin*

De Probatissima Arte Oculorum

Glasgow, GUL, Hunter MS 513, ff. 2r–37r

10 a·morter | grynde hem in maner
of sauce and medle hem | well to
geders so that they welle
dissoluid | that tuti w*ith* that wyne
and after do putte it | in a·newe
potte and w*ith* hem medle ℥ ·j· &
ß· rede | rose levis dried and and
15 sethe hem w*ith* the for|saide wyne
and tuti ouer the esy fire til the |
wyn be halfe wasted and than
thorwe a ly|nnen clothe clense it
and kepe hit in a viole | of glas
and putte twies in a day ther of in |
the eyȝe .s. erly at morwe and late
20 at euene | do so all a·weke and
withe this medecyne | we haue
cured men and women oute of
number | And natheles er we do
eny cure to hem ¶ First | we laten
hem blode of the mydell veyne in |
the forhede yef they be yong and

---
10 grynde] colere *added in outer margin in a late hand*

Oxford, Bodleian Library, Ashmole MS 1468, pp. 1–6

Basel, Ö.B.U., MS D.II.11, ff. 172r–177v

aquel colliri per una | senmana.
epueis meti lon en .i^a. | ampolha. e
uncha ne los uelhs | delmalaute
lomatin el uespre | e de dins una
senmana sera gue|ritz los ma- 20
lautes. et anos recor|da que pus
demil malautes a|uem gueritz am
aquest colliri | bon |
¶ Efau uos saber que enans | que
uos metatz daquest colli|ri als 25
uelhs uos los deuetz far | sancnar
delha uena del front mi|ggana si
son joues oson uielhs | purgatz
enans loseruelh am | nostras
pillulas que son contr*a* | la-
maluestat dels uelhs. aques|ta 30
recepta receph. aloe epatico |
scandali rubey. esuli reubarbe |
ana .℥ .ß. turbis minoris. cata|pucia
agarici. ana ℥ .i. fay cofie|g. am 35
suc deartemisa. edisem uo*s* | per
serth que tan solament no | ual ala
prusor dels uels ans | uos dic que
ual aquest engue*nt* | ala prusor del

Biblio.-Médiathèques de Metz, MS 176, ff. 1r–16r

pruritum: ℞ aloe epatica, sandali rubri, | esule, reubarbi ana ʒ ß, turbith et cata|pucie minoris et agarici ʒ quartam | partem, et conficiantur cum succo arthe|me-
30 sie, et recipiatur de eis secundum | vires pacientium. Dicimus uobis uere | quod non tantum ad pruritum oculorum valent | sed etiam ad omnem pruritum et sca|biem tocius cor-
35 poris de quocumque hu|more sit. Et vocamus pillulas has | Beneuenuti, nomine compositoris sui, | et tunc dabitis ipsas ad honorem | Dei nostri. |

Glasgow, GUL, Hunter MS 503, pp. 1–135

pacyent yf he be yong to blede. | on the veyne yn the myddys of   15
the || hede. yf he be agyd. purge   [33]
hys brayne | wyth. Pullyalys or peletys. made ayen | ycche. Thus made. Take Aloes epatyk. | sandalys rubeus. esule. rubarbe. ana half | ann vncer. turbiter.   5
catapucie minoris & | agaryk. ana a quarteron of ann vncer. and | confect hem with the Jus of mugworte. | And lete the pacyent resceyue therof | after þeir strength. And truly þies pe|letys ar   10
not good only for ycche of eyon. | ¶ But also for all maner ycche. and | skabe of what humor þat euer yt be | causyd. And thies arnn clepyd. Pil|lule bennemici.

---

15 the] hede. *added in lower margin*
2 ayen] pile for ycche *added in outer margin in a late hand* 3 epatyk] Pillulae, | Beneue|nutae. *added in outer margin in an Italic hand*

London, British Library, Sloane MS 661, ff. 32r–46r

Esula, Rubarbe ana ʒ ß. Tur|bith, Caputie minoris, Agaricke ana ʒ ij, | and make them   5
vpp into a mass with the Juyce | of Mugworte. and let the patient be | purged with these pills accordinge to his | strength And trulye these pills are not | good onlye for the ytch   10
of the eyes: but allso | for all manner of ytch. by what humor | so euer yt be caused. and theye be called | Pillulæ Beneuenutj.

---

4 Turbith] Pills against | the Itch called | Pilullæ Beneuenutj   7 of] mog *deleted*

Glasgow, GUL, Hunter MS 513, ff. 2r–37r

9r   yif they be ‖ olde folke we yeue oure pill the which ben a yen|st 3eyche of the ey3en and they clensen the hede and | the brayne · ℞ aloes epatik Sandal rubie esule Reubi*um* | an*a* ·℥· iiij turbith cathapuc*es* mi agarici an*a* ·℥ q·
5   make | hem vp with the iuse of arche*mesia* and late the seke take þ*er*of | after his myght ¶ And we saye you that these pil*u*llis | ben gode nought only ayenst 3eiche of the ei3en but | also ayenst all maner 3eiche of all the bodye and | scabbe it is worthilich good for
10   allmaner humour | and we clepen these pil*u*llis compositoris sui is

Basel, Ö.B.U., MS D.II.11, ff. 172r–177v

cors etala ronha | fortment.   40
dequalque humor | que sia. dona pueyssas al malau|tes segon que sera lamalautia ‖ elausan dieus   174rb
nostre senhor et | yeu ben uenguth quar ten ey a|mostrat tant gloriosa cura la | qual tedic per serth que uos auez | proada motas ue-   5
gadas |

---

24 be] olde *added in lower margin*
6 pilullis] pelles *added in outer margin in a late hand*

Oxford, Bodleian Library, Ashmole MS 1468, pp. 1–6

Biblio.-Médiathèques de Metz, MS 176, ff. 1r–16r

27. Docuimus causam accidencia
40 et signa de | pruritu oculorum qui
uenit ex humore | sanguineo, et
notauimus vobis glo|riosissimam
curam secundum expertissimum |
magisterium nostrum et Artem
Nostram | Probatissimam Ocu-
45 lorum. Adhuc doce|bimus uos
5rb alias infirmitates que || procedunt
ex habundancia sanguinis | et in
quo tempore magis superhabun-
dant | et nocent oculis. Et dicimus
quod hee | magis accidunt in fine
5 Augusti | usque ad exitum
Septembris quam in | alijs tempo-
ribus, et similiter accidunt
propter | mutacionem aeris. Vnde
propter obtalmie | dominantur
temporibus illis et eciam propter |
commestionem diuersorum
10 fructuum | qui tunc comeduntur,
et occasione ob|talmie inueniuntur
panniculi in o|culis.

Glasgow, GUL, Hunter MS 503, pp. 1–135

Also ther ben other | sekenes of   15
eyon causyd & engendrede || of   [34]
blode. as obtalmies &
panniculus. | and thyes happyn to
be engendred mo|re a bowte the
ende of august & so forth | to the
ende of septembre more thanne
in | oþer tymes of the yere. for by   5
cause of | chaungyng of the eyre. ¶
Obtalmies | comunly haue þer
domyne or power þat | tyme. for
by cause of dyuersytees of |
frutees þat be eten at that tyme. & |
by occasyonn of obtalmyes be   10
founde | yn the eye pannycles.

London, British Library, Sloane MS 661, ff. 32r–46r

[27]   Allso there be other | syckenesses of the eyes caused & bred of blood | as Ophthal-   15
mia & Paniculus. And these doe | happen to faule out especiallye about | the end of
August, & so continuew to *the* ende | of September more then at any other tyme | of the
yeare, by reason of the chaunginge of | the ayre. Ophthalmia are moste commonlye | at   20
that tyme of the yeare; because of the | diuersityes of ffrutes that be eaten at that | tyme,
and after the Ophthalmia doe often | follow Paniculus.

---

16 to] fore *deleted*

Glasgow, GUL, Hunter MS 513, ff. 2r–37r

And | yit we shull tech of other infirmitees the which | comen of the habundance of blode and tho maladies | fallen in the ende of Auguste till the ende of Sep|tember more than in any other tymes of the | yere ¶ And also they comen fro the mutacions of | the aer and ther fore obtolime hauen dominiou*n* in | tho tymes / And by cause of obtolmeis paninculis | ·i· litell westis ben engendred in the ey3en

Basel, Ö.B.U., MS D.II.11, ff. 172r–177v

¶ Encaras te uuelh mai mos|trar dautras enfermetatz que | uenon per gran abundancia de | sanc et enqual temps uen mais | efa mal als uelhs. ¶ Don uos | dizem ques abundan pus en | lafin daosth edura entro setem|bre ¶ Etaquesta enfermetat ue | per trop maniar. toi frucha diu|ersa que mania hom pus en a|quel temps que en autre. eue | atressi per so que om muda day|re ¶ Eper so en aquel temps uen | pus obtalmia que no fa en au|tre temps. et aquelh pannicu|li uenon trop fortment als ue|lhs enaquel temps eperso ieu | uos uuelh dire que enfermetat | es obtalmia.

Oxford, Bodleian Library, Ashmole MS 1468, pp. 1–6

Biblio.-Médiathèques de Metz, MS 176, ff. 1r–16r

28. Explanare vobis volumus | quid est obtalmia. Dicimus vobis quod | obtalmia quidam sanguis
15 corrup|tus generatus ex humo‑ ribus calidis | et ponatur super albedinem oculorum, | id est circumcirca tunicas et nigre‑ dinem | oculorum. Et ascendit in oculis cum | magno furore et
20 ardore et cum | magna habun‑ dancia lacrimarum, | et subito ueniendo tumescunt oculi | tali modo quod ab illa hora inantea | paciens non potest dormire nec quies|cere, ideo quia apparet sibi
25 sentire | quod oculi sint pleni harena, spinis, | et fumo. Explana‑ uimus vobis | causam accidencia et signa de obtalmia, | et docuimus uos quid est obtalmia | secundum rei ueritatem. Ammodo doce‑
30 bimus | vos curam quam facere debetis omnibus | pacientibus hanc infirmitatem, | tam juuenibus

Glasgow, GUL, Hunter MS 503, pp. 1–135

Than yt ys con|uenyent to tell what ys obtalmye. | And what ys a pannycle. Obtalmye, | ys a corrupte blode gendryd of hote | humurs. and communly yt   15
stondyth || of the whyte of the   [35]
eye. and rownde | a bowte the tonycles. and the blaknes | of the eye. and yt commyth with a grete | furour and brynnyng. and habun|dance of terys þat a noon   5
the eyn bolne. | And on such wyse þat from þat tyme | forth. the pacyent may haue no reste | nor slepe. For euer yt semyth to hym þat | hys eynn were ful of grauel or thornes. | or smoke. ¶ To thys   10
maner of sekenes | be yt yn yong folkys or aged. thys | ys the cure.

---

14 ys] obtalmia *added in outer margin in a late hand* 11 thys] Pulvis Be|nedictus *added in outer margin in an Italic hand*

London, British Library, Sloane MS 661, ff. 32r–46r

[28] Therefore I will nower | tell yow, what Ophthalmia & Paniculus is | Ophthalmia is   25
a corrupte blood engendred | of hoate humors, and yt is commonlye oppon | the white of
the Eye. And round about the | tunicles and the blackenes of the Eye, and | yt commyth   30
with a great feruor & burninge with | abundance of teares swellinge the Eyes: In | sutch
sorte, that the patient can take no rest | and yt semeth to the patient as though his | eyes
wer full of gravell, or smoke, or thornes | To this disease be yt in younge, or aged | 35
people this is the Cuer. Take of white Sar||cocoll and beat yt well to powder in a brasen | 37v
mortar, & fill the eye full of this powder | and let him lye wydeopen till the powder | be
consumed, and in the meane tyme make | a plaister of towe, and wet them well in | 5

---

26 engendred] Ophthalmia | what it is 36 Sarcocoll] cocoll *lower margin*; The Cuer of | ophthalmia *outer margin;* Puluis Bene|dictus *outer margin*

De Probatissima Arte Oculorum

Glasgow, GUL, Hunter MS 513, ff. 2r–37r

¶ wher|for knowe ye that obtolmia
20 is maner of corupte | blode
engendred of hote humorus and y
sett on | the white of the ey3en and
dessendethe in to the | ye3en w*ith*
grete wodenes and w*ith* grete
brynnyng | and w*ith* moche
habundance of teres and they
soden|ly comyng that the ey3en to
9v swelle that they may ‖ leue none
heres and the pacient may nought
slepe ne | rest for hym semithe
that is ey3en were full of sonde |
or full of thornes or smoke ¶ The
Cure of this mala|die is bothe to
yonge folke as to olde folke ¶ ℞
5 sarco|colle white pulueri3ed right
well in a morter of | bras and do
of that poudir in the ey3en of the
pacient | w*ith*yn and putte in well

---

3 or¹] C *added in outer margin*
3 maladie] ℞ *added in outer margin*
7 withyn] pouder *added in outer margin in a late hand*

Basel, Ö.B.U., MS D.II.11, ff. 172r–177v

¶ Obtalmia es una | mala|utia
laqual sengenra als | uelhs per 25
abundancia desanc co|rompuda
loqual sanc cengenra | delas
humors caudas emet sen | aquel
sanc corru*m*puth sobre lo bla|nc del
uelh emonta als uelhs | amgran 30
furor et amgran ardor |
sobiranament am gran abun|dancia
delagremas esoptament | los uelhs
enflon enon romano*n* | aqui ges
depelhs el malaute no*n* | pot 35
dormire nipauzar et aparli | sentir
als uelhs arena et espi|nas fum |
¶ Aras uos uelh dire las mala|utias
elas medessinas elas curas las cals
auem faitas epro|uadas per mot 40
detemps dela | obtalmia las quals
sepodonfar | ad homes ioues et a
uiels. ℞. ‖ angelot. ʒ .i. esia blanc. 174va
esarcocol|li. ʒ .i. efay poluera ben
en .i. mor|tier decoyre epueis met
daque|lha poluera als uelhs ben ed
a|ias pueis destopa mulhada en | 5

Oxford, Bodleian Library, Ashmole MS 1468, pp. 1–6

Biblio.-Médiathèques de Metz, MS 176, ff. 1r–16r

quam senioribus et econtrario. |
Pro obtalmia: ℞ anzarut al|bum id
est sarcocollam, et puluerizetur |
35 optime in mortario eneo, et de |
puluere illo in oculis pacientis
pona|tis – et bene impleatur oculus
puluere | predicto, et paciens
iaceat supinus | donec puluis
40 consumatur. Ex alia | parte
habeatis stuppam lini, et in aqua |
frigida balneetur. Postea expri-
matur | et super oculos clausos
ponatis il|lam plagellam, ipso
infirmo iacente | supino, cum
45 medicina, et ab illa hora | inantea
5va videbitis mirabilia – quod ‖ pa-
ciens qui non poterat die noc|tuque
requiescere ita subito cum
po|sueris puluerem predictum in
oculis sta|tim incipiet dormire et
5 requiescere | a languoribus suis.
Et prouidi | medici Salernitani
vocant infir|mitatem istam obtal-
miam, et hoc | secundum Ypocra-

Glasgow, GUL, Hunter MS 503, pp. 1–135

Take sarcacollum album, | and
bete yt wele to pouder yn a
bra|sym morter. And of pouder put
the eye | ful. and lette hym ley 15
wydeopyn. tyll | the powder be
consumed. and yn the ‖ meane [36]
tyme make a plaster of flaxen |
herdys. and wessch þem welle to
gyd|der yn colde water. And presse
oute all | the water yn thyn honde.
and thenn | ley yt on the seke ey. 5
the pacyent ly|yng alwey
wydeopyn. And a noon | thow
schalt see þat he schal begynne | to
rest. and to sclepe. ¶ Thys maner |
of infirmyte. the grete lechys of
sa|lerne clepyd. Obtalmyam. But 10
I | quod Benuomicius calle yt.
Torturam | tenebrosam. For so
much as it commyth | with so
greet a torment þat it makyth | the

---

12 album] here | note *added in outer margin in a late hand*

London, British Library, Sloane MS 661, ff. 32r–46r

coulde water, then wringe them out harde, | and applye them vppon the sore eye, and
yow | shall see yt in short tyme to bringe him to reste. | This manner of infirmitye the
great letches | of Salerne called Obtalmiam. But I call | yt Torturam tenebrosam. ffor so 10
mutch as | yt cometh with so great a torment, that yt | maketh the Eye dym and darke and
the | foresayde medicine is called Pulvis Bene|dictus, the blessed powder. ffor with that | 15
powder without any other bloodlettinge or | purgation or Oyntment, I have holpen |
manye of this manner of syckenes,

---

11 yt] Tortura Te|nebrosa *outer margin* **14** foresayde] Pul: Benedic|tus. *outer margin*

De Probatissima Arte Oculorum 271

Glasgow, GUL, Hunter MS 513, ff. 2r–37r

    of that forsaide poudir in | the ey3en and lete the pacient lye vp right w*ith* that | medecyne / and in that other p*ar*tie haue a·stupe of |
10 lyne herdes ·i· of towe y bathed in colde water and y |wronge oute that shall be laide on the ey3en yshitte | of the pacient / And whiles he lyeth vp ryght w*ith* | the medecine for that houre after thou shalt see | wonder and meruelous
15 thing ¶ That the pacient | the which myght afore this medicyne nought slepe | ne reste anone ryght he shall begynne to reste and | to slepe for his penaunce ¶ Leches of Saleren clepe*n* | this infirmite obtalmia ¶ And we clepen it tortu|ram ·i· torment · For whi hit comethe dou*n* so w*ith* grete |
20 torment that the ey3en ben all forderked ¶ And þe | medicyne forsaid we clepen the blessed

Basel, Ö.B.U., MS D.II.11, ff. 172r–177v

aygua fregga el malaute estia | euers los uelhs clauses efaita | una ora lo pacient siueyra me|rauelhas car el se repauzara ben | edormira. 10
e. nos auem guerit|das motas gens am baquesta | poluera egasanhat debon arge*n*t | per la gratia dedieu |

Oxford, Bodleian Library, Ashmole MS 1468, pp. 1–6

Biblio.-Médiathèques de Metz, MS 176, ff. 1r–16r

tem et Galienum, mira|biles
medicos; nos autem vocamus |
10   ipsam   torturam tenebrosam, ideo
quia | cum descendit in oculis ita
descen|dit cum magna tortura quod
oculi | tenebrantur. Et medicinam
voca|mus puluerem benedictum,
15   quia cum | intrat   oculis ab illa
hora inantea | paciens habet
requiem et recepit sani|tatem,
benedicens Deo et predictum
pul|uerem benedictum. Et cum ista
cura | sine aliqua minucione et
20   purgacione | et   sine ulla unctione,
innumerabiles ho|mines libera-
uimus, et infinitam | pecuniam de
ea lucrati fuimus. Vnde | uos
similiter faciatis cum benedictione
mea. |
   29. Adhuc dicemus uobis pessima
25   et | diuersa   genera infirmitatum
que ge|nerantur in oculis occasione
obtal|mie, ob hoc quia non fuerunt
bene | curati a principio, sicut

Glasgow, GUL, Hunter MS 503, pp. 1–135

eye dymme and derke. And the |
forseyd medycyne ys callyd.   15
Pul||uerem benedictum, the   [37]
blessyd powder. | For w*ith* þat
powder wyth oute ony oþ*er* |
blode lettyng or purgac*i*on. or
oyne|ment. I haue holpyn many of
thys | man*er* of sekenes.   5

¶ Knowe ȝe þat | euyl curyng. euyl
kepyng. vnknow|yng lechys
folowyng errors. for lak | of dewe
crafte wyth theyr Imp*er*tyne*n*t |
medycynes. addyn sorow vpon

London, British Library, Sloane MS 661, ff. 32r–46r

[29] Knowe | ye that many vnskillfull lechys. followinge | Error, for lacke of dew   20
knowled: w*ith* there | impertine*n*t medicines, add sorrow vppon Sor|row, and paine vnto
paine by occation where | of many of there patien*tes* doe neu*er* recou*er* | health. and in
some by reason of there | contrarye remodyes, the whole Eyes doe | swell w*itho*ut the   25
lydd*es*, and be mutch disfi|gured, & there sighte lost. and when theye | are broughte to
this plighte, there will no | medicine helpe them, for as mutch as *the* Eye | is dissevered   30
& come out of his inward & | propper seate, and in a manne*r* mortified | in all his
substance. And yet some there be, *that* | by occation of the Ophthalmia, are greatly
tro|bled in there eyes w*ith* fumes, and often wepynge | through there owne disorder ffor   35
that theye || eate meates that are contrarye, and hurtfull | vnto them But yet theye are not   38r
vncurable | wherefore if any sutch come to yo*r* Cuer ffirst | purge his braine w*ith* these

Glasgow, GUL, Hunter MS 513, ff. 2r–37r   *Basel, Ö.B.U., MS D.II.11, ff. 172r–177v*

pouder For | ther thorugh the
pacient hathe geten grete rest |

¶ Nowe tell we of the kyndes of   Encaras uos uuelh ensen|har   15
maladies þat | ben engendred in   diuersas enferme|tatz que uenon als
the ey3en thorowe accacioun of || uels | per aquesta obtalmia. quar
10r obtolime · For so moche that it   al|cus son megges que uolon cu|rar
was nought cured at | begynnyng   eno podon eson fols car els |

Oxford, Bodleian Library, Ashmole MS 1468, pp. 1–6

Biblio.-Médiathèques de Metz, MS 176, ff. 1r–16r

scripsimus | in Arte Nostra Proba-
30 tissima Oculorum. | Vnde sciatis
karissimi quod propter malam
cus|todiam et propter malam curam
quam mul|ti stolidi medici faciunt,
ignoran|tes Artem et sequendo
errorem cum | medicinis suis,
35 addunt dolorem super | dolorem.
Et ab illa occasione oculi de|al-
bantur tali modo quod multi de
pa|cientibus istis nuncquam ad
pristinam | sanitatem reuertuntur,
et in quibusdam | humores ocu-
lorum dissoluuntur propter |
40 magnum dolorem qui accidit
propter | medicinas contrarias. Et
eminent | cum tanta concauitate
extra pal|pebras, et pacientes
apparent de|turpati et nichil vident.
45 Vnde dici|mus de talibus quod
postquam venerunt ad illum
5vb statum, nulla medicina || potest
eos liberare, ideo quia oculus est
li|beratus a suis nutrimentis et est

Glasgow, GUL, Hunter MS 503, pp. 1–135

sorow. | and peyn opon peyne. by 10
occasyonn wher|of many a pacyent
comme neuer to helth. | and yn
sum occasyon of suche
contra|ryous medycyns. the eyon
with all þeir | concauytee. apeerun
wythout the lyd|dys. that þei be 15
foul disfygurde and || dyshonurde. [38]
and yit þei see not. And | when þei
ar come to the plyte. þere | may no
medycyne helpe þem for as|muche
as the eye ys dyssauerd and
depar|ted from hys Inwarde sy3te. 5
or place. | and mortyfyed yn all
hys substance. | And yit sum oþer
ther be. þat by occasy|on of
obtalmie ar gretly troublyde | yn
þere eyen. fumous & Oftenn
wepyng | for evyll keepyng. And 10
for that they | ete contraryous
metys. but yit þei arnn | not
vncurable. wherfor. yf ony such |
come to your cure. Fyrst pourge

London, British Library, Sloane MS 661, ff. 32r–46r

pills. Take Polipodye | Esula Mirabolanes cytrine Rubarbe ana ʒj. Masticke | Qubibes, 5
Saffron Spygnarde Nucis Indice Cynamon ana | ʒj. Powder them and mingle them with
mylke, ma|kinge them vpp into pills, and geve vnto the pati|ent sutch quantitye as his
strength will beare. | And after he is thus purged geve him, of the | Electuarye called 10
Diaolibanum Salernitanum. as | yt is before sayde in the Cuer, of the thirde Cura|ble
Cataracte., and let him take yt morninge | and Eveninge. And in the morrowe
followinge | put into his Eyes of the powder, called Puluis | Nabetis. The makinge there 15
of and the virtew | shalbe here after shewed. in the Cuer of the three | Panicles And at

---

4 Polipodye] Pills to purge | the Heade. *outer margin*

Glasgow, GUL, Hunter MS 513, ff. 2r–37r

    as we haue saide ¶ wherfor dere
wor|thi frendes knowe ye that for
wycked and euyll | kepyng and for
euyll cure of vnwise leches as
5 ma|ny donn that ben nought
knowyng in this crafte | and ther
for they may sorowe on sorowe
and ther|for the ey3en ben made
white in soche maner þat | neuer
efte may come a yene to her
former helþe | ¶ In the which
10 maner humours of the ey3en | ben
dissoluid for her grete anguysshe
and sorowe | and for her contrarie
medicynes ¶ And the ey3en |
shewen hem w*ith* all the
holowenes w*ith* outen the | ey3en
liddes and the pacient is ben so
dissowlid | and for blemysshed
15 and nought mowyn see ¶ wher|for
we sayne of suche pacien*tes* after
that they ben | brought in to soche
state / no medicyne may helpe
hem | ne delyu*er* ther afterward ¶

Oxford, Bodleian Library, Ashmole MS 1468, pp. 1–6

Basel, Ö.B.U., MS D.II.11, ff. 172r–177v

meton alcunas medescinas | que 20
fan mai de mal que de ben | eper
aquesta mala cura los ue|ls tornan
grosses esonfora de | lor loc
natural et esta mal | al malautes. 25
et aquestz uelhs | no cen poyrian
curar per totas | las medecinas del
mon quar | los uelhs son fora
delors locs | naturals et es
mortificat |
Encaras uos uulh | mot dire es 30
ensenhar de | motas emfermetatz
que | uenon per aquesta malautia |
ques anom obtalmia. motz | son 35
que se trobon als uels et | anlos
fort torbatz et an los | clars ebelhs
enon ueson res | ¶ Et aisso uen per
mala garda | car els manion
uiandas con|trariosas quant 40
anlomal. et | aquest es losenhal
que hom a | la ma*l*utia quar tot

---

24 natural] il *expunged* **42** malutia] l *added over the line*

Biblio.-Médiathèques de Metz, MS 176, ff. 1r–16r

mor|tificatus cum sua tota sub-
stantia. Et | dicimus vobis adhuc
5   quod occasione obtal|mie multi
conturbantur oculi et non | clare
uident sed habent oculos fumo-
sos, | et accidit eis propter malam
custodiam – ideo | quia semper
comedunt contraria quando
paci|untur, et remanet eis illud
10 vicium | quia oculi eorum semper
lacrimantur. Vnde | si aliquis
istorum uenerit in cura uestra, |
prius purgetis ei cerebrum cum
pil|lulis istis: ℞ polipodion, esule,
mi|rabolani citrini, reubarbi ana
15 ʒ 1, masticis, cubebe, | croci,
spice nardi, nucis indie, cina-
momi | ana ʒ 1 et cum lacte
sicomori confi|ciantur et recipiat
paciens secundum vi|res suas de
istis pilullis. Facta pur|gacione
20 detis ei ad sumendum mane | et

Glasgow, GUL, Hunter MS 503, pp. 1–135

hys | brayne w*ith* þies peletys.
Take poly|podye. esule   15
myrabolanys cytryne. || rubarbe.   [39]
an*a*. ʒ. I. Masticys. Cubibys. |
saferon. spygnarde. Nucys
Indicem. | Cynamo*n* an*a* adrame.
And þan me|dyll them w*ith* mylke
and yeue to the se|ke aft*er* hys   5
strength. And after thys |
purgac*i*on. yeue hym morne &
yeue | of the electuarie.
Dyolibanu*m*. or saler|nitanu*m*. os
yt ys sayd be forn in the | cure of
the .iij. curable cat*er*acter. And |
on the morn*n* put yn hys ey. of   10
the | powder callyd. Puluis
nabetys, | The makyng therof and
the vertu | yt schal be tauȝt

---

14 brayne] brain*n* *added in outer margin in a late hand*
7 salernitanum] pag. 22 *added in outer margin in an Italic hand*
11 nabetys] pag: 53 *added in outer margin in an Italic hand*

London, British Library, Sloane MS 661, ff. 32r–46r

Even put there in of the pow|der called Puluis Alexandrinus as is before sayde. | and this   20
must be continued till the patient be | p*er*fectlye cured. com*m*aundinge him all this |
whyle to eschu those meat*es* that be hurtfull. |

---

18 powder] He hath not | spoken of this | powder before | excepte he meane | his Puluis Be|nedictus. for by | this name he | hath not spoken | of yt. *outer margin*

De Probatissima Arte Oculorum 277

Glasgow, GUL, Hunter MS 513, ff. 2r–37r

        And that the ey3en is | separat and departed fro his noursshynges and y |mortified with all his substance
20 ¶ Also thorwe the | accasion of obtolmie the ey3en of many ben trub|led and they sein nought clerely ¶ But they haue | her ey3en full of smoke and it is comen to hem | for her euyll kepyng / for whi they wole ete & | drinke all that is to hem contrary whan the ||
10v penaunce was comen to hem and this vice leuyþ | with hem that her ey3en alway teren and wateryn | wherfor yif any such come to oure cure ¶ First | we purge hem with
5 these pil*u*llis that purgeþ | her brayn ¶ ℞ polipodij esule mirabal*an* atrine reubi*um* | · ℨ·j· w*ith* mele acermu be they made and yeue hym | therof after her

---

5 her] ℞ *added in outer margin*
7 therof] pelles *added in outer margin in a late hand*

Oxford, Bodleian Library, Ashmole MS 1468, pp. 1–6

Basel, Ö.B.U., MS D.II.11, ff. 172r–177v

iorn los | uelhs lui lagremeggon Et si | tu uoles guerir daquest malh ||
fay aital maneyra prumeyra|ment   174vb
purga lo ceruelh am las | pillulas.
℞. polipodij esuli. mi|rabolis
citrini. reu -barbe. ana ℨ. | ij. efay 5
cofiment am lait des | succamors esegon que sera lo | malaute dona li delhas pillu|las ¶ Ecant loceruelh serapur|gatz donali amaniar matin e | uespre del nostre lectoari 10
ieroso|limitano loqual atrobaras | enlaterssa espessia delas caractas | ecura las epois mete dintre los | uelhs dela poluera del angelhot | sobre dit fin quesia ben gueritz | 15
aras uos auem complidas | las enfermetatz dela obtalmi*a* |

---

17 obtalmia] a *added over the line*

Biblio.-Médiathèques de Metz, MS 176, ff. 1r–16r

[sero] de dyabolano nostro
Iherosolomita|no sumendo, sicut
habetis in tercia specie | catharac-
tarum curabilium. Et intus po|natis
de puluere nabetis in mane, et | in
sero de puluere alexandrino
25 donec | deliberentur ad plenum
– et iterum custo|diant se a rebus
contrarijs. |
30. Iam expleuimus vobis trac-
tatum | de obtalmia et docuimus
uos di|uersa genera infirmitatum
30 que procedunt | occasione sui et
scripsimus uobis probatissi|mam
curam pro vnaquaque infir|mitate
per se secundum magisterium
nostrum | et Ars Nostra
Probatissima demonstrat. | Am-
modo incipiamus in nomine
35 Domini | nostri Ihesu Christi de
panniculis qui generantur | in

---

20 sero] M loco, VP2 (f. 296r), VR
(f. 38v) sero

Glasgow, GUL, Hunter MS 503, pp. 1–135

hereaft*er* yn the cu|re of the iij
pannycles. And at eve | put theryn   15
of the powder callyde. || Puluis   [40]
Alexandrini. As it ys | seyd a lytle
before. And thys do | tyll the
pacyent be ful hoole. And | yn
meane tyme kepe hym from |
contraryus metys. | 5

Now after the Obtalmie. | I wyll
speke of pa*n*nyclys | and her curys.
whych | be gendryde of
sup*er*habundance of | blode. as   10
Obtalmies be In dyu*er*se | wyse. In
tyme of euyl keepyng. | and after
by grete peyne fallyng | yn the
heede ys causyd the mygre|ym.
wherthrugh the peyne descen|dyth   15
yn to the templys. & yn to the ||
browys. And makyth the veynes | [41]
to bete. of whych peynful betyng. |
the eyon arn*n* trowblyd. ¶ The |
pannyclys arn*n* gendryd yn the
eyon*n* | yn .iiij. wyse as thus. The   5

London, British Library, Sloane MS 661, ff. 32r–46r

[30] Now havinge spoken de Ophthalmia I will | proced to speake of the Panicles and
there Cures. | whitch be engendred of Superabundance of | bloode as Ophthalmia is.   25
↓By↓ vsinge disordred | and evell dyett is caused great paine in the | head, and there w*ith*
is caused the megreym, & | from thence the paine fauleth downe into the | temples, and 30
into the forehead. and maketh the | vaines to beate, through w*hitch* paine full beatinge |
the eyes be trobled. And the Panicles are | ingendred in the Eyes fowre mann*er* of
wayes | The first manner of Panicle appeareth in the | Eye as a sede of the graine called 35
Millium | and this groweth in the Cote called Saluatrice. || and in some places there are 38v
called Guttaticj and | in other places Pedacelle. and in Naples. theye | are called Creature.

---

24 Cures] Cap. 4°. *outer margin* 26 By] for *deleted,* By *added over deletion* 36 Saluatrice] i:
Cornea. *outer margin* 3 are] 2 *outer margin*

Glasgow, GUL, Hunter MS 513, ff. 2r–37r

myght ys and whan they be so y
|purged yef hem erly and at euen
de olibano nostro | ierusali*mi*tanus
the whiche was saide afore ¶ The |
10 ·2ᵉ· kynde of catarac*tes* curable
putte w*ith*in the ey3e | pouder of
Alexandrine till they be fulliche
delyiu*e*red | and yet lete kepe hem
fro contrary metes ·/·
**Of þe | first pa*n*nicle enge*n*dred
i*n* þe ey3en & þe cure of it |**
Of pannculis of ey3en ben
15 engendred on many ma|ners
vid*elicet* of euyll keping and ofte
tyme for mo|che hede ache
comyng in to the hede as whan |
ther cometh an emigrayne and
Descendethe to the | templis and
vnder the ey3e liddes and makethe
to | powsi ·i· meue as dothe a pows
20 and by suche maner | powsyng
the ey3en wateryn and ben

—————
13 first] 6 *added in outer margin*

Oxford, Bodleian Library, Ashmole MS 1468, pp. 1–6

Basel, Ö.B.U., MS D.II.11, ff. 172r–177v

Aras uos | uuelh dire enom dieu |
nostre senhor delas em|fermetatz 20
dels paus o dels panni|culi que
cobron los uelhs co|ma drap delin
subtil. et enge|nron se per gran
abundancia | desanc et engenron 25
se en mo|tas maneyras.
prumeyra|ment per mala garda.
segon|dament per mota dolor dela |
testa don uos dic que per aque|sta 30
gran dolor dela testa. uen | una
enfermetat en la testa q*ue* | anom
emigranea que hom | agrandolor
alfront et als so|sobrescils epres
delas aurelh|as efa batre las uenas 35

Biblio.-Médiathèques de Metz, MS 176, ff. 1r–16r

oculis similiter ex habundancia san|guinis. Dicimus autem quod panniculi | oculorum multis modis generantur: primo | per malam
40 custodiam, secundo per | multos dolores accidentes in capite – vnde | pro illis doloribus uenit emigra|nea, et descendit in timporibus et | supercilijs, et facit pulsare uenas, et | pro illa pulsa-
45 cione oculi conturbantur. | Vnde panniculi generantur et apparent in
6ra || oculis diuersimodi. Primus panniculus, | dicimus, est ille qui apparet in oculo [ut] grana | milij super tunicam. Et in multis locis | vocantur isti panniculi gitatici, et |
5 in alijs pidatilere, et in Pulia creature | – et certe satis bene dicunt quia propter dolorem | capitis et superfluitatem sanguinis | creantur in oculis cum

Glasgow, GUL, Hunter MS 503, pp. 1–135

fyrste | pannycle apperyth yn the ey as the | seyd of a corne clepyd In laten. Mi|llys. And yn ynglych. Myleseed. | Thyes greynes or cornellys of my|le growun yn the 10 tonycle. Saluatri|ce. And In sum place they arnn cle|pyd. Guttatici. And yn oþer places. | Pedacelle. And yn Naples þei ar | callyd. Creature. ¶ The secunde | pannycle ys that whych 15 apperyth || on the tonycle [42] saluatryce lyke a spotte | yn the face. or lyke a frakyn. or the | scale of a fysch. ¶ The iij^d apperyth | on that on partye of the ey. as a flake | of snowe when yt 5 snewyth. ¶ The | iiijth. ys when all the ey aperyth white | and no blaknes aperyth. neþer on the | tonycle nor on the ly3te.

---

2 oculo] VR (f. 39r) ut *added*

London, British Library, Sloane MS 661, ff. 32r–46r

The second Panicle is | that whitch appeareth on the tunicle Salvatrice | like a spott in 5 the face. or like the scale of a fish | The thirde appeareth on the syde of the Eye | like a flake of Snowe when yt snoweth. The | ffourth is when all the Eye appeareth white, | and noe blackenes appeareth.

---

6 The] 3 *outer margin* 8 ffourth] 4 *outer margin*

Glasgow, GUL, Hunter MS 513, ff. 2r–37r
   disturbled wher|for paninculi ben
   engendred in dyue*r*s maners

Basel, Ö.B.U., MS D.II.11, ff. 172r–177v
fort. e | per aquel batement delas
ue|nas los uelhs lagremeggon | ese
torbon eperso sengenro*n* als | ulhs
los pannicli etapareysson | als   40
ulhs endiu*er*sas maneyras |
Prumeyrament seengenron | als
uelhs coma gran de mil de | sota
las tunicas. emotz dizon q*ue* | es
gota pa*n* euen als uelhs amgra*n* ||
dolor. losegon apar sobre   175ra
latunica | ques es amaneyra
descata faita | coma lentilha. loters
apar en | launa part del uelh coma
floc d*e* | neu. lo quart es que   5
cobre la | pupilla et es blanc eno*n*
es nie*n*t |

Oxford, Bodleian Library, Ashmole MS 1468, pp. 1–6

Biblio.-Médiathèques de Metz, MS 176, ff. 1r–16r   *Glasgow, GUL, Hunter MS 503, pp. 1–135*

    dolore mixto. Secundus panni-
    culus, dicimus, est ille qui |
10 apparet in oculo super tunicam ad
    mo|dum lenticule siue lentiginis
    uel | ad similitudinem squame
    piscium. Tertius | panniculus
    apparet ab vna parte oculi | ac si
    esset vnus floccus de niue quando |
15 ningit. Quartus panniculus est
    quando | totus oculus apparet
    albus et nulla | nigredo apparet
    ibi, | neque de tunica neque de
    luce.

    31. Narrauimus uobis | qualiter   ¶ The cure | of the fyrst ys. put no
20 panniculi generantur in oculis | et   medycyne | nor wyth yn. nor   10
    quot sunt species eorundem. Inde | wyth oute. For þis | Infirmytee
    docebimus vos de vnoquoque   may not be curyd wyth | laxatyvs.
    secundum | magisterium nostrum   nor wyth pouders. nor | wyth
    probatum per | longum tempus et   coleryes. nor wyth electuary|es.
    per longum exer|citium et Artem   nor wyth cauteryes. For all þies |
    Nostram Probatissimam | Ocu-   raþer noye þan helpe. For thys   15
25 lorum, et primo incipiamus ad   maner || of pannycle ys curyd   [43]
    primum. | Dicimus ergo quod   wyth thys. | Precious oynement,
    quando videtis in ocu|lis hec signa,

London, British Library, Sloane MS 661, ff. 32r–46r

[31] The Cure of | the firste is: that yow put no medicine nether | with in nor with out   10
for this infirmitye maye | not be Cured with laxatiues, nor with Powders | not with
Colleryes, nor with Electuaryes nor | with Cauteryes: ffor all these doe rather hurt | then   15
good But this manner of Panicle is cu|red with this pretious Oyntment Take fortye |
tender Croppes of Bramble and stampe them so | smalle as possible yow can, with a good
handfull | of Rewe and halfe a pound of Alabastere, and | ffenell seedes powdred halfe   20
an ownce Of | Oyle of Roses on pounde incorporate all | these together put them in a new
Earthen pott | with a quarte of white wyne. And to all these | put fowre owmces of dryed
flowers of Cha|momile. and on ownce of waxe. Then boyle | them on a softe fyer till all   25

---

10 the] The Cuer of | the first pa|nicle *outer*   *margin*   17 tender] Vng: Alabas|trinum. *outer*
margin

| Glasgow, GUL, Hunter MS 513, ff. 2r–37r | Basel, Ö.B.U., MS D.II.11, ff. 172r–177v |

	¶ The	first panniculi we saye that apperethe in the ey3e	is as it were and corne of milesede ¶ ware you	ther of that ye putte none	Aras uos auem dith	del *p*anncli en qualmaney	ra se engenron. Aras uos	direm en lo nom dedieu delas	curas de cascun las quals	10
25	medycyne w*ith*in the ey3e	for	nos uos	dizem persert eper	
	whi in this first panniculi it nedith	ueritat que	nos auem prouadas	
11r	nought but ‖ make we this glorius cure in this cause ¶ ℞·xli tallos	or croppes of rede breres xl· the	per lonc	temps ¶ E prumeyrameyrame*n*t	uos uuelh dire dela prumeyra	ques es en luelh comagran de	milh ¶ E dic uos que quant uos	auretz en luelh	15

―――――――――――

1 tallos] ℞ *added in outer margin*

Oxford, Bodleian Library, Ashmole MS 1468, pp. 1–6

Biblio.-Médiathèques de Metz, MS 176, ff. 1r–16r

    id est ut grana milij, ca|ueatis ut nullam medicinam ponatis | in oculis uel extra, ideo quia ista
30 in|firmitas non potest curari cum medi|cinis laxatiuis, aut cum pulueribus, | collirijs, electuarijs, aut cauterijs – quia | nocent eis; sed faciatis eis hanc | curam que est gloriosissima pro istis |
35 panniculis qui apparent in oculis ut | grana milij: ℞ xl tallos siue cimas | intibi bene teneros, et pistetis eos | ad modum salse; ex alia parte habeatis | 2 libras boni
40 vini albi et ponatis | hec in simul in olla noua, et cum eis pu|gillum rute et 4 ʒ flore camomille | sicce uel uiridis, et de lapide qui dicitur | alabaustrum ℔ ß, seme feniculi ʒ ß, olei | rosacei ℔ 1, cere ʒ 1. Hec

---

37 intibi] N (f. 57v) tales uel cimas rubi, VP2 (f. 295r) calos seu timas rubi, VR (f. 39v) tallos siue cimas rubi

Glasgow, GUL, Hunter MS 503, pp. 1–135

Take xl tend*er* | croppys of bremell & stampe hem | as smale as sause. and a goode hand|ful of   5
rewe. and powd*er* of alabastre. | halfe a pownde fenkyl seed pondered. | halfe an*n* vnce. Oyle of roses a pounde. | all thyes encorp*er*ate to gydder. put | þem yn a new erthen pott wyth a | quarte of whyte wyne. And to all | 10
thyes. put iiij. vnc*er* of drye floures | of Camamyl. and of wexe. an*n* vnc*er* | Then boyle yt wyth easy fyre. tyll | all the wyne be consumed. and was|ted so   15
ferforth that yt semyth to frye. ||
After thys a non*n* put þerto the   [44]
whyte | of vj. Eggys. And always stere. tyll | þei be yncorp*er*ate. to gydd*er*. Thanne | str*e*yne yt þorugh a lynnyn cloyth. | and thys   5

---

2 tender] vng: Ala|bastrinu*m* *added in outer margin in an Elizabethan hand*

London, British Library, Sloane MS 661, ff. 32r–46r

the wyne be con|sumed and wasted so farr forth that yt semeth | to frye. And after this put there to the whites | of vj Egg*es*. and Allwaise stirr yt till yt be in|corporate together Then   30
straine yt through | a lyninge cloth, and kepe yt to yo*r* vse. And | w*ith* this annoynt the temples of the patient | and the forehead downe to the browes, w*hitch* only | will cuer this panicle, that is like to the | graine of Millium.   35

De Probatissima Arte Oculorum

Glasgow, GUL, Hunter MS 513, ff. 2r–37r

    lengthe of thyn hand | and that
they ryght tendre and grynd hem in
the | same as it wer Sauce than in
5 the tother partie ha|uethe ·℔·ij of
gode white wyn and putte hem to
ge|ders in a newe erthen potte and
w*ith* hem putte an | handfull of
rewe and ℥·iiij of drie or of grene
ca|mamille floures and of
alabaustre stone ·℔·ß of þe | sede
of fenell ·℥·ß and of oyle of Roses
10 ·℔·j alle þes | grynde hem and
putte hem in the forsaid wyn ta|ke
the floures of camamille and wexe
·℥·j and | and in that potte lete hem
boyle at a softe fire | and lete hem
sethe so ouer that esy fire till all |
that wyn forsaid be all consumed
15 first that it | seme that it
begynnethe to frie / And after
that | hauithe sixe white of eyryn

---

4 hauethe] A oynt|men̄te *added in outer margin in a late hand*

Oxford, Bodleian Library, Ashmole MS 1468, pp. 1–6

Basel, Ö.B.U., MS D.II.11, ff. 172r–177v

aquelh gran del | milh gardatz uos
que neguna | medescina non
metatz de dins | lo uelh ni 20
deforas quar aquesta | enfermetatz
no cen deu curar | am medecinas
am*m* laxatiuas | ni ampolueras ni
am lectoaris | ni am cauteris. car
totas aque|stas cauzas lin nozon 25
persert | Mais uos faretz aquesta
cura | la qual yeu uos persert que
ela | es gloriosa fort per aquest
pan|niculi ques aparon com*a* gran |
de milh et aquesta es la cura e | 30
uos faretz .i. enguent lo qual | non
ual tant solament en aqu*e*|st
panniculi ans persert ual | atota
dolor decors en qual que | part 35
com laia et es enguent | pus
glo*r*ios que nos aiam enca|ras uos
dic que non es pretz en | el. Recep
.xl. tauls de romze | epiza los ben

---

29 coma] a *added over the line*
38 romze] pus uermels que poyras trobbar *expunged*

Biblio.-Médiathèques de Metz, MS 176, ff. 1r–16r

45   omnia pistentur | et in predicto
vino ponantur preter flores ||
6rb camomille et ceram, et postea
po|natur olla super lentum ignem
cum | predictis rebus ut bulliat
donec to|tum vinum consumetur ita
5   quod videa |tur frigide. Postea
habeatis vj | albumina ouorum, et
in olla cum predictis | rebus
misceantur donec bene
formentur; | deinde habeatis
pannum lini et intus | ponatur et
10 peroptime coletur, et | exiet inde
preciosum vnguentum alabas|trum.
Et vocamus ipsum preciosum | a
precio, quia non est precium in
mundo | quod ei assimilari possit:
vnde preciosum, | id est
virtuosum. Et dicitur alabastrum |
15 ab alabastro, quia componitur |
ab alabastro lapide. Et de isto
preci|oso vnguento vngatis ei

Glasgow, GUL, Hunter MS 503, pp. 1–135

Oynement ys callyd. Pre|ciosum
vnguentu*m* alabastri, the
pre|scyous oynement of alabast*er*.
wyth | thys anoynt the temples of
the pacy|ent and the forhede
down*n* to the browys | which   10
oonly curyth thys pannycle. | þat
aperyth as greynes of milie, |

---

5 frigide] VP2 (f. 295r) frangere

London, British Library, Sloane MS 661, ff. 32r–46r

Glasgow, GUL, Hunter MS 513, ff. 2r–37r

    and in to that potte | wethe the forsaide thinges medle hem till thei | be right well medlyd and than hauythe a lynn|en clothe and lette it renne thorowe and so lete |
20 clense it thorowe that clothe where the best and | moste p*re*cyous of oynement*es* passed forthe // And | of p*re*cyous oynement we haue delyu*ere*d these ma|ner panniclis that apperen in the ey3en in ma|ner of a corne of milesede

Basel, Ö.B.U., MS D.II.11, ff. 172r–177v

en maneyra | desalsa edautra part   40
aias doas | liuras de bon uin blanc
emeto | tot en cemps en una ola
noua || sobre lo foc. emeti .i. plen   175rvb
poinh de | ruta. e .iiij. ʒ. de
camamilla dela flor | o uerda
osecca. esi podes met i del | pols
duna peyra ques a nom a|labaustro   5
mieia liura. de semen|sa defenolh
.ʒ .ß. doli rosath. iª. liu|ra. de sera.
ʒ .ij. totas aquestas cau|zas piza
enans que tulas metas | aluin
exceptat las flors dela ca|mamilha   10
sci era efay o tot bolhir | alfoc
suau tant entro quel ui | sia
co*n*sumatz que aparera quela | ola
uuelha rompre. epueis aias | .vj.
albums duous emescla los | ben   15
am totas aquelhas causas | finque
sian ben en corporatz emes|clatz
am baquelhas causas epu|is aias .i.
drap delin ecolhatz tot | aisso

---

11 suau] en *expunged*

Oxford, Bodleian Library, Ashmole MS 1468, pp. 1–6

Biblio.-Médiathèques de Metz, MS 176, ff. 1r–16r

timpora | et frontem usque ad supercilia, et | cum ista sola vnctione liberabitis | istos panniculos qui apparent ut | grana milij.

32. Certe karissimi postquam | placuit Deo ut ego componerem | librum istum, [nolo] vobis occultare | que erant mihi secreta, quia nisi | sciencia philosophorum testaretur per scriptum, | nunquam possent uera discerni a fal|sis nec vlla ratio esset in mundo. |

33. Adhuc dicimus vobis de predicto | vnguento alabastro multas alias | virtutes quas habet. Vnde dicimus | vobis vere quia non tantum valet | in istis panniculis ut grana milij, sed |

———

23 nolo] M volo, N (f. 58r), VP2 (f. 295r), VR (f. 40r) nolo

Glasgow, GUL, Hunter MS 503, pp. 1–135

¶ Thys precyous oynement hath ma|ny grete vertues. for not oonly yt ava|lylyth for thys manner of pannycle þat | apperyth as grene of milie. But also ‖ where any mann fele any dysease yn | the body. let hym anoynte hym þere|of. and he schal fynde ease. And yf | a mann haue a wounde.

15
[45]

London, British Library, Sloane MS 661, ff. 32r–46r

[33] This pretious Oyntment | hath manye great vertewes ffor not onlye ‖ yt avayleth for this manner of panicle, that doth | appeare like a graine of Millium. But allso | where a man feeleth any disease in the Bodye. | if he annoynt him there with. he shall finde ease. | And if a man be wounded let him dresse the wound | with this Oyntment, and yt shall both clense yt, and | close yt. And for the touth atch, annoynt the Cheke | on the place againste the touth, and yt will slake *that* | paine. Allso if a woman have paine in the Matrix | let her eate of this in manner of an Electuarye, and | she shalbe freed of her

39r

5

10

———

36 onlye] yt *lower margin* 5 wound] for a wounde *outer margin* 7 the[2]] for the touthatch *outer margin*

Glasgow, GUL, Hunter MS 513, ff. 2r–37r

Basel, Ö.B.U., MS D.II.11, ff. 172r–177v

egardatz pueis aquel en|guent. 20
edaquest enguent unchatz | las
templas el front al malau|te am
baquest enguent uos | gueriretz
aquel pannicli que | es coma gran
de milh.

11v ¶ And we saye you ‖ nought o*n*ly
these panniclis this medicyne is
gode | for ¶ Butt where euer in the
body is any sorowe | that is in any
partye of the body or in the hede |
other in the fete or in any other
5 place yef the pa|cient be anoynted
ther withe anone he shall be |
delyu*e*red fro that·Ache and

¶ En|caras uos uuelh dire autras | 25
uertutz ques a aquest engue*n*t |
precios car el es aissi pressios. |
que non a el mon negun tant |
pressios que se puesca compar|ar 30
ad aquest enguent car si | tu ten
unchas am aquest en|guent qualque
dolor que tu a|ias al cors. o al pe. o
a la testa. o | al estomac. o als

Oxford, Bodleian Library, Ashmole MS 1468, pp. 1–6

Biblio.-Médiathèques de Metz, MS 176, ff. 1r–16r

```
      ubicumque est dolor in corpore |
      et paciens invnxerit se, statim
35    li|berabitur ab illo dolore, et si
      pona|tur super plagam facit
      ipsam | consolidare. Et hec duo
      facit, scilicet | mundificat et
      consolidat, et subito expellit
40    dolorem. Et si quis | patitur
      dolorem dentium aut gin|giuarum
      et inunxerit se, statim li|berabitur.
      Et quando inueniebamus |
      mulieres habentes dolorem et
      torsi|ones matricis, dabamus eis ad
45    com|medendum   ac si esset
6va   electuarium, || et   statim erant
      liberate. Et quando | inueniebamus
      aliquos febricitan|tes fortiter,
      faciebamus eos ungere | stomacum
5     pedes et manus et renes, | et
      statim requiescebant a languo|ribus
      suis. Valet eciam ad emigra|neum
      dolorem et ad omnem egri|tudinem
      oculorum, facta inunctione | ex eo
```

Glasgow, GUL, Hunter MS 503, pp. 1–135

let hym ley | of thys onement 5
þertoo. and yt schal | clense yt. &
close yt. Also for the tooth|ake a
noynte thy cheke þer ayenst. & | a
non*n* yt slakyth the payne. Also
yf | women haue payn yn ther
matrice. | ete of thys oynement as 10
a lectuarye | and a noon*n* schalbe
delyu*er*d of ther | payn. Also men
In axesse. ymade | to be anoynted
on the stomake. on | the hondys.
and on*n* the feete. and | the 15
Reynes. And a noon*n* to be
dely||u*er*d and releuyd. Also thys [46]
oyny|ment ys for eu*er*y mygryme.
and for | eu*er*y payne of the ey. yf
the pacyent | be anoynted
therwyth. the forhede. | the 5
templys and browys.

London, British Library, Sloane MS 661, ff. 32r–46r

paine. Allso if men in the | axesse be annoynted there w*ith* on there stomake, and | on there handes, ffeete, and Raynes theye shalbe deli|vered.

---

11 the] what he meaneth | by Axesse. I doe | not knowe excep | yt be the Agens | or Hiccofe. *outer margin*

Glasgow, GUL, Hunter MS 513, ff. 2r–37r

  sorowe and yf it be | laide on
a·wounde it mundifiethe it and
consolidiþ | it and sodenly it
swagethe the anguysshe and that |
sorowe ¶ Also who so hathe any
10 sorowe or ache jn | his tethe or in
his gomys and he be anoynted
w*ith* | this oynement anon he is
delyu*er*d ¶ And whan | we fonde
any women that hadde corrupciou*n*
or pe|naunce in her marice we yeue
hem to eten in | maner of a·letuar
and a non*n* they wer delyu*er*ed | ¶
15 Also yif we fonde any that hade
feuerys | we made hem to be
anoynted on the stomake | on her
fete on her Reynes a none they
rested | fro her langure ¶ Also this
medecyn is gode | for almaner
emigrayn and sorowe and ache of |
20 ey3en and for almaner maladies
of the ey3en | wethe anoyntyng
made in the forhede and on | the
templis and on her browis and on

Oxford, Bodleian Library, Ashmole MS 1468, pp. 1–6

Basel, Ö.B.U., MS D.II.11, ff. 172r–177v

roinhos. o a la | camba el gueritz 35
en contenant | ¶ E faute saber que
nos nauem | donat amaniar motas
uega|das amaneyra de lectoari
alas | femnas quel auian mal ni
do|lor en la mayre. eper lo sert 40
nos | las gueriam tost. eual
encaras | a dolor emigranea. et
atota dol|or de uelhs es amalautia
sol | que tu ne unches lo front
elas || cilas elas templas | 175va

Biblio.-Médiathèques de Metz, MS 176, ff. 1r–16r

10   super frontem, in timporibus | et
supercilijs.

Glasgow, GUL, Hunter MS 503, pp. 1–135

34. Audiuistis diuer|sas virtutes preciosi vnguenti alaba|ustri, compositi a nobis, et curam | primi panniculi secundum Artem Nostram | Probatissimam
15   Oculorum. Ammodo | procedamus de secundo panniculo qui | apparet super tunicam ad modum | lentiginis uel ad similitudinem squame | piscium. Secundus panniculus est ille | qui apparet

¶ The | secund panycle I wyll ȝe knowe. | but yf yt be curyd a non yn the be|gynnyng of the growyng þereof. | yt wyll not be curyd after the pacy|ent schal wele se. For   10
when yt ys | incarnate & hardened vpon the to|nycle. þow ȝe wolde wyth your twyc|chys lyft it vp and

---

7 but] The seconde | pannicle *added in outer margin in an Elizabethan hand*

London, British Library, Sloane MS 661, ff. 32r–46r

[34]   The second Panicle muste be cured at | the begininge of the growinge there of   15
Otherwise | yt will not be cured. ffor when yt is incarnate & | hardned vppon the Tunicle, when yow woulde with | yor twytches lift yt vpp and cutt yt w*ith* a rasor | yow can not so subtillye cutt yt but that yow shall | cutt the tunicle there w*ith*, and so destroye all the | 20
substance of the Eye. wherefore I councell yow | that when yow see this manne*r* of Panicle not new | but incarnate and hardned vppon the tunicle of | the Eye meddle not w*ith* the Cuer there of. ffor | there will nether come worshipp nor creditt there | by: but   25
hurt to yo*r* name and fame amongst the | people.

---

16 incarnate] The Cuer of th*e* | second Panicle. *outer margin*

Glasgow, GUL, Hunter MS 513, ff. 2r–37r

    her ey3e |liddes and so in diu*er*se maners approued is the | vertues of this gloriouse and virtuose
12r oyneme*n*t || Alabastri / and it is gode for the pannicle that appereþ | in maner of a·corne milesede the which may nou3t | w*ith* pouders ne w*ith* cautaries ne withe none elect|uaries be holpen but this p*r*ecious oynement
5 ala|baustri best and all other forsaid is noying saue | that precious oynement ·/·

Of ·2· secunde | pannicle and the cure of it. |
Of the ·2· pannicle is that the whiche appe|rethe on the tonicle in
10 the maner of a·|vecche or in the maner of ascale of a·fissh | the whiche maladie yif it be nought holpen | whiles it is newe and or that it be harded or | endured on

---

6 secunde] 7 *added in outer margin*

Oxford, Bodleian Library, Ashmole MS 1468, pp. 1–6

Basel, Ö.B.U., MS D.II.11, ff. 172r–177v

Aras uos uuelh dir enom | de iesu crist del segon | panniculo que apar sobre | latunica del uelh 5
amaneyra des|cama depeis coma es una lenti|lha edic uos que aquest panni|culo si alcomensament cant el | uenc non es curatz am aquestas | curas que yeu tediray 10

---

3 segon] manda *expunged*
9 aquestas] *final* s *added over the line*

Biblio.-Médiathèques de Metz, MS 176, ff. 1r–16r

20 super tunicam oculorum | ad
modum et similitudinem supra |
dictum; vnde dicimus uobis vere
quod si | iste panniculus a
principio generaci|onis sue non
fuerit curatus cum | istis curis quas
25 dicam, nunquam | poterit postea
curari ad plenum, | ita quod bene
videat, ideo quod incar|natur et
indurescit super tunicas |
oculorum. Et si uelletis ipsum
ele|uare cum uncino et incidere |
30 cum rasorio, non potestis sic
in|cidere subtiliter quod non
incidatis | tunicam. Et si ita est,
tota substantia oculi | destruitur.
Vnde karissimi moneo vos | quod
cum videritis tales panniculos |
35 non recentes sed induratos super |
tunicam oculorum, non recipiatis
eos | in cura uestra quia non
possetis | inde habere honorem, et
bona fa|ma vestra diminueretur.
40 Igitur di|mittite errorem et

Glasgow, GUL, Hunter MS 503, pp. 1–135

kut yt wyth a | rasoure. 3e mowe
not so sotyllye | kut yt. but þat 3e   15
shuld kut the | tonycle therwyth.
wyth whych || kut. all the   [47]
substance of the ey. shuld | be
dystroyed a noon. wherfore I
coun|sel yow that when 3e se thys
man*er* | of pannycle. not new. but
incarnate | and harded vpon the   5
tonycle of the eye. | take yt not in
cure. for 3e may haue | no
worschype þerof. but hurtyng |
your name & fame among*is* the
peo|ple.

London, British Library, Sloane MS 661, ff. 32r–46r

Glasgow, GUL, Hunter MS 513, ff. 2r–37r

    the tonicles of the ey3en and that |
    with our cure the whiche that
15 folwithe neuer | after it worthe
    helpen ne cured at the full | that
    they euer shall see wele after ¶
    For | yf ye wolle withe an hoke
    lifte it vp and | cutte it withe
    a·Rasour it may nought so lig|htly
    be cutte that þat ye shull kutte the
20 sub|staunce of the ey3e is loste ·
    wherfor Derworþe | frendes we
    comaunde you whan ye sein any |
    suche pannicles after that they ben
12v nought || newe and indurati and
    harded ouer the tonicles of þe |
    ey3en ne take hem nought in to
    your cure for ye mowe | haue of
    hem no woship

Oxford, Bodleian Library, Ashmole MS 1468, pp. 1–6

Basel, Ö.B.U., MS D.II.11, ff. 172r–177v

iamais | planament no sen poyra
curar | ni enteyrament. per que se
en|carna esi torna dur. Et situ lo*n* |
uolias curar am croc dargent |
epueis lon osteces am lo razor | 15
non sepoyria far. que tu non
o|stesses atressi las tunicas delh |
uelh esi latunica era ostada la |
tunica del uelh seria destrucha |
¶ Don uos assaber amix meus | 20
efils atotz que cant uos ueyretz |
aquest panniculi endurat. efer|mat
que negun non recepiatz | en
uostra cura car per sert nol |
poyriatz guerir ni auer honor | e 25
uostra fama nesceria merm|ada.
eper aquo anatz perlauia |
deu*e*ritat elaissas falssas errors |
de mals megges efaitz obras | de 30
piatat edieus cera am uos |
elausatz lon totz temps car el | uos
afayt uenir auia de u*e*ritat |

28 falssas] *final* s *added over the line*

Biblio.-Médiathèques de Metz, MS 176, ff. 1r–16r

timorem, et | caueatis uobis ab ipso ut non | nominemini stolidi medici.

35. Postquam | habetis ueram et certam noticiam de | vnaquaque egritudine oculorum secundum |
45   magisterium nostrum et Artem
6vb   Pro||batissimam Oculorum, operamini ipsam cum | salute. Et non medicetis egritudines | malas et incurabiles — itote per viam | veritatis et date honorem Domino
5   Deo | nostro Ihesu Christo cum laudibus, et se|quamini ipsum operantes opus misericordie et | pietatis. Vnde antequam incarnetur super | tunicam saluatricem curabitis eam. | Cura hec est:
10   faciatis cauterium in tim|poribus cum cauterio rotundo sicut | demonstrauimus in cauterijs nostris, ideo | quia ignis contrahit, dissoluit, et con|sumit, et non permittit ipsum incarnari | super

Glasgow, GUL, Hunter MS 503, pp. 1–135

¶ Neuer the lesse yf ȝe comme þer|to. while yt ys new growe. and   10
not | incarnate vpon the saluatryce. cure | yt onn thys wyse. ¶ Fyrst yn the | the begynnyng make a Cauterye | in the templys wyth a rownde Cau|tarye. whych as I   15
schal shew you || afterwarde   [48]
among my Cautaryes. | for fire | drawyth and dissoluyth and con|seruyth. and suffryth no pannycle | to be Incarnate vpon   5
the tonycle. | And so by drawyng dyssoluyng | and consumyng by þat place cau|teryzed. thys maner of pannycle | ys consumyd wasted & dystroyed. | and the ey able to   10

---

12 the[1]] The cuer ther|of. *added in outer margin in an Elizabethan hand* 1 Cautaryes] whych as I schal shew you. *deleted*

London, British Library, Sloane MS 661, ff. 32r–46r

[35] Neuerthelesse if yow come to yt, while | yt is newlye growen and not incarnate vppon | the Saluatrice cuer yt on this manner. ffirst | in the begininge make a Cauterye in   30
the temples | with a rownde Cauterye, whitch I shall shew | yow after amongst my Cauteryes ffor fyer | draweth, and dissolveth, and consumeth, and | suffereth no panicle to be incarnate vppon | the tunicle But by drawinge, dissolvinge and | consuminge by that   35
place cauterized This | manner of Panicle is consumed, wasted & | destroyed, and the Eye maye be clarified with || the medicines followinge. When this Cauterye is | made as   39v
before is sayde: put into the pacientes | eye lyinge wide open, of the powder called | pulvis Nabetus. whose makinge shalbe toughte | here after And whilst he lyeth with the   5
powder | in his Eye Take fowre Crabbes and rost them | then take the skynn from the

---

31 whitch] as *deleted* 38 with] the *lower margin*

Glasgow, GUL, Hunter MS 513, ff. 2r–37r *Basel, Ö.B.U., MS D.II.11, ff. 172r–177v*

¶ And be ware you that ye tech | it nought to vnkunyng leches lest he lese all that he | dothe for in vnexperience and his vnkunyng wherfor | we saye you eftsones that such a·pannicle shulde be | holpen for whan it is cornned inharded and Joked on þat | tonnicle that Johannicius clepethe Saluatricem For | after it is so waxen harde for none cure it worthe neuer | helpen ¶ The Cure of this is to make a·cauterie in | the templis withe a·rounde cauterie of hote Iren y fyred | ¶ for fyre dissoluethe and drawethe and consumethe & | suffreth nought it to wexe croked on the tonicle and | that Dothe fire whiche drawyng to

5

10

10 helpen] C *added in outer margin*

Oxford, Bodleian Library, Ashmole MS 1468, pp. 1–6

¶ Doncas nos uos uolem dire | la medecina elacura daquest se|gon panniculi edic uos que | uos locuretz alcomenssament | quant el se comensa ad en|carnar sobre latunica quar | cant es endurat noia concel | sensa perilh eperso enans que | sia dura tu faras .un. cauteri | lo qual se fay am foc tira e con|suma coma nos auem mos||trat motas uegadas car lo foc tira | motas econsuma edisol enonlo | layssa encarnar sobre latunica | per so car tira edisol e consuma | per aquelloc cauteriat. et aquel | panniculi se consuma per lo foc. | elo uuelh esclariseis el fa clar | am aquestas medecinas quetu | lin aiudaras ¶ Tu penras quatre | pomas emetras las sota las sen|res caudas. equant ceran cuy|tas

35

40

175vb

5

10

Biblio.-Médiathèques de Metz, MS 176, ff. 1r–16r

    tunicam, quia sic attrahendo, |
15 dissoluendo, et consumendo, per illum | locum cauterizatum, consumitur ille | panniculus et clarificatur oculus per ipsum | cum additis medicinis subscriptis. | Facto cauterio mittatis in oculo de
20 pul|uere nabetis, et ex alia parte habeatis | 4 poma acerba et sub cinere calido co|quantur. Hoc facto mundentur a cortice | exteriori et medulla, pistentur et cum | eis admisceatur clara vna oui. Et |
25 tantum ducantur poma illa cum clara oui | quousque fiat quasi vnguentum, et de isto | emplastro ponatur super stuppam et pona|tur super oculum, oculo ipso clauso, et | bis in die mutetur emplastum
30 illud. Posi|to tamen puluere illo prius in oculis, pos|tea emplastrum

Glasgow, GUL, Hunter MS 503, pp. 1–135

be claryfyed w*ith* | the medycyns folowyng when | thys Cauterye ys made lyke as I | seyd. a noon put In to the pacy|ent ey lying wydeopon of the pow|der callyd.   15 Puluis nabetus. whych || schal be [49] tau3t aft*er*. And whyle lyeth | wyth the powder yn hys ey. take iiij. | Crabbys and rost þem. doo awey the | pyllys wythoute. and the coore wyth|yn. and incorp*er*ate   5 them wyth the | whyte of an egg. in man*er* of a oyne|ment. and ley yt on a plaster of | clene flexen herdys. and bynde yt | to the eye. wyth a lynnen*n* cloyth. & | so let   10 yt be. from morn*n* tyll yeue. | And þen make a new plaster. fro | yeue tyl the morn*n*. And thus shall | 3e

---

15 whych] shal be. *added in lower margin* **3** the[1]] plast*er added in outer margin in a late hand* **4** wythyn] of Crabbs *added in outer margin in an Italic hand*

London, British Library, Sloane MS 661, ff. 32r–46r

outsyde, and the | core from w*ith*in, and incorporate them w*ith* | the white of an egg in the manner of an oynt|ment, and laye yt vppon a pledget of | fyne towe and bynd yt to the   10 Eye. w*ith* a lyninge | cloth and so let yt rest from morninge till | Eveninge. and then renew yt and let yt | rest vntill the nexte morninge. And thus | shall yo*w* cuer all these   15 manner of Panicles | while theye are new, and the Patient shall re|cou*er* syght and lyghte. to the glorye of God. |

---

9 oyntment] w *deleted* **13** renew] l fourth Panicle *outer margin*   *deleted* **15** shall] He speaketh no|thinge of the thirde & fourth Panicle *outer margin*

De Probatissima Arte Oculorum

Glasgow, GUL, Hunter MS 513, ff. 2r–37r

15 & dissoluyng | and consumyng
itte by cauterie and that panicle
shall | be wasted and claryfieth the
ey3en withe medecyns | I· added
afterward wreten ¶ whan the
cautarie ys | made putt wi*th*yn the
ey3e of pouder nabat*is* ir 3uccr*e* |
candi ¶ And on the other p*a*rtye
20 take 4 applis y rosted | vnder
hote eu*er*y and do a·way her
barkes of the ou|temeste of tho
apples and grynde hem in A
morter | of bras and w*ith* hem
putte the white of ·4· eyren & | so
longe bete hem gedres till it be as
it were lich | a noynement and
than the poudir of nabotis in the |
25 ey3en putte the pacient shall shitte
13r his ey3en and || on the ey3en lay
that emplaster of the forsaid applis
on | herdes of flexe and bynde it

Basel, Ö.B.U., MS D.II.11, ff. 172r–177v

mondalas dela escorssa de | foras
episza ben la substancia en | .i.
mortier de eram emeti una | clara 15
duou emescla tant entro | que sia
coma enguent o empla|ustre emeti
destopa. epueis tu | met dedins lo
uelh depoluera de nabet. fay aisso
meti destopa | sobrel luelh claus
emuda do|as uegadas dedias al 20
matin | et al uespre eligua pueis
am|buna plecha o pausa de drap |
delin en aquesta man|eyra segura
aquest sego*n* | panniclu*m* ¶ 25
Edaquesta | gloriosa cura uos faitz
gra|cias adieu pus que ami |

---

22 of] plaster *added in outer margin in a late hand*

Oxford, Bodleian Library, Ashmole MS 1468, pp. 1–6

Biblio.-Médiathèques de Metz, MS 176, ff. 1r–16r

superligatum cum segmenta lini, |
et ita maneat de sero usque in
mane | et a mane usque in sero. Et
sic cum | istis curis curabitis tales
35 panniculos | dum sunt recentes,
et pacientes recu|perabunt lumen
usque ad plenum, lau|dantes et
benedicentes Deum et studium |
nostrum. Non nobis sed Domino
Deo Nostro | demus gloriam et
referamus gratias. |
40 **36.** Tertius autem panniculus est
ille qui ap|paret sub tunica oculi
sicut flos ni|uis quando ningit, et de
ipso faciatis cu|ram secundi
panniculi sicut fecisti cum |
cauterio in timporibus, et in oculis
45 po|natis de puluere nabetis. Sed
7ra tamen || adiungatis cum eo istam
medicinam que | valet contra

Glasgow, GUL, Hunter MS 503, pp. 1–135

cure almane*r* of pannycles. whyle |
they ar new. and the pacyent
schall | recou*er* ly3t pe*r*fy3tly to   15
the louy*n*g | ¶ of gode. ||

---

31 segmenta] Al stuppa, P fascia, VR
petia

London, British Library, Sloane MS 661, ff. 32r–46r

Glasgow, GUL, Hunter MS 513, ff. 2r–37r

ther to // And whan nede | ys
assonys Doith othir applis on the
same maner erly | and at ny3te ¶
Thus thou shalte cure all such
manere | pannicles whiles they
be newe and they shull reco|uer her
hele praisyng and worshipping
almy3ty god |

Of the therd pannicle & the cure of it |
Of the thridde maner of panincle ys that the | whiche apperethe fro the on partye of the ey3e | as it were whan it snowyth a fleke of snowe | ¶ And we sayne that same Cure ye shull do as we | haue saide in the·2ᵉ· pannicle as ye haue afore / þat | is to saye with atuterye in the templis and ye shull | putte in the

---

7 it] 8 *added in outer margin*

Oxford, Bodleian Library, Ashmole MS 1468, pp. 1–6

Basel, Ö.B.U., MS D.II.11, ff. 172r–177v

Aras uos uuelh dir delater|sa
maneyra delpanniculo | edic uos
que el secura en | aquelha maneyra
quefalose|gon. empero aiustatz i
aquesta | medescina que ual fort
contra | la blancor del uelh car fa
tornar | negra latunica egasta la
macu|la blanca. Recep .iiij. ʒ. de
bon | ligno aloes et aias .iª. ola
noua | et ompletz lan de carbos
uius | emetez loligno aloes sobre
los | carbos. e pueissas aias .i.
bassi | bel enet ecobri laolla en

Biblio.-Médiathèques de Metz, MS 176, ff. 1r–16r

[albedinem] oculorum, ideo quia |
nigrescit tunicam destruendo
maculam, | id est albedinem
oculorum. Hec est: accipit 4 ʒ
5   boni | ligni aloes, et interim
habeatis parapsi|dem nouam, et
impleatis eam carbo|nibus viuis.
Postea ponatis lignum | aloes
super carbones illos, et ex alia |
parte habeatis vnum [bacile]
10   mundum et | magnum, et
parapsidem cooperiatis de
car|bonibus ita quod totus fumus
ille recipi|atur in bacile. Recepto
fumo habe|atis ʒ ß de puluere
nabetis et in fumo | predicto
misceatur et cum pistello ereo |
15   ducatur donec in subtilissimum

Glasgow, GUL, Hunter MS 503, pp. 1–135

---

2 albedinem] M albuginem, N (f. 59r) albedinem, VP2 (f. 298v), VR (f. 41r) albugineum   9 bacile] M batile, VV (f. 173r) baccile, VR (f. 41r) Berger (p. 27) bacile   14 ereo] VP2 (f. 298v), VR (f. 41r) eneo

London, British Library, Sloane MS 661, ff. 32r–46r

Glasgow, GUL, Hunter MS 513, ff. 2r–37r

    ey3e of the pouder nabatis ¶ But
15 na|theles putte ther to with hym
this medicyn the whi|che Also is
gode ayenst the whitenesse of the
ey3en | for whi it blakethe the
tonicle and it distroiethe the |
spotte and the whitenesse ·i·
webbes of the ey3en | and this is
the medicyne ¶ Take ·ℨ·q· of fyne
20 tree | of gode aloes and also
hauethe a·newe platter of | stonye
erthe full of firy colys than lay that
aloes | tree on the quyk colys And
on that other side haue | ye a
moche clene basyn that maye ouer
keuery þat | stonen plater withe
25 the colys So that it may take | all
that smoke and reseyue it in to the
13v basyn And ‖ that fume y reseyued
than haue ye anabiatis ·2·q· |
poudred and in that bacyn where
that the fume | of Aloes ys

Basel, Ö.B.U., MS D.II.11, ff. 172r–177v

aques|ta maneyra que lo bassi
recepi|a tot lo fum. epueis aias. ℨ
.i. de ‖ pols denabet emescla lon   176ra
am lo | fum delbassin ben pistat
am .i. | pistador decoyre etrissa
ben en|tro que sia ben poluerizat
emes|clat am lo fum efay aisso   5
met daquesta poluera dedins | los
uels epueis met desob|bre lo uelh
claus lo emplaus|tre delas pomas
ayssi coma es | dit desobre edelha
poluera a|tressi mudaras aytantas   10
ue|gadas es aquesta es lacura: |
amlaqual motas uegadas per|sonas
auem curadas |

---

19 tree] ℞ *added in outer margin*   5 dedins] edefo|ra *expunged*

Oxford, Bodleian Library, Ashmole MS 1468, pp. 1–6

Biblio.-Médiathèques de Metz, MS 176, ff. 1r–16r

pulue|rem reducatur. Facto puluere bis in die | in oculis mittatur et desuper oculos | emplastrum pomorum sicut docuimus vos in | tractatu secundi panniculi. Et ita
20 ligetis | cum fascia bis in die sicut superius dictum | est. Et cum istis curis curabitis tercium | panniculum et non cum alijs. Et magis | inuenimus de istis tercijs panniculis in | Tuscia quam in alijs prouincijs.

25 37. Dice|mus de qua specie fit puluis nabetis | postea narrabimus virtutes quas | habet contra pannum oculorum sed tantum | propium suum est liberare secundum et tercium | panniculum.

Glasgow, GUL, Hunter MS 503, pp. 1–135

*And thys preciosus powder we calle. | Puluis nabetus, And yt ys [53,11]

---

11 And] *This paragraph (§37) appears after §40 in the MS*

London, British Library, Sloane MS 661, ff. 32r–46r

[37] *And the powder I spake | of is called Puluis Nabetus. And yt is made of | Sugar 40r,25 whitch in the Arabicke tounge the Sarazins | call sugr. gelyppm. And Christien men call yt | Sugar Candye of Alexandria. This powder is | good to heale all diseases of the 30 Eyes. |

---

25 And[1]] *This paragraph (§37) appears in the MS after §40*

Glasgow, GUL, Hunter MS 513, ff. 2r–37r

    receyued medle hym theryn hym |
    theryn w*ith* a·brasyn pestell till it
5 be made in to | a   right sotill
    pouder with that forsaide fume of |
    the poudre medle hem well to
    giders ¶ whan | this poudre ys y
    made þus as y haue asayde | than
    do of this poudre twyes a·day
    naturall | that is at the morwe and
10 at euen in to the ey3e | and
    a·boue that laye a·plastre y made
    of applis | as I haue taught you in
    the secunde pannicle þan | bynde
    it to withe a bonde till it come to
    his hele | ayen and we haue
    delyiu*e*red and y cured many |
    folke w*ith* these cures withe outen
    numbre
15 ¶ Nowe | we   shull teche you of
    what spice ye shull make | poudre
    nabat*is* of whiche is the p*r*operte to
    deliuer | the secunde and the·iij^{de}

Oxford, Bodleian Library, Ashmole MS 1468, pp. 1–6

Basel, Ö.B.U., MS D.II.11, ff. 172r–177v

¶ Encaras uos uuelh dir las |
uertutz delapoluera del nabet | 15
eprouensals lo apelhan succre |
candi dalissandria e prumey|rament
mollifica lo pannicu|lo deluelh
segondament miti|ga   ladolor 20

Biblio.-Médiathèques de Metz, MS 176, ff. 1r–16r

  Dicemus ergo quod puluis |
30 nabetis fit de zucaro nabetis
secundum | arabicam linguam
– Sarraceni et Bar|barici uocant
ipsum zucarum gilleb. | Nos autem
Christiani secundum medicos
vo|camus ipsum candi alexandri, et
35 de isto fa|cimus puluerem nabetis,
qui puluis | facit multa mirabilia
ad pannum | oculorum: primo quia
mollificat pannum | oculorum,
secundo quia mitigat ipsorum |
dolorem, tertio quia destruit
40 rubo|rem ipsorum, quarto autem
quia corrodit | totum pannum et
totam maculam, quin|to quia
confortat oculum et acuit visum, |
sexto uero quia lacrimas
constringit | si hee sunt de humore
45 frigido. Et est ita | securus puluis
quod ad omnes infirm|itates
oculorum prodest et nulli obest. ||
7rb Adhuc dicemus uobis de
puluere | nabetus quare mollificat:

London, British Library, Sloane MS 661, ff. 32r–46r

Glasgow, GUL, Hunter MS 503, pp. 1–135

mayd | of sugyr. whych Im arabyk
tong. | the sarasyns calle sug*er* 15
gelypp*m*. And | crysten men cal yt [54]
sug*er* candy of alex||and*er*. Thys
powd*er* ys goode and syker | to
hole al sekenes of eyon.

---

12 mayd] sug*er* *added in outer
margin in a late hand* **14** And]
puluis | nabetus | quid *added in
outer margin in an Italic hand*

Glasgow, GUL, Hunter MS 513, ff. 2r–37r

    pannicle the zuere nabatis | ys
made after arabie tung and
saracenys speche | and turkes
clepen it zucre gylope we cristin
20 men | clepen it zucre nabatis and
Also zucre candi of | Alexandri of
these zucre candi of Alisaunder
we | make poudre nabatis ¶ The
whiche poudre | doithe many grete
14r merueiles to the pannicles || of the
ey3en First it makethe nesshe that
pannicle | for his grete moystenes
¶ Secunde it swagethe | the ache
for his swetenes and his mekenes
3ᵉ it | Distroiethe redenes of ey3en
5 for his purite of is | hete qᵉ· it
fretethe the webbes in the ey3en
for is | hardenes / for whi or that it
be dissolued and it be | y brought
in to water myghtly it fretethe the |
webbe ·5· it comforthe the sight for

Basel, Ö.B.U., MS D.II.11, ff. 172r–177v

deluelh. terssament | gasta
edestruis la rossor el uer|melh del
uelh ¶ Quarta|ment coros lo
panniculo. lo sin|quen es quar
conforta luelh. | ¶ E lo set 25
restreinh las lagremas | si son de
la humor fregga ¶ En | aquesta
maneyra uos dic que | atotas las
emfermetatz aiu|da et en deguna
non notz |

---

18 ys] pouder | nabates *added in outer margin in a late hand*

22 del] uou *expunged*

Oxford, Bodleian Library, Ashmole MS 1468, pp. 1–6

Biblio.-Médiathèques de Metz, MS 176, ff. 1r–16r   *Glasgow, GUL, Hunter MS 503, pp. 1–135*

dicimus | propter humiditatem quam habet, secundario mi|tigat propter suauitatem sue
5 dulcedinis, | tertio destruit ruborem puritate | caliditatis sue, quarto corrodit pan|num propter duriciem suam – quia antequam | dissoluatur et reuertatur in aquo|sitatem, potenter corrodit
10 pannum | oculorum – quinto confortat quia si aliqua | calligo est in oculis, purifi|cat et clarificat oculum et visum ocu|lorum et viuificat spiritum visibilem, sex|to
15 constringit lacrimas si ipse lacri|me sint de humore frigido, quia propter | caliditatem suam contemporat illam frigiditatem. |
38. Docuimus uos quomodo debetis illum | puluerem componere cum fumo de | ligno aloes pro tercio panniculo,
20 secundum | Artem Nostram Probatissimam Oculorum. |

London, British Library, Sloane MS 661, ff. 32r–46r

De Probatissima Arte Oculorum

Glasgow, GUL, Hunter MS 513, ff. 2r–37r

    yeff any hete | be in the ey3en it
10 purifiethe it and also it clereþ | the
    sight and it quickethe the visible
    spirit ·6· fore | for it constraynethe
    teres yef the teres were of | colde
    humours for thorugh his hete it
    w*ith* tempere|the the coldenes of
    humours ·/·

Basel, Ö.B.U., MS D.II.11, ff. 172r–177v

Of the ·4·þ*e* **| pannicle and the cure of it.** |
15 Of the ferthe pannicle ys whan the ey3e appe|rethe all white and

¶ En caras uos uuelh dire | del 30
quart panniculo que es | cant luelh
apar tot blanc e deg|una negror no
y apar aqui ni | delha tunica nidela
lutz don uos | fau saber que uen 35
pergran dol|or dela testa que

———

13 ·4·þe] 9 *added in outer margin*

Oxford, Bodleian Library, Ashmole MS 1468, pp. 1–6

Biblio.-Médiathèques de Metz, MS 176, ff. 1r–16r

    Dicimus quod quartus panniculus
est quando | totus oculus est
dealbatus et nulla | nigredo videtur
ibi de tunica neque | de luce. Vnde
sciatis quod accidit propter |
25 magnum dolorem uenientem per |
medium capitis cum magno
furore | et circumdat totum
oculum circum|circa, et propter
illum dolorem oculus | dealbescit
30 et apparet in colore | lucidi
alabastri, et paciens non videt | sed
dicit quod totus mundus videtur |
ei esse albus, et non potest discer-
nere | vnam rem ab alia, et oculi
semper | lacrimantur, et tota
35 naturalis albedo | oculi apparet
rubea circumcirca tu|nicam deal-
batam. Audiuistis | signa, hec est
cura: primo faciatis | pacienti
cauterium in mollicie | capitis
40 sicut videbitis in cauterijs | nostris;
facto cauterio habeatis xii
albu|mina ouorum et ponatis ea in

London, British Library, Sloane MS 661, ff. 32r–46r

Glasgow, GUL, Hunter MS 503, pp. 1–135

Glasgow, GUL, Hunter MS 513, ff. 2r–37r

      none blake ys ther y |seyn neyþer
      no thinge of the tonicle of the |
      ey3en neither of the sight ¶ Than
      wetethe well | that þat fallethe fore
20 the moche akthe that is | comen
      doun by the mydward of the heuyd
      w*ith* grete | wodenes and furosite
      and it enclosethe the ey3en | all
      aboute and for that grete anguisshe
      of Akþe | the ey3e wexethe white
      and apperethe in colour | as
      shynyng alabaustre and the pacient
14v fro þens || forward seethe nought
      or yif any of lyght shewe yit | he
      seeth but feblyche For hym
      semethe that all the | worlde ys
      white and he may not knowe ne
      shewe o | thing from a nothir
5   thinge / and his ey3en ben | alway
      wateryng and all the naturall white
      of þe | ey3en appereth rede all
      aboute the tonicle y whited | ¶ The

---

7 The] C *added in outer margin*

Oxford, Bodleian Library, Ashmole MS 1468, pp. 1–6

Basel, Ö.B.U., MS D.II.11, ff. 172r–177v

dechen per mie|g eua en torn luelh
eper aque|lha dolor uenc aquelh
blanc | al uelh et apar lo uelh
lusent | de color delapasso el   40
passient no*n* | pot pus ueser mais
que ditz q*ue* | tot lomon li apar
blanc. eno | pot diuisar. una cauza
dautra || elos uells lilagremegon   176rb
tot iorn | etota lablancor li apar
entorn | latunica em blanquesida.
aras uos ey dit la cauza els
accidens | daquest quart
panniculo |
¶ Aras uos uulh dire las   5
medesci|nas nostras proadas
atotas | prouas proadas adonar ¶
Don|cas aquesta es lacura que
uos | uos faretz en aquesta ma-   10
lautia | vos faretz vn cauteri en lo
suc | delatesta. equant auretz fait |
aiatz .xij. albums duous e faitz |
los ben batre en una scudelha | am
bunfust en tro que tornon | en   15
escuma. epueis laissatz los |

Biblio.-Médiathèques de Metz, MS 176, ff. 1r–16r

    vna | parapside noua et cum vno
    stipite | ducantur illa albumina
    donec re|uertantur in spumam, et in
45 illa aqua | intingatur bombax,
    postea dimitta|tur aliquantulum
7va residuum et proiciatur || spuma.

Glasgow, GUL, Hunter MS 503, pp. 1–135

    Et in illa aqua intingatis |
    bombacem, et oculis clausis
    super|ponatis decies in die et
    similiter | in nocte usquequo
5   paciens peruenerit | ad perfectam
    sanitatem. Et cum hac | cura
    curabitis quartum panniculum | et
    non cum alijs. Vnde moneo uos |
    karissimi ut caueatis uobis ne in
    is|tis 4 panniculis aliam
10 medicinam | ponere presumatis,
    nisi secundum quod uobis |
    prescripsimus hic supra, quia non |
    debent curari cum pulueribus
    corro|siuis neque cum alijs medi-
    cinis uio|lentis, quia si poneretur
15 dolor super | dolorem augmen-

London, British Library, Sloane MS 661, ff. 32r–46r

Glasgow, GUL, Hunter MS 513, ff. 2r–37r

  Cure of this ys first ye shull make a
cauta|rye in the neysshe of the
heued as ye shull see in | our*e*
cauterijs ¶ And whan ye haue y
10 made a cau|tery take to whites of
eyren and putte hem in | a disshe
that is newe and swynge hem till
they | make skume and afterward
lete it rest ¶ And | after that kest
away that skume and that clere |
water putte theryn a pece of clene
15 cotun & the | ey3en y shitte lay
ther abouen ·x· tymes in the | daye
and ·x· sithes in the nyght till the
pac*ient* be | parfitely hole with this
cures we haue y cured | to the
Fulle the ·I*e* pannicle ¶ For why it
is y pro|uyd and parfitelich it
20 worshippithe the leches craf|te ¶
Wherefore bethe well ware in
these foure | pannicles and bethe
nought bolde to putte other |
medicynes in to the ey3e but thoo
that we haue | wreten to you ¶ For

Oxford, Bodleian Library, Ashmole MS 1468, pp. 1–6

Basel, Ö.B.U., MS D.II.11, ff. 172r–177v

pausar efaita una ora ostatz | la
scuma etaiatz de coton emu|latz
lon en aquelha dels uous | que
roman en aquest emplaus|tre uos 20
mudas .x. uegadas el | jorn e .x.
alanuyt en tro que | sia gueritz ¶
Complit es delaqua|rta maneyra
eson causas proa|das per nos don
uos disem per | sert que nos ne 25
auem assatz cu|ratz daquesta en
fermetat per | gracia dedieu ¶ Et
yeu ben uen|guth uos prec amix
meus e | filhs cars que uos autres
fass|atz segon la mia medescina 30
ese|gon las mias curas prouadas |
eiamais non poyretz errar |

Biblio.-Médiathèques de Metz, MS 176, ff. 1r–16r

taretur et sic | magis obesset quam
prodesset. |

Glasgow, GUL, Hunter MS 503, pp. 1–135

39. Expleuimus uobis tractatum | 4
panniculorum qui generantur in |
oculis ex habundancia sanguinis. |
20 Modo incipiamus, in nomine
Ihesu Christi | et Beatissime Marie
Virginis ac Lu|cie Virginis, de alijs
infirmita|tibus uenientibus in oculis
occa|sione flegmatis. Vnde dicimus
25 quod propter | occasionem
flegmatis in multis hominibus |
superueniunt lacrime in oculis de |
quibus lacrimis generantur tres |
diuerse infirmitates: prima
scilicet | quod propter nimium
30 cursum lacrimarum | mollificantur
palpebre superiores | et in
intrinseca parte palpebrarum |
nascuntur pili, et illi pili pun|gunt

Off the Infyrmitees of flewme, | [50]
And lyke as blode arne | gendryd
obtalmyes | and pannycles. ry3te
so | by occasyon of flewme arnn 5
gendrid | oþer dyuerse sekenes.
and specyally. iiij. | Of whych the
fyrst ys habundance | of terys. by
whos grete fluxe. the | ey lyddys
arnn so molifyed and ma|de soft. 10
þat withyn grow herys. whych |
pryk the balle of the ey con-
tynuelly. | Of whych prykkyng.
the eyon be | so troubled þat the
pacyent may | not opon hys eyonn.
Som boystious | & vnconnyng 15
leches pullen a wey || the herys. [51]

London, British Library, Sloane MS 661, ff. 32r–46r

[39] Here my Author left of to speake any further of | the other 2. panicles. And   39v,18
begineth to speake | of the other infirmityes caused of flegme. | 20
Now like ⌊ as ⌋ of Bloode are ingendred Ophthalmia & | Panicles Even so by occation of
fflegme are in|gendred other diuers syckenesses. and especially | fowre, Of the whitch the
first is abundance of | Teares by whose great fluxe the Eye liddes | are so mollified and   25
made softe, that within them | growe heares, whitch doe continuallye prycke | the Balle
of the Eye Through whitch pryckinge the | Eyes be so trobled, that the patient can not
open | them Some boystarous vncunninge leetches doe | offer to pull them a waye, and   30
the patient fee|leth ease for a tyme: but when the heares | doe growe againe, then the
patient is worse | then before, ffor the more that those heares | be pulled, the greatter and   35

21 Now] Cap. 5° | Of diseases | caused of fflegme.   25 Teares] Of Teares *outer margin*

De Probatissima Arte Oculorum

Glasgow, GUL, Hunter MS 513, ff. 2r–37r

    I do you to vndirstonde þat | these
panincles were neuer withe none
15r other || medecyns that ben violent
but rather they egreg|gyn sorowe
and woo & akthe more on a noþer
woo·/· |

**Of 4 sikenesse þat comeþ of
flume & þe cure of þe** | **first·** |
5 Nowe in the name of criste
begynne we of | the sekenesse that
cometh thorough the ac|casion of
fleume ¶ And we sayne that
tho|rugh accasion of fleume that
teres comyn in | many folkes as in
10 to her ey3en of the which te|res
thre diuers maladies ben
engendred ¶ Wher |for we wole
teche you of the firste ¶ Wherfor |
we saye you that for the grete
cours of teres þe | ouer ey3eliddes
ben ouer moche y neysshed
aboue | that in the ware party

---

3 þe²] **10** *added in outer margin*

Oxford, Bodleian Library, Ashmole MS 1468, pp. 1–6

Basel, Ö.B.U., MS D.II.11, ff. 172r–177v

¶ Aras uos auem dich de la car|ta
especia del panniculi aras | es tot   35
complit del panniculi | Aras uos
uuelh dire delas | autras en fer-
metatz que ue|non als uelhs per
flecma car | perocasion deflecma
motas la|gremas sengenron als   40
uelhs | delas quals lagremas sen
en|genron tres enfermetatz. ¶ Aras
uos uuelh dir la prumey||ra   176va
emfermetatz la qualh sengen|ra per
aquestas lagremas et es | trop mala
es escontra natura | don uos disem
que per las lagre|mas atrops que   5
son laspalpel|as tornon molhas so
es las | sobiranas ededins
naysson | pels efan ponhidura de
dins | los uelhs edaquelha pon-

Biblio.-Médiathèques de Metz, MS 176, ff. 1r–16r

  pupillam oculorum, et pro illa |
  punctione oculi totaliter
35 contur|bantur quod paciens non
  potest | oculos aperire donec pili
  ex toto | eleuentur et extrahentur
  cum | pici cariolis. Vnde aliqui
  stolidi | medici eradicant pilos et
40 illi | vident, sed quando re-
  nascuntur ue|niunt ad deteriorem
  statum, quia | quanto magis
  extrahuntur | tanto magis in-
  grossantur, et pro vno qui ex-
45 trahitur 4 renascuntur et | pungunt
  tanto plus super pu|pillam ocu-
  lorum ut si essent pili por|corum.
7vb Et ex illa punctura oculi || contur-
  bantur et rubescunt tali modo |
  quod paciens non potest aperire
  oculos propter | frequentem
  puncturam pilorum, et | multi sunt
5 qui amittunt lumen cum | tota

---

39 illi] VP2 (f. 298v) patientes *added*

Glasgow, GUL, Hunter MS 503, pp. 1–135

And þan pacyent seeth | for a
tyme. but whenn the herys | growe
a yenn. thann commyth they to |
wors astate. for the more þat þei |
be pullyd. the gretter and the 5
harder | they waxen. And sum
tyme for | oonn growyth .iij. or iiij.
And tho | pryk the eyon as swynes
brystyllis | And trouble so the
eyon that the | pacyent may not 10
vpon hys eyon. | And many lesen
her syght. wyth | all the substance
of þer eyon. by occa|syon of such
heyres. wherfore þis | dyssease
must be cured oþer wyse þan |
thus. 15

---

1 seeth] heares on the | eyes. *added in outer margin in an Elizabethan hand* **14** þan] The cuer *added in outer margin in an Elizabethan hand*

London, British Library, Sloane MS 661, ff. 32r–46r

the harder theye | growe againe, & cause farr more greatter paine || and some tyme for 40r
on groweth .3. or .4. And those pricke | the Eyes like swines bristles. and doe so offend |
the Eyes, that the patient is not able open them | and many doe lose there sighte, with all
the substance | of the Eyes, by occation of those heares. and there|fore this disease muste 5
be otherwise cured.

---

36 paine] and *lower margin*

De Probatissima Arte Oculorum 317

Glasgow, GUL, Hunter MS 513, ff. 2r–37r

15   wexen heres tho that | priken the
balle of the ey3en ben disturbled in
soche | maner that the pacient may
nought open his ey|3en till the
heres be don all away and y
pluc|ked a·way w*ith* smalle
pynsours ·i· whynders ¶ But |
vnderstonde that by suche heres
20   the state of þe | pacient ys moche
y febled in p*ro*cesse of tyme for
|whi the more that the heres ben y
drawyn vp | withe suche
wyndresse so moche the gretter
heres | ther wexen there as they
weren drawyn vp | ¶ And for one
here ther wexen foure or mo that |
25   is so y drawen vp / And thoo
15v   prilken euer more || the balle of
the ey3e as thoughe it were hogg*es*
bris|till so sharpe the be and
sokene // And that for | suche
heres prickyng the ey3en ben
disturblid | and wexen rede in
5   soche maner that the pacient | may

Basel, Ö.B.U., MS D.II.11, ff. 172r–177v

chu|ra los uelhs se corompon el | 10
malautes non pot obrir los | uelhs
entro que los pels ne sian | ostatz
amponcha de agulha e | fam uos
saber quel malaute | torna apeior 15
estament et el sa|peiora entro que
los pelhs sian | natz ¶ Doncas si li
fora melhor | si non agues traitz
los pels | ¶ Don uos fau saber que
aita*n*t | quant los pells son 20
arabatz | aitant tornon pus
grosses. | eper .vn. com ne tratz ne
nays|son quatre ¶ E ponhon los
ditz | pels. los uels coma si erant |
pels deporc. et en la ponchura | 25
dels pels los uelhs si torbon |
etornon fort uermels en aq*ue*s|ta
maneyra que los uelhs | non pot
obrir per lagran pon|chura dels 30
pels de sus ditz E | son trops quen
perdon los ue|lls del tot per la gran
ponchura dels pels. |

Oxford, Bodleian Library, Ashmole MS 1468, pp. 1–6

Biblio.-Médiathèques de Metz, MS 176, ff. 1r–16r

substantia propter occasionem
puncture pilorum. |

Glasgow, GUL, Hunter MS 503, pp. 1–135

40. Audiuistis signa istius egri-
tu|dinis – modo audiatis curam:
Accipi|atis duas acus longas ad
mensu|ram digiti minoris, et
10 habeatis vnum | filum et ponatis
ipsum per foramina | ambarum
acuum, et ligetis bene adinui|cem.
Postea subleuetis palpebram |
superiorem cum digitis uestris et |
accipiatis de corio palpebre cum
15 predictis | acubus, tali modo
quod oculus possit clau|di et
aperiri. Postea ligetis bene acus
ab | utraque parte et dimittatis
donec ca|dant per se cum corio
palpebre. Et | in cicatrice quam

¶ Take ij nedyll of the len||gth of   [52]
thy lytyll fynge*r*. and put a | threde
thorugh the eyon of boyth. & |
bynde þem wele to gydder. than
w*ith* | thy fyngers lyfte vp the
ower ey lyde. | and w*ith* these   5
nedyllys. take so of the | ledder
where theys herys growe þat | the
pacyent may opon & schyt hys |
eyon. And þan bynde wele thyse |
nedlys to gydder at boyth endys, |
And so lett it be tyl the nedyls   10
fall | a way by þem selfe. wyth the
pese | of ledder that was be
tweyne þem. | The whych doon.
put no medycyne | yn the wonde

London, British Library, Sloane MS 661, ff. 32r–46r

[40] Take | 2. nedles of the length of thy little finga*r*, and | put a thridd through the Eyes
of both the nedles | and binde them well together. then w*ith* thy fingars | lifte vpp the   10
over Eye lidd, and w*ith* these medled | take so of the leather where these heares growe |
that the patient maye open and shutt his Eyes: & | then bynde both these together at both
the endes | fast and so let yt rest, till the nedles faull a|waye of them selves. w*ith* the pece   15
of leather *that* | was betwene them The w*hitch* done put no medicine | into the wounde
that the nedles have made, for yt | will heale well of yt selfe. But if any panicle or | other
ranckelyn be bred in the Eye, by reaso of the | paine, that wilbe cured by the powder   20

---

9 fingars] Note here howe | w*ith* out sence Bar|rowe hath penned | yt in his booke wil|linge to
binde the | Needles at both the | endes, before yo*w* | take vpp the skynn. *outer   margin*
20 powder] c *deleted*

De Probatissima Arte Oculorum

Glasgow, GUL, Hunter MS 513, ff. 2r–37r

    nought open his ey3en for the contynuall | prickyng of the heres ¶ And in sum*m*e men the | heres for nemyn lyght w*ith* all the substaunce of | the ey3en For the ofte pricking & many ben of wha*m* | the ey3en thorowe suche occasion ben Distroyed |

10 ¶ And nowe shull teche you of cure after oure | doing moste approuyd and this is the cure // | ¶ Take two long nedill*es* in the lengthe of thi litil | fynger and on the tother side hauethe a threde | and putte it in the two holes of the

15 nedill*es* | and bynde hem well to giders by the holes | ¶ And afterwarde lifte vp the ouer ey3e lid w*ith* | your twey fyngers and ye shull taken of | the hide of the ey3e liddes w*ith* the forsaide | nedill*es* and than bynde hem well to

-----

12 Take] C *added in outer margin*

Oxford, Bodleian Library, Ashmole MS 1468, pp. 1–6

Basel, Ö.B.U., MS D.II.11, ff. 172r–177v

¶ Aras uos auem ditas las en|fermetatz daquesta money|ra delas 35
lagremas e de fleuma | ¶ Aras uos direm las curas | daquesta enfermetat sobre | dicha las quals nos auem fay|tas e prouadas per lonc tem|ps per gracia dedieu. | 40
Prenetz doas agulhas que sian | ayssi longas coma lo det me|nor. edautra part aias filh e || passe 176vb
perlotrauc delas agulh|as. elia ben las agulhas am | lo filh launa apres lautra ep|ueis leuatz ab una man las | palpelhas de sobre. e- 5
prendetz | del angelhot edel canton de la | palpelha am las anguilhas.

319

Biblio.-Médiathèques de Metz, MS 176, ff. 1r–16r

20   acus facient nullam | medicinam
ponatis quia per semetipsam |
saluabitur. Et si pannus in oculis |
fuerit generatus et non fuerit
destructus, | medicetis ipsum cum
puluere nabetis | bis in die usque-
25   quo sanentur et cla|rificentur oculi
pacientis – quia li|berabunt ad
plenum. Et plures inue|nimus de
ista infirmitate in Callabria | quam
in alijs prouincijs et magis reg|nat
in mulieribus quam in hominibus. |

Glasgow, GUL, Hunter MS 503, pp. 1–135

þat the nedlys haue | mayd. for yt   15
shall hele wele ynowe. || by yt   [53]
selfe. but yf any pa*n*nycle or |
rankyll be gendyrde on the ey by
vy|olence of the peyn. And þat
schall | be curyd w*ith* the powder
callyd. Pul|uis nabetus. put yn the   5
ey twyes | on the day tyl the ey be
claryfyed and | ful helyd. And
wyth thys sekenes | of eyon q*uod*
my autor I founde moo | ywoxen
yn Calabur. þen yn ony | oþ*er*   10
pr*o*uynce. And specyally of
wome*n*. |

---

10 women] *§37 follows in the MS*

London, British Library, Sloane MS 661, ff. 32r–46r

called Pul|uis Nabetus. put into the Eye twice everye daye | till yt be healed. And w*ith*
this syckenes of the | Eyes I found more trobled (quoth my Autho*r*) in | Calabria then in
any other province, and especi|allye amongst women.   25

---

25 women] *§37 follows in the MS*

Glasgow, GUL, Hunter MS 513, ff. 2r–37r

20   giders | the ends of thoo nedill*es*
sotilliche in seche | maner that the
ey3en of the pacient may | open
and shitte and afterwarde bynde
hym | well the tone fro the tother /
And thoo ned|ill*es* so y knytte be
16r still till they falle be hem || selfe
w*ith* the skyn of the ey3e lid ¶ And
after | that thoo nedill*es* ben so y
falle doo no medicyn | therto ·i· to
that woundes that the nedill
hauen | y made for it wole hele by
5   hym sylfe / and asonu*s* | or
afterwarde that ey3e that is hirt of
the pric|kyng of thoo heres hele it
w*ith* a wexed clothe | w*ith* the
poudre nabat*is* twies aday till the
ey3e | of the pacient ben y clarified
/ And w*ith* this cure | infinite men
we haue delyu*e*rid and we haue y
10 |wonne herw*ith* moche mony ¶
And many of suche | maladies we
fonde in calebre mo than in any

Basel, Ö.B.U., MS D.II.11, ff. 172r–177v

e | liatz en tal maneyra lacarn | am
las agulhas. que puesca | claure 10
los uels es obrir | es sian las
agulhas ben de cas|cuna part liadas.
elayssas las | agulhas liadas am
baquelh*a* | part carn delas pal-
pelhas en|tro que caian dels uelhs. 15
am | la carn os am lo cuer. e
qua*n*t | seran casutas neguna
mede|cina en aquelha nafra que |
auran faitas las agulhas. | car per 20
se meteis se curara. | ¶ Esi lo
panniculo que sengen|ra de dintre
los uelhs per oc|cayson del
mouement e delh | batement dels
pels non sia | destruc. megga lon 25
am la pol|uera del nabet doas
uegadas | en lo jorn en tro quesian
los | uelhs clars. et am baquesta |
cura nos ne auem geritz motz |
malautes emalautas egasa|nhatz 30

9 puesca] trayr *expunged* **12** las] *final* s *added over the line*
13 baquelha] a *added over the line*

Oxford, Bodleian Library, Ashmole MS 1468, pp. 1–6

Biblio.-Médiathèques de Metz, MS 176, ff. 1r–16r

30 41. Dicimus quod secunda infirmitas est illa quando | oculi apparent turbati et pleni ve|narum et sunt pannosi et paciens non | clare videt. Infirmitatem istam pannum | rubeum vocamus.
35 Audiuistis signa | et hec est cura: primo faciatis ei totum | caput radi et cum cauterio rotundo fa|ciatis ei cauterium in mollicie capitis | et in tymporibus cum cauterio longo | sicut demonstrabimus vobis in
40 cauterijs | nostris. Factis cauterijs mittetis in oculis | de puluere nostro alexandrino semel in | die donec recipiat lumen usque ad ple|num. Et bis in mense purgetur cum | pillulis nostris iherosolomi-

Glasgow, GUL, Hunter MS 503, pp. 1–135

¶ The | second sekenes cawsyd of flewme i*n* | the eyon. ys when þei appere trobled | and ful of venys closed w*ith* a pa*n*nycle | so that the pacyent may not wele | se. And thys sekenes we calle. Pan|nu*m* vitreu*m*. Off whych thys ys the | the cure. ¶ Fyrst at the be-gynny*n*g | doo shaue of all the hede. And than | cauterye hym w*ith* a rounde cauterye | yn the soft of hys hede. And w*ith* a long | caut*er*ye yn hys templys. whych so | doon. put yn hys eyon oonys

[54,2]

5

10

---

4 the] vaines in the | eyes *added in outer margin in an Elizabethan hand*
7 Pannum] The cuer *added in outer margin in an Elizabethan hand*

London, British Library, Sloane MS 661, ff. 32r–46r

[41] The second disease caused of fflegme. in the Eyes | is when theye appeare trobled and full of vaines | closed w*ith* a panicle so that the patient can not | well see, and this disease we calle Pannu*m* vitreu*m* | of w*hitch* this is the Cuer. ffirst at the begininge | shave of the Heare from the head, and then cau|terize him in the softe of the head w*ith* a | rounde Cauterye || and w*ith* a longe cauterye in his temples. w*hitch* done | put into the corners of his Eyes of the powd*er* | of Candye once in the daye till he receave | againe his full sighte And twise in the Mo|neth purge him w*ith* Pillulæ Jerosolomitane | and when

40r,31

35

40v

5

---

31 of] Pulvis Nabetus | what yt is *outer margin* Eyes] The second | disease cau|sed of fleg|me. *outer margin* 35 begininge] The Cuer: *outer margin*

De Probatissima Arte Oculorum 323

Glasgow, GUL, Hunter MS 513, ff. 2r–37r

oþer | coumce & more it wexethe
in wymmen than in men |

**Of þe secunde infirmite & þe
cure therof** |
The secunde infirmite that
15   happethe torugh | the habundance
of teres and by the accasion | of
fleume is this whan the pacient
seiþ | his ey3en apperen trobly and
full of vaynes | and they ben of
smale weystes and the pacient |
seithe nought clereliche ¶ This
20   sikenes we cle|pen pannum
vitreum the glasyn webbe
netheles | ye haue y· herde his
accidence / And the cure of | it is
this First late shaue all his hede

---

13 therof] 11 *added in outer margin*
21 ye] C *added in outer margin*

Oxford, Bodleian Library, Ashmole MS 1468, pp. 1–6

Basel, Ö.B.U., MS D.II.11, ff. 172r–177v

assatz de bos deniers. | ¶ Et auem
ne atrobatz mais. | demalautes de
aquesta malau|tia en la calabria.
que en deguna | part euen plus   35
alas femnas | que non fa als
homes |
¶ Aras uos auem ditas las cu|ras
dela prumeyra enfermetat | que
uen als uelhs per ocasion |
deflecma ede grant habundan|cia   40
delagremas |
¶ Aras uos uuelh dire dela
sego|nda enfermetat que es quant |
los uelhs aparon torbatz eples || de   177ra
uenas eson ples de petitz pan|niculi
el pacient non uetz clar | ¶ Enos
appelham aquesta em|fermetat
panno uitreo. so es | drap de   5
ueyre opanno de ueire | aras uos
auem dit dela segon|da maneyra de
la emfermetat. ¶ Aras uos uuelh
dire lacura | que hom ydeufar.
anaquesta | segonda emfermetat

Biblio.-Médiathèques de Metz, MS 176, ff. 1r–16r

45   tanis et cum | ibit cubitum
recipiat de dyaolibano | nostro. Et
8ra cum istis curis curabitis ||omnem
infirmitatem que procedit ex |
habundancia lacrimarum occasione
flegmatis, | et magis inuenimus de
ista infir|mitate in Tuscia et in
5   Marchia An|chone quam in alijs
prouincijs.

Glasgow, GUL, Hunter MS 503, pp. 1–135

of þis | pouder of candye. onys of   15
the daye. || tyl he receyue ayen ful [55]
sy3te. And | twyes yn the monyth
pourge hym | wythoute wyth
pelett*is* callyd. Pulu|le Jherosolo-
mitane. And when he | goyth to   5
bede. lete hym resceyue of our |
electuarye clepyd. Dyaolibanu*m*
saler|nitanu*m*. tyl he be hole. And
of thys | sekenes. we founde many
mo pacyent*is* | yn tuscia marchia.
þen yn ony oþ*er* | contreys.   10

London, British Library, Sloane MS 661, ff. 32r–46r

he goeth to bedd let him receave of | our Electuarye called Diaolibanu*m* Salernitanu*m* |
till he be well.

---

8 till] Carnositye | in the Eyes | the thirde in|firmitye of | flegme *outer margin*

De Probatissima Arte Oculorum 325

Glasgow, GUL, Hunter MS 513, ff. 2r–37r

    and w*ith* | a longe cauterye as we
16v haue y saide in oure cau||terijs do
to hym the whiche y do putte in to
his ey3e | of oure poudre of
Alisaunder onys in the day till |
the pacient take is sight at the Full
And twyes | in the monthe he shall
be purged w*ith* oure pill | Jersi-
5 tanis whan he shall goo to his
bedde yif | hym of our*e* diaolibano
we haue Cure w*ith* these | thing*es*
moche folke and this euyll
regnethe moste | in tusky and in
marche more þan in any oþ*er*
pr*o*uince |

Basel, Ö.B.U., MS D.II.11, ff. 172r–177v

que uen | per occayson de- 10
lagremas |
¶ Dic uos prumeyrament que |
quant uos ueyretz los malau|tes
ques an aquesta en ferme|tat
segonda. Prumeyrame*n*t | uos lin
fays trayre lo cap efa|itz lin .i. 15
cauteri redon per lo | mal delatesta
eper las temp|las pres delas
aurelhas. cau|teri lonc. e del cap
redon quan | uos auretz los
cauteris. me|tetz de dins los uelhs 20
de la pol|uera nostra alexandrina
ques | fa am bangelhot esarcocolli
co|ma es dich de sobre enla*s*ca-
rac|tas vna uegada lo jorn en|tro 25
que sia gueritz ben euna ue|gada
lomes donatz lin delas | nostra
pillulas ierosolimita|nas sobre
ditas. et am baque|sta cura uos
curatz las emfer|metatz de las 30

---

23 enlascaractas] s *added over the line*

Oxford, Bodleian Library, Ashmole MS 1468, pp. 1–6

Biblio.-Médiathèques de Metz, MS 176, ff. 1r–16r   Glasgow, GUL, Hunter MS 503, pp. 1–135

42. Tercia | infirmitas est illa quando totus oculus | apparet carnosus, et si illa carnosi|tas apparet super oculum indurata | per vnum annum uel per duas uel per | tres uel per plures, non oportet eos me|dicare cum pulueribus neque cum col|lirijs, quia non prodesset ei. Sed prius | faciatis ei radi caput, postea faci|atis ei cauterium sicut fecistis in se|cunda infirmitate. Factis cauterijs in | sequenti die aperiatis oculum pacientis | cum digitis uestris et cum rasorio to|tam illam carnosi-

¶ The thyrde Infirmytee | caused of flewme. when the eye appe|ryth carno*us* or fleshly. whych carno|syte or fleshelynes. yf yt be woxen | harde vpon the eye. a yere. or ij. or | mo. yt may not be

11 apperyth] Carnosity | in the eyes added in outer margin in an Elizabethan hand

London, British Library, Sloane MS 661, ff. 32r–46r

[42] The thirde infirmitye cau|sed of fflewme is when the Eye appeareth | carneous and fflleshye, w*hitch* carnositye & | fflesshines if yt be waxen harde vppon the | Eye a yeare or towe or more It can | not be cured, nether w*ith* powders, nor | Colleryes ffor theye will nothinge avayle. | wherefore as I sayde in the cuer before | the patient*es* heades must be shaved and cau|terized ffirst as I sayd before let him be | cauterized, and the next daye after, open | the Patient*es* Eyes w*ith* yo*r* fingars, and w*ith* | a sharpe Rasor cut of all the carnositye | so warelye that yo*w* toutcht not the tunicle | Salvatrice w*hitch* Johanitius calleth the Con|iunctiue. But rownde about the tunicle | betwixte the blacke nd the white, verye | warelye cutt awaye all the carnositye | whitch done fill the Eye full of the pow|der of Sugar Candye w*ith*out any other | thinge: then let the patient shutt his | Eyes. and laye there on a boulster of | towe wet in the whites of Egg*es*. and for | xv. dayes

Glasgow, GUL, Hunter MS 513, ff. 2r–37r

Of þe maladie of fleume & þe cure of it |

10   THe thride maladye that comethe þourʒ | the accasion of fleume & it is that whan | all the eyʒe apperethe full of Flesshe and | it is in the eyʒe endurid by a yere or to or more | than it behouethe nought
15   to helpe w*ith* poudres | ne w*ith* coll*ir*is for they helpen nought ¶ But first | lete shaue all his hede and afterwarde make | cauterijs as I haue taught in the ·2ᵉ· infirmite |

---

9 Of] 12 *added in outer margin*

Oxford, Bodleian Library, Ashmole MS 1468, pp. 1–6

Basel, Ö.B.U., MS D.II.11, ff. 172r–177v

lagremas dels u|uelhs las quals uenon per | gran flecma Mais quant el | anara dormir manie cascu|na nueitz del nostre lectoari | ques a nom diaolibano. lo | qual   35
atrobaras en lo capitol | delas caractas ¶ E daquesta | emfermetat auem assatz a|trobat en toscana et en la | marca dancona |

¶ E   la terssa emfermetat es | 40
quant lo uelh apar trop carn||os esi   177rb
aquelha carnositat es | de sobre lo uelh eque sia en du|resit. per .i. an o per dos o plus. | nol nos couen a meggar. am | pillulas ni am   5
colliris quar | aprofiecha donc uos lin faretz | rayre latesta prumeyra- ment | epueissas faytz lin .i. cauteri | coma es dit de sobre ¶ Et en lo segon jorn. uos li obretz los | uels al malaute am vostres | detz.   10
etota aquelh carnositat | uos subtilment talharetz en | aital maneyra que non talhes | la tunica

Biblio.-Médiathèques de Metz, MS 176, ff. 1r–16r

tatem eleuetis; et | incidatis ita subtiliter quod tunicam sal|ua-
20 tricem quam Iohannitius vocat coniunctiuam | non tangatis, sed circumcirca tunicam | inter albedinem et nigredinem pau|latim incidatis donec totam carnosita|tem eleuetis. Hoc facto de puluere
25 alexandrino | habeatis et totum oculum sine aliqua | admixtione impleatis, et paciens | claudat oculum et bombacem cum | clara oui superponatis. Deinde usque ad | xv dies cum clara oui bis
30 mutetur | in die. Finito numero dierum dimitta|tis claram oui et superponatis ei em|plastrum de ista herba sanctissima factum, quam | vocamus cardellam – Sarraceni et | Arabes vocant ipsam tusesam,
35 Greci | autem vocant ipsam zucu, Apuli car|ducellum, Salernitani lucucellam, Ro|mani vero vocant ipsam crispignam, | Tusci uero

Glasgow, GUL, Hunter MS 503, pp. 1–135

cured. neiþer wyth || wyth [56]
pouders. neþer coloryus. for it
shuld | no thyng a vayle. wherfore
as I sayd | be fore. the pacyentis
hede must be sha|uynn and
cauteryzede. ¶ Fyrst as | I sayd yn 5
the cure be fore. and on the | nexte
day after. opynn the pacyentis
eyon | wyth your fyngurs. And
with a rasure | cut all the carno-
sytee. so warly and | so sotylly þat

---

15 wyth¹] This kinde of a puste flesshye swellinge | vppon the lower parte of the Eye, vppon | the Coniunctiua, beneth the Cornea: I | hauinge vsed manye remedyes for the | remouinge, or asshawayginge there of | and all in vaine was after cured by | section as our Author sayth. *added in lower margin in an Italic hand* **3 shauynn**] The Chy|rurgicall | Cuer. *added in outer margin in an Italic hand* **8 cut**] NB. *added in outer margin in an Italic hand*

London, British Library, Sloane MS 661, ff. 32r–46r

after chaunge the plaister twice | everye daye. and after xv. dayes make this | plaister
Take a handfull of an herbe cal|led Cardus Benedictus in English Sowthistle | stampe yt
well and mingle yt with halfe the || white of an Egg. and make a pledgett of towe | and 41r
laye yt there on, and applye to the Eye | 3. dayes. Everye daye dressinge yt twice And |
after 3. dayes, leave of all plaisters, & let | the Patient lye with his Eyes open. and 5
everye | daye in the morninge put into the sore Eye of | the Powder called Pulvis
Benedictus. And in | the Eveninge of the powder called Pulvis | Nabetes. till he be
perfectlye well And in | the meane tyme let him abstaine eatinge of | Eeles, Onyans, and 10

---

34 the] white of *lower margin* **7 Pulvis**] It is the powder | of sarcocoll as | before in the | Cuer of Oph|thalmia *outer margin (cross-reference indicated with the astronomical sign of Piscis (♓) in the body of text)*

De Probatissima Arte Oculorum 329

Glasgow, GUL, Hunter MS 513, ff. 2r–37r

¶ whan thoo cauterijs ben y made
in the secu*n*de | day open the ey3e
20 of the pacyent w*ith* your fyn|gres
and kutteþ a way all that Flesshe so
sotil|lyche and so wyseliche· that
the tonicle saluatilla | that
Iohannicius clepethe coniunct*inam*
that it | be nought touched ¶ But
17r all aboute the blake || tonicle
alitill and alitill begynnethe to
kutte and all | that carnosite
holiche lifte hit vp and whan that |
this is y do hauethe of the poudre
of Alisaundre | and all the ey3en
w*ith* outen any other amixtiou*n* |
5 fille it full / and lete the pacient
shitte his ey3e and | lay ther
anoward cotou*n* y wette in the
glayre of | a naye twyes in Aday
and that shall be y conte|nued
fiftene dayes ¶ And whan thoo

Basel, Ö.B.U., MS D.II.11, ff. 172r–177v

la qual apelhon alcus | megges 15
co*rn* iunctiua et entorn | la pupilla
elo blanc de luelh | uos talhares
aysi subtilmens | e pauc epauc en
tro ques aq*ue*|la carnositat sia de
tot ostada | equant aquesta causa 20
auretz | faita metetz de dins lo uelh
d*e* | ben plen delapoluera ale-
xan|drina sensa autra mescla la |
qual es sobredita epueis aiaz |
destopa mulhada o coton e sia | 25
banhatz en clara duou eme|tes de
sobre luelh claus del | malaute.
efay aysso per .xv. | jorns doas
uegadas lo dia:- ¶ E complitz los
jorns. ostan | lo coton desobre los 30
uelhs ¶ E | pueis aias erba sanc-
tissima. | la qual nos apelham
cordelha | episatz lan ben. e-
mesclatzi. una | glayra duou.
emetetz lo | de sobre luelh am 35

---

23 blake] tonicle *added in lower margin*

16 luelh] u *expunged* 34 lo] uel *expunged*

Oxford, Bodleian Library, Ashmole MS 1468, pp. 1–6

Biblio.-Médiathèques de Metz, MS 176, ff. 1r–16r

  vocant ipsam citebitom, Sar|di
uocant ipsam lammomiam. Vnde |
40 dicimus vobis: ℞ de ea manipulus
1 et piste|tur bene et cum ea
misceatur me|dia clara oui et
ponatis super bom|bacem uel super
stuppam, et super oculum | ponatis
bis in die scilicet mane et [sero] |
45 usque ad 3 dies. Et sic dimittatis
em|plastrum et paciens semper
maneat oculis | apertis. Sed tamen
8rb deinde curatur cum istis || pulue-
ribus usque ad sanitatem, scilicet
de | puluere alexandrino in mane
et | puluere nabetis in sero, et
interim | custodiat se a cibis
5 contrarijs sicut sunt | anguille
fungi carnes bouine hir|cine
caprine salatine, a caseo et| cepis et
allijs acruminibus et legumini|bus
et sic de similibus. Et cum istis |

---

44 sero] M loco, VP2 (f. 296r), VR
(f. 38v) sero

Glasgow, GUL, Hunter MS 503, pp. 1–135

ȝe touche not the tony|cle. Salua- 10
tryce. whych iohannyci*us* | clepyth
the co*n*iunctyfe. but rounde | a
bowt the tonycle be twene the
blak | and the whyte soft and
sotylly cut | yt tyll ȝe haue reysed
all the carno|sytee. whych so 15
doon. fyll the ey ful || of the [57]
powd*er* of Candie wi*th*out ony |
oþ*er* thyng. then doo the pacyent
shitt | hys ey. And þ*er*on ley a
plaster of | coton or of flaxen
herdys wyth | the whytte of an 5
egg. And xv days | after chaunge
the plaster twyes | on a day. And
aft*er* xv. days make | thys plaster.
¶ Take and hand|ful of an herbe
callyd. Cardus be|nedictus. Sow- 10
thystyl yn englych. | stampe yt
wele and medyl yt wi*th* | halfe the
whyte of an*n* egg. and | make a
plaster of coton or flaxen | herdys.
and ley yt on the ey iij. | days 15
remeuyng the plaster eu*ery* || daye. [58]

London, British Library, Sloane MS 661, ff. 32r–46r

Beefe. and all other quesye | meates. and w*ith* these manner of medicines | quoth my
Autho*r* I have cured a great nu*m*ber. | of people.

De Probatissima Arte Oculorum 331

Glasgow, GUL, Hunter MS 513, ff. 2r–37r

    dayes ben | fulfilled leue that
10 glaire of the ay and takethe | this
holy herbe that is y clepit Cardus
benedict*is* | Romayns clepen it
Crispinam with glaire of a·naye |
stampe it and grynde hem as a
plaster and leye it | on coton or
flexe and do it on the ey3e twyes
on | the daye ·s· erliche and at
15 euen And than do yn | of this
poudre till the pacient be alsso hole
as | he was that it is to saye of the
poudre of Alysaun|der at the
morwe and of the poudre nabatis
at | euen ¶ And ferthermore kepe
hym from contra|rie metes as from
20 elys conger beef bere flesshe | and
gotys and from chese and from
rawe oynons | from potages / And
w*ith* these curis we haue he|led
moche folke ¶ And this infirmite
17v habundeþ || moste in sardine in
poile than in any oþere prouinc*es*
·/·

Basel, Ö.B.U., MS D.II.11, ff. 172r–177v

coton o am | bestopa. doas uega-
das en lo | jorn. elo matin el
uespre. epu|eis meti dedins lo uelh
dela | poluera sobre dita alexan-
dri|na en lomatin. e de la pol- 40
uera | del nabeth al uespre egarde
se | decausas contrariosas so es
a||saber danguilhas. edecebas. 177va
ede | legums. ederbas uertz. E de
car|n de buou ede carn deboc ed*e*
ca|bra. ede totas autras malas
ui|andas. edaquesta enfermet|tat 5
an mais en serdenha que | en autra
part enos auem ne | assatz
gazanhat da questa en|fermetat |

Oxford, Bodleian Library, Ashmole MS 1468, pp. 1–6

Biblio.-Médiathèques de Metz, MS 176, ff. 1r–16r

    curis infinitos homines curauimus |
10 et liberauimus, et magis inue-
nimus de | ista infirmitate in
Sardinia quam in | alijs prouincijs.

43. Dicimus quod quarta | infir-
mitas est illa quando oculi semper
apparent inflati et semper lacri-
15 mantur | et paciens non potest
aperire oculos propter | pondero-
sitatem palpebrarum superiorum. |

Glasgow, GUL, Hunter MS 503, pp. 1–135

eche day twyes. morn & yeue. |
And after iij. dayes complete.
leue | all plasters. and lete the
pacyent | lye wyth open ey. And
eue*ry* daye | at morn. put yn the   5
sore eyon. of | the powd*er* callyd.
Puluis bened*ic*tus. | And at eue. of
the powder callyde. | Puluis
nabetus. tyl he be p*er*fy3tly | hoole.
And yn the meane tyme. let | hym   10
abstene hym from elys. oyne|ones.
& befe. and all oþ*er* queysy
metys. | And w*ith* thys man*er* of
medycyne q*uo*d | my*n* autor. I
haue holpen & curede | wi*th*out
nombre. of people. Of thys |
sekenys q*uo*d he I fonde mo In   15
sardo||nia. than yn oþ*er* countrees.   [59]

¶ The | forth sekenes causyd of
flewme yn | the ey. is when the
eyon epere bolle|yn. and be all

---

3 bolleyn] swollen eyes | with
weping *added in outer margin in an
Elizabethan hand*

London, British Library, Sloane MS 661, ff. 32r–46r

[43] The fourth syckenes caused | of fflegme in the Eye, is, when the Eye | appears   15
swollen and all waise weepinge, & | the patient can not open his Eyes for the |
ponderousnes and heavines of the vpper Eye | lydd*es*. And if yow will trulye vnderstand |
of this sickenes, turne vpp the ou*er* Eye | lidd w*ith* yo*r* fingu*r*, and yow shall see yt to | 20
appeare all fattye. and the fattnes wille | like vnto the graines of Milliu*m* And this |
disease is called the scabb ˪in˩ the Eye. And | is caused of abundance of Salte flegme | 25
ffor the Cuer where of yo*w* must first | purge the stomacke and the Braine w*ith* this |

---

14 caused] The fourth | disease of the | Eye caused | of Flegme *outer*   margin **15** when] *a
elongated minim like that frequently used at the beginning of an* n *or an* m *is deleted after this
word* **18** Eye] Teares *outer margin* **24** in] off *deleted*, in *added over deletion* And] The Scabb
in | the Eye *outer margin* **26** first] p *deleted*

Glasgow, GUL, Hunter MS 513, ff. 2r–37r *Basel, Ö.B.U., MS D.II.11, ff. 172r–177v*

Of | the ·4· maladie of fleume &   ¶ Oras uos uuelh dir dela quar|ta   10
the cure of it | emfermetat que uen perla | flecma
THe ferthe infirmite that comethe   efa lagremeiar los uels | la carta es
thorugh | occasiou*n* of fleume   cant los uelhs son | efla ttz
  elagremeggon el malau|tes non   15
─────────────   pot ben obrir los uels | per la
2 the] 13 *added in outer margin*

Oxford, Bodleian Library, Ashmole MS 1468, pp. 1–6

Biblio.-Médiathèques de Metz, MS 176, ff. 1r–16r

    Vnde quando vultis certificari de ista | egritudine, reuersetis palpebram | superiorem cum digitis
20 uestris sursum | et videbitis eam quasi pinguem, et | illa pinguedo apparet quasi caracta|rata et graciosa sicut grana milij, | et Arabes et Sarraceni vocant infir|mitatem istam iarafimnaxin, id
25 est | scabies in oculis. Vnde sciatis quod hoc | accidit ex habundancia flegmatis | salsi, et cum videbitis talem infir|mitatem: primo purgetis ei stomacum | et cerebrum cum rebus istis: ℞
30 turbit, | aloe, epatici, reubarbi, ana ʒ 1, ex alia | parte habeatis sucum radicis ebuli | ℔ 1 et dissoluatur in simul cum | predictis rebus et dimittatis sic | stare
35 per totam noctem et in sum|mo

---

24 iarafimnaxin] VP2 (f. 300r) raxasumicaxin

Glasgow, GUL, Hunter MS 503, pp. 1–135

weys wepyng. and | the pacyent   5
may not opyn hys eyon. | for the
ponderosyte and the heuynes | of
the ouerlyddys. and yf ȝe wyll |
quod he be verryly certyfyed of
thys | sekenes. turne the ouerlydde
of the ey. | with your fyngers.   10
And ȝe schal se yt ap|pere all fatty.
And the fatnes shall | be greynous
asmuch as the greynes of | myle.
whych sekenes sarasyns and | yn
arabye ys callyd. Iherafrumax|yn,   15
þat ys to sey. scab yn the eye. ‖
And thys sekenes ys gendred of   [60]
super|habundance of salt flewme.
To why|ch sekenes. do thys cure
fyrst. ȝe must | pourge the stomake
& the brayn of | the pacyent. with   5
þis resceyte. Take | turbyt. Aloes.

---

6 heuynes] teares *added in outer margin in a late hand* 10 appere] fattines *added in outer margin in an Italic hand* 6 turbyt] Johan *added in outer margin in a late hand*

London, British Library, Sloane MS 661, ff. 32r–46r

medicine followinge Take of Turbith, Aloes, | Rubarbe of etch ʒ j. of the Juyce of ↓ the roote of ↓ walworte | a pounde let the foresayde things be powdred | and verye well   30
mixed with the sayde Juyce | & let yt so stand all nighte, and be tymes | in the morninge straine yt and let the ‖ patient take there of fastinge a good quantitye | and on the nexte   41v
daye after, with yor fingars | torne vpp the Eye liddes, and with a hooke or a needle and thridd lifte vpp the Carnositye & | then with a Rasor cutt of that flesshye | fattnes from   5
vnder the Eye liddes, Even from | the on lacrimall to the other. whitch beinge done | laye vppon the Eye a pledgett of towe wett in | the whites of Egges. and renew yt twice eve|rye daye. for the space of nyne dayes. And | then for the spare of 3. dayes followinge   10

---

33 the¹] patient *outer margin* 5 cutt] y *deleted*

De Probatissima Arte Oculorum

Glasgow, GUL, Hunter MS 513, ff. 2r–37r

5   enchesonde in to the ey3en | is
    whan the ey3en apperen for swolle
    and | ben alway Full of teres and
    the pacient may no|ught open his
    ey3en for the heuynes of the ouer
    |brouys wherfor we shull teche you
    whan ye | wole be y certefied of
10 this maladie ouer turne | the ouer
    ey3e liddes w*ith* your fynggres
    vpward | and ye shall y see it as it
    were fattynes and þ*at* | fattynes is
    y warred and kyrneled as it were |
    kyrnell of myle sede wherfore my
    dere frendes | ye shull wetyn that
15 it happethe of the habundau|nce
    of salte fleume ¶ And yef ye seyn
    suche a ma|ladie First ye doo
    purgen the stomake and the bray|ne
    w*ith* these thing*es* ¶ Take turbit
    aloes epat*icus* reu|barbe ana ·℥·iiij·
    and on that other side hauethe |
    drie rotis of walworthe ·℔·j· and

15 maladie] ℞ *added in outer margin*

Oxford, Bodleian Library, Ashmole MS 1468, pp. 1–6

Basel, Ö.B.U., MS D.II.11, ff. 172r–177v

greuesa dels palpelhas | ques
aparon greuas epesans | equant uos
uolretz esser sertz | da quelha en
fermetat tenesi | assatz las   20
palpelhas de sobre | am uostres
detz. e uos uenrez | desobre
desobre coma vn gras | et aquel
gras apar quassada | e carnosa
coma gran demilh | et anom   25
ronha delhs uelhs | e dic uos que
quant uos uey|retz aquesta enfer-
metat uos | lon purgaretz en
aquesta ma|neyra. quar uen de
flecma | salsa ¶ Tupren turbis   30
aloe ep|aticum. reubarbaro. ℥ ·ß. e
da|utra part aias desuc de ebuli |
vna liura efay disolure am
a|quelhas cauzas sobre ditas |
elayssa o estar en tro almati | 35
epueis colatz o. epueis prenga |
lacolha dura et al segon dia |
obretz los uelhs ereseruatz | las
palpelhas am uostres | detz etota   40
aquelha carnosi|tat uos lin curaretz

Biblio.-Médiathèques de Metz, MS 176, ff. 1r–16r

  mane coletur, et paciens su|mat de
illa colatura et in sequenti | die
aperiatis oculum pacientis et |
reuersetis palpebram cum digi|tis
uestris. Et tota illa carnositas |
40 cum uncino et rasorio eleuetur |
et incipiatis incidere ab vna parte |
lacrimalis usque ad aliam, et
totam | illam pinguedinem in-
tegram eleue|tis, scilicet que est
45 sub palpebra et ap|paret grossa. Et
leuata carnosita|te bambacem
8va intinctum clara oui su||perponatis
oculo bis in die usque | ad ix dies
et postea de nono die in|antea
ponatis de emplastro grosso | bis
in die usque in tercium diem.
5 De|inde semper maneat tamen
oculis aper|tis et semper in sero
ponatis in o|culo de collirio nostro
alexandrino | usque ad perfectam
firmitatem et sani|tatem. Et cum
10 hac cura innumerabiles | homines
curauimus et liberauimus. | Et

Glasgow, GUL, Hunter MS 503, pp. 1–135

epatyk. Rubarbe. lyche | of ycche
an vnc*er*. then take the Juce | of
the roote of walworte a pounde |
and the forseyd thyng*is* pond*er*ed
& resol|uyd yn the sayd Jus. And 10
let yt stond | all a nyght. and be
tyme or the morn*n* | clense yt. and
lete the pacyent ta|ke þ*er*of fastyng
a good quantite. and | on*n* the
nexte day after that wyth y*our* |
fyngurs tornyth the ey lyddys. 15
And || softly w*ith* a twycche lyft [61]
the carnositee. | And w*ith* a rasure
be gynne to cut the | greynes yn
fatnese tha ys vnd*er* the | eyelede.
euyn from that oon lacrymal | to 5
the tooþ*er*. whych doon. plaster
the | eye wyth herdys. & the
whytte of | an egg. And so do ix
days eche daye | chaungyng the
plaster twyes. And | after the ix
days. lay þ*er*to the playst*er* |
graciou*s* a forseyd. twyes on the 10
daye. | iij days foloyng. after

London, British Library, Sloane MS 661, ff. 32r–46r

applye | vnto yt the plaister Gratious afore Sayde, re|newinge yt twice everye daye. After
whitch | tyme let the patient have his Eye open And | allwaise at Even to put into his 15
Eye of | our powder called Colleriu*m* Alexandrinu*m* | (w*h*itch is taughte before in the
Cuer of the .3. | panicle.) till he be p*er*fectlye holle. And w*ith* | this sayth my Author I
have cured mutch | people 20

---

12 plaister] I thinke he | meaneth that | of Cardus Bene|dictus w*h*itch he | Englisheth Sow| thistle *outer margin (cross-reference indicated with the astronomical sign of Mars (♂) in the body of text)* **17** whitch] My booke from | whence I tooke | this coppye, did | want the tracte | of the .3. and 4. | panicle: And [the *deleted*] | therefore I doe | not vnderstand | what he meane|th. by his Colle|riu*m* Alexandri|nu*m*. And Bar|row in his Method, of Phisike, | stealinge all | out of this Au|thor, w*ith* out once | naminge him, paßeth maye | of these faulte*s* | & doth seme | not to vnder|stand them. *outer margin*

De Probatissima Arte Oculorum 337

Glasgow, GUL, Hunter MS 513, ff. 2r–37r

20 dissolue hem to |geders w*ith* the
    forsaide thinges w*ith* ℔·ß of hote
    wa|ter and lete hem stonde so all a
    nyght and erliche | clense it and
    yif to the pac*ient* to Dryngke that |
    pocou*n* of this colature and on the
18r secunde daye || ye shull open the
    pac*ient* ei3e and ouer turne the
    ey3e |liddes withe your fyngers and
    all that fattnys ye | shull lifte it vp
    withe a ku*t*tyng rasour and ye
    shull | begynnen at the on
    lacrimall place and kutte to þe |
5   tother lacrimall place all holiche
    all that fathede | a way the whiche
    duellethe and apperethe corny wiþ
    |in forthe and putte on the ey3e
    w*ith*outforthe cotun y wet|te in
    glayre of aneye twies on aday erly
    and late ·ix | dayes ¶ And when all
10 this is don after þe ix day|es laye
    on the eye of oure plastre graciose
    the whi|che ys y made of Cardus
    benedictus w*ith* the white | of

Oxford, Bodleian Library, Ashmole MS 1468, pp. 1–6

Basel, Ö.B.U., MS D.II.11, ff. 172r–177v

am lo ras|or ben afilat etalan
ecome*n*salo | atalhar am lorasor
delapart | lacremal so es delblanc
de ues || laurelha en ro alautra   177vb
part | etota aquelha gra*y*ssa ostatz
lan | enteyrament la qual esta
sota | lapalpelha delapart carnosa
e | quant uos auretz leuada la | 5
carnositat metetz din sobre | luelh
de coton mulhath en cla|ra duou
emetetz |

2 grayssa] y *added over the line*

Biblio.-Médiathèques de Metz, MS 176, ff. 1r–16r

magis inuenimus de ista infir|mitate in Hobaria inter saracenos | quam in alijs prouincijs.

Glasgow, GUL, Hunter MS 503, pp. 1–135

whych tyme. | lat the pacyent haue hys eyon opyn. | And alwey at yeven. put yn hys ey | of oure colerye callyd, Colerium alex|andrinum, whych ys tau3t before yn || the cure of the thyrde pannycle tyl he | be perfytely hoole. And wyth thys quod | he I haue curyd muche people. and | of thys sekenes sekenes I founde mo|yste yn barbarye a mong the sara|syns.

15

[62]

5

44. Et quando fui|mus in partibus illis inuenimus | feminas Sarracenicas que faciebant | istam curam hoc modo: accipiebant | frondes arbore ficuum et reuer-

And when I was þer quod he. I | fonde women vsyng thys cure. They | tooke the braunches of the fyg tree. | and turnyd the eye lyddys. And with | the leuys they

10

London, British Library, Sloane MS 661, ff. 32r–46r

[44] I have allso knowne sayth he wo|men for this Cuer to take of the Braunches | of the figg tree, and torned the Eye liddes | And with the leaves theye rubbed the sore place | till the Eye liddes wer all blodye & manye | wer amended there by but yt lasted not | longe but yt reversed againe And some | did rubb that fattines with Sugar, ₁ & ₁ for a tyme | theye wer amended but yt did quickelye | after retorne into the pristine estate.

25

---

21 to] ta *deleted*

Glasgow, GUL, Hunter MS 513, ff. 2r–37r

aneye as it is y saide in the Chapitre afore & | conteyne this twies aday by thre daies y con|teyned · and in the ey3e putte
15 of oure collerie of | Alisaunder as it is said a fore at begynnyng of | the first chapitre of the maladies of blode and | as we shulle writen in the ende of this tretise | of the collerijs of ey3en and of the ey3e liddis | ye shull fynde the whiche
20 all they reseyue to|thie of Alisaundre and of this collerie the pac*ient* | shall vsen till he be hole at the Fulle and de|lyuered · and of this maladie ye shull fynde moste | in barbarie and amonge sara3eyns
18v mo of hem || than in any other prouinc*es*

Basel, Ö.B.U., MS D.II.11, ff. 172r–177v

[...] per cantas uegadas lanafra *sera* [...] |

Oxford, Bodleian Library, Ashmole MS 1468, pp. 1–6

Biblio.-Médiathèques de Metz, MS 176, ff. 1r–16r

sa|bant palpebram sursum et frica|bant donec palpebre erant
20 sangui|nolente. Et multi de illis preualebant | tamen non diu permanebant in eodem | statu. Et multi alij accipiebant | zucarum et fricabant super illam | carnosi-
25 tatem et conualescebant, | sed deinde tamen in paucis diebus reuer|tebantur in eodem statu – ideo quia | non erant curati secundum Artem Nostram | Probatissimam Oculorum.

45. Docui|mus uobis causam et
30 curam istius | quarte infirmitatis que prouenit | occasione lacrimarum habundantium in | oculis ex flegmate. Modo docebimus | vos mirabile electuarium pro illis | dictis lacrimis: ℞ olibani, castorei,
35 nu |cum muscatorum, nucis Indie, gariofili, cubebe | ana ʒ 1, folij lauri, spice narde, croci, | cardamomi ana quartam partem ʒ,

Glasgow, GUL, Hunter MS 503, pp. 1–135

rubbyd the sore place | tyl the ey ledys weren all blodye, | and many were amendyd þerby. | but yt lastyd not long. And som | rubbyd þat fatnes wyth suger for | a tyme 15
þei were a mendyd. but soon ||
after yt tornyd ayen into the [63]
fyrste | estate,

¶ And now I wyl teche yow | practysers a merveilous and a prescious lec|tuarye for the forsayd terys. and | yt ys thys. Take ¶ 5
Olibani castorij. | Nootmyggis. nucys Indie. Clouys. | Cubibes. ana an vncer. And of the | leuys of laurei. spynarde. saferon. |

---

3 lectuarye] againste | teares *added in outer margin in an Elizabethan hand*

London, British Library, Sloane MS 661, ff. 32r–46r

[45] And | now (sayth he) I will teatch yow practizers | a mervelous & a pretious 30
Electuarye for | the fooresayd teares, and yt is thus made | Take of Olibanum of
Castoreum, of Nut|megges, of Nux Indica, of Cloves of || Cubibes of etch ʒ j. of the 42r
leaves of Laurej. | of Spignarde. of Safforne of Cardamomi | ana ʒ ij of Seedes of dill of
Smalage of Ba|silicon of Alexanders of Aniseedes & of ffe|nell seedes of etch ʒ ß. Pulyal, 5
Hysope Seedes | of Rewe ana ʒ iiij Sede of Henbane white | Poppye Muske Camphere
ana ʒ j. Beate all | these to powder & searse them verye finelye | except the Olibanum
ffor that must be boy|led in clarified Honye till yt be thorowlye | melted & dissolved. 10

---

34 of^t] Cubibes *lower margin* 1 Laurej] An excellent | Electuarye for | teares in the | Eyes. *outer margin* 5 Seedes] This recept don [dot *a. corr.*] | mutch differ | from that set | out by Barrow | in his Method | of Phisicke. *outer margin*

Glasgow, GUL, Hunter MS 513, ff. 2r–37r   *Basel, Ö.B.U., MS D.II.11, ff. 172r–177v*

¶ Of the meruelous electu|chi for teres of ey3en the whiche comen thorowe oc|casion of fleume and it is y made thus ¶ Take oli|bani castor notemug*es* notis of ynde
5   clowys safrou*n* | cardamo*n*i an*a* ·ℨ·j folia lauri spice nardi ana | semen aneti apij basilico*n*is carui

2 occasion] ℞ *added in outer margin*
5 ana] *a word, now effectively effaced, follows*

Oxford, Bodleian Library, Ashmole MS 1468, pp. 1–6

Biblio.-Médiathèques de Metz, MS 176, ff. 1r–16r

  seminis | aneti, seminis apij,
seminis basiliconis, carui, | anisi,
seminis alexandrini et feniculi
40 ana | ʒ ß, nepitelle sicce, pulegij,
ysopi, | seminis rute ana ℈ 4,
seminis iusquami, | papaueris albi,
musci, camphore, ana | ℈ 1, et hec
omnia puluerizentur et cri|bellentur
45 subtiliter. Ponitur olibanum | quod
debet bullire cum bono melle |
despumato; liquefacto olibano cum
8vb || melle, remoueatur ab igne et
reuer|setur in vna magna parapside
cum | alijs speciebus et ducantur
bene quousque | cum melle
incorporentur, et in pixide |
5 reseruetur et semper cum medica-
ueritis | infirmos uestros, in sero
detis de hoc ad | commedendum
cum iuerint dormitum | ad modum
et quantitatem vnius castanee. |

Glasgow, GUL, Hunter MS 503, pp. 1–135

Cardomomi. ana a quartron.
halfe | ann vncer seedys of dylle. 10
of sma|lache. basylycon seede. of
alexandre. | of annes. and of fenel
ana halfe | an vncer. drye neppe.
pulyal. ysop. | sede of rewe. ana
iiij drammes. se|ed of henbane. 15
whytte popee. muske. || Campher [64]
ana a dram. bete all thyes | to
powder. and sotylly sarce them.
sa|ue the olybanum. þat must be
boylyde | wyth claryfyed hony tyl
yt be moston. | Than take yt from 5
the fyre. and pow|er yt yn to a feir
plater large and of | tree. wyth the
oþer powders. and wyth | a lytyl
ladyl styre yt to gyddyr. tyll | the
spycys be yncorperate wyth the
ho|ny. And lete yt be kept styll yn 10
the | same plater. And ȝe shall
cure your | pacyentis. yeue them at
yeue. when | þei goo to bede of
thys lectuarye the | quantite of a
chesteyne.

London, British Library, Sloane MS 661, ff. 32r–46r

Then take yt from | the fyer & power yt into a fayre plattar. | verye large And mixe there
with the other | powders stirringe them verye well together. | and let yt be kepte still in 15
the same plattar | And at nighte when yor patientes goe to bedd | geve them the quantitye
of a Chestnutt of | this Electuarye

Glasgow, GUL, Hunter MS 513, ff. 2r–37r   *Basel, Ö.B.U., MS D.II.11, ff. 172r–177v*

    macedonici fen*iculum* ana |
quarter·ʒᵉ·j se*m*is papau*er*is allse
iusq*u*iami al an*a* ʒ·j muske |
camphor an*a* ·ʒ·ß· all these sotil-
liche shull be grounde | to right
sotill poudre and w*ith* a sotill sarce
10 hem on|taken   olibanu*m* the
whiche shall be y soden in good |
clene skemed hony and whan that
olybanu*m* ys y |lequefied w*ith* the
hony Do it in to aplater and | ther
the spices forsaide medle hem to
geders and | well encorp*a*re hem
& kepe w*ith* the hony that
15 oliba|nu*m*   was relented yn and
than doo it in to a· | boxe & kepe it
to thi store and yeue of this
letua|rye the mou*n*taunce of a
chestayne at ones

Oxford, Bodleian Library, Ashmole MS 1468, pp. 1–6

344　　　　　　　　　　　　　　　　　　　　De Probatissima Arte Oculorum

Biblio.-Médiathèques de Metz, MS 176, ff. 1r–16r

     46. Scripsimus uobis mirabile
10 electuarium | pro lacrimis que
semper habundant in ocu|lis, et ita
vocamus ipsum quia mirabi|lia
facit mirabiliter: lacrimas constrin-
git, | flegmata destruit, cerebrum
calefacit, dolorem | emigraneum
15 expellit, oculos aperit, su|percilia
releuat, lumen clarificat – et eti|am
valet ad illos qui paciuntur para-
li|sim et amittunt loquelam et
impedite | loquuntur. Et nos
probauimus et sicut scrip|simus
inuenimus, quia innumerabiles
20 ho|mines cum ipso liberauimus et
curauimus. |
     47. Modo incipiamus in nomine
Ihesu de | aliis infirmitatibus que
ueniunt | in oculis occasione
colere, et inde sciatis | quod sint
due. Dicimus ergo quod prima
25 in|firmitas accidit ex fumositate
colere super|habundantis in
stomaco, vnde resoluitur | ex ea

Glasgow, GUL, Hunter MS 503, pp. 1–135

And thys lec|tuarye. q*u*od he ys   15
callyd meruelo*us* || and p*re*scious. [65]
For yt doth many p*re*sciou*s* |
m*er*uele*us*. hyt dystroyth the teres
& | flewme. yt warmyth the brayn.
it | puttyth a wey the peyne of the
my|greyme. It openyth the eyon. It   5
re|leuyth the ey lyddys and
clarifyth | the syght. It ys also
good for th*e* eyon | þat haue the
gowte and the palsye. | Item for
them þat haue loost their | speche. 10
or haue impedyment yn | spekyng.
Althyes I haue p*re*uyd | q*u*od he.
And as I here wryte. so ha|ue I
founde & manny haue I holpen. |
Off the infirmytees causyd of |
Coolore. || 15

---

15 meruelous] & p*re*sciou*s* *added in*
lower margin 7 the[1] e *added over*
the line 8 palsye] gout and | palsi
and for | the eyes *added in outer*
margin in an Elizabethan hand

London, British Library, Sloane MS 661, ff. 32r–46r

[46] And this Electuarye is | quoth ↓ the ↓ Author called mervalous & pretious | for yt 20
doth destroye the teares, and flegme, yt | warmeth the braine yt putteth a waye *the* paine |
of the Megrim, yt openeth the Eyes, yt releveth | the. Eye lidd*es* and clarifieth the sighte
It | is allso good, for the gowte, and the paulseye | in the Eyes, and for them that have 25
loste | there spetch All these (sayth my Auth*or*) have | I proved, and have holpen
manye./ |
[47] Cap. 6°. of Infirmities caused | of Choller. |
Now will I intreat of those diseases of | the Eyes caused of Choller w*hitch* be towe in | 30
number, And the first is caused of super|abundance of Choller in the stomacke, from ||

---

22 releveth] releceth *before the correction* 23 It] ffor the Gowte | & Paulseye in | the Eyes.
outer margin 28 caused] Cap. 6°. *outer margin* 33 from] whence is *lower margin*

Glasgow, GUL, Hunter MS 513, ff. 2r–37r

    And | we clepe it meruelous For it
dothe many woun|dres it
constraynethe and stoppethe teres
20 it dis|troieth fleume / it hetethe
the brayne it fordothe þe | akþe
and the penaunce of the mygrayne·
· It opo|nethe the ey3en it releuyght
the brouwis and clereþ | the sight

**Of ·2· maners of occasiouns of |
coler & the cure of the first** ||
19r THorowe the accasion of colre two
sekenesses | fallethe in the ey3en /
And we sayen that | the first
infirmite the whiche that falleþ |

Basel, Ö.B.U., MS D.II.11, ff. 172r–177v

---

23 coler] 14 *added in outer margin*

Oxford, Bodleian Library, Ashmole MS 1468, pp. 1–6

Biblio.-Médiathèques de Metz, MS 176, ff. 1r–16r

quedam fumositas et ascendit ad | cerebrum cum magno furore et dolore. | Et propter illum dolorem
30 oculi conturbantur | tali modo quod inter oculos pacientis et | rem visam apparet quasi vmbra, sed | tamen oculi apparent clari ita quod non | videtur intus nec extra aliqua | macula in oculis. Sciatis
35 ergo karissimi quod | peccatum non est in oculis sed in stomaco. Igitur | karissimi si oculi sunt clari in intrinseca | parte nulla medicina in oculo talium | valet – quia si puluis esset corrosiuus, cor|roderet tunicam, et collirium si esset |
40 corrosiuum excitaret reuma per totum | cerebrum.

Glasgow, GUL, Hunter MS 503, pp. 1–135

Now after thys quod the autor | I [66]
shall trete of the sekenes | of the
eyon causyd of co|ler. whych byth
ij. wherof. the first | ys causyd of 5
superhabundance of co|ler yn the
stomake. Of the whych | ys
resoluyd a corrupte fumosytie | þat
ascendyth vp to the brayn with |
greete furowre & pyne. wherof
the | eyon be so troublyd þat be 10
twene | þem and their obiecte. þat
ys the | thyng. ys yn the maner of
ashadowe | or a clowde. and yit
the eyon a|pere feire & bryght.
And neiþer yn | the eyon. nor 15
wythoute. ys no spot. || aperyng. [67]
and þerfore. the defaute of | thys
ys not yn the eye. but in the |
stomake. and þerfore no
medycyne | schalbe put yn the ey.
but in the | stomake. And the cure 5

1 Now] of sicknes of the eies caused of | Collor *added in upper margin in an Elizabethan hand*

London, British Library, Sloane MS 661, ff. 32r–46r

whence is resolved a corrupte fumositye that | ascendeth vpp to the braine with great 42v
furye | and paine whitch doth so troble the Eye, that | betwene them and there obiecte,
there doth ʟ seme to ˩ ap|peare as yt wer a clowde or a shadowe, | to the Patient, and yet 5
the Eyes appeare | fayre and brighte, and nether within the | Eyes, nor without, there is
no spott appea|ringe, and therefore the fault of this is | not in the Eye: but in the 10
Stomacke, and | therefore no medicine is to be put into the | Eyes but to the stomacke.
whitch shall swage | the paine, & open the opilations of the sy|nowes, that the visible
spiritt maye the | more freelye passe. 15

5 shadowe] & *deleted*

Glasgow, GUL, Hunter MS 513, ff. 2r–37r *Basel, Ö.B.U., MS D.II.11, ff. 172r–177v*

    of the fumosite of colre whiche is
5   in the stomake of | the pac*ient*
    where of a·maner of fumosite ys
    resolued | and it ascendethe in to
    the brayne w*ith* a grete wode|nes
    and brennyng and fore that
    penaunce the | ey3en ben dis-
    trobled in so moche that it
    shewithe in | the pacientes ey3e as
10 it were ashadowe ¶ But | whan
    the ey3en of suche ben y opened
    we se no|ught w*ith* inne ne w*ith*
    oute to haue any spotte ·i· ma|cu*l*la
    in the ey3e But in the stomake and
    in the bray|ne ys the cause of that
    maladie and the mat*er*ie | ther of
    wherfor my dere frendes whan ye
15 fyn|de suche and the ey3en ben
    clere w*ith*ynforthe and | w*ith*oute
    none poudres ne colleries ben for
    suche | maladies

Oxford, Bodleian Library, Ashmole MS 1468, pp. 1–6

Biblio.-Médiathèques de Metz, MS 176, ff. 1r–16r

48. Audiuistis signa prime | infirmitatis et hec est cura: primum oportet | purgare cerebrum et stomacum ab illo hu|more vnde venit illa obumbracio, quia |
45 cessante causa cessant accidencia. ℞ reubarbi, | esule minoris, san-
9ra dali, mirabolanum || citrini ana ʒ iiij, radicis feniculi, brusci, sparagi, | petrosili, apij, siccutelle, cicoree, [capilli | veneris] M ana 1, in aqua bulliant et | cum eis adiungantur ʒ ij polipodij | quar-
5 tum et tantum bulliant ut aqua reuer|tatur ad medietatem. Postea coletur | et in illa colatura ponatis

---

46 sandali] M reubarbi *expunged*
3 capilli veneris] M capilie ana, VP2 (f. 301r), VR (f. 46r) capilli ueneris

Glasgow, GUL, Hunter MS 503, pp. 1–135

þerof shalbe | w*ith* a electuarye mytigatyf & ap*ery*|tyf. whych shal swage the peyne | and opyne the opylate holes ner|uys þat þe uisible spyryt maye | frely passe þereby. 10
And þus shalbe | the lectuarye made. ¶ Take ru|barbe. esule minorys. rede sawn|ders. mirabolys. cytrine. an*a*. iiij. | vnc*er*. the rotys of fenel sp*aragus* brusc*us* | p*er*cely smalach. 15 [68]
sicacelle. cycorye. || capyllys vener*is*. an*a* of eche an hand|ful. polypody of the oke. ij. vnc*er*. boyle | all thies herbys yn feir water. to the | halfe be wasted. And þen clense | yt. than take the 5
for seyd spycys | wele powderd. And put þem to the | seyd lycour. wyth ij pounde of su|ger. And

---

11 rubarbe] An Electuarie | Againste da|sselinge and | mistes Rising | before the | eyes *added in outer margin in an Elizabethan hand*

London, British Library, Sloane MS 661, ff. 32r–46r

[48] And yo*w* shall make | an Electuarye to that purpose after this | sorte. Take of Rubarbe of Esule minoris, | redd Saunders, Mirabolens citrines, ana ʒ iiij | the root*es* of ffenell of A speragus of Brus|cus of Parsleye of Sonaloge of Sico|celle, of Chicorye, of 20
Capillis veneris ana | M.j. of Polipodye of the Oke ʒ ij Boyle all these | herbes, in fayre

---

16 an] An Elect: for daslings and | mistes rysinge | before the | Eyes. *outer margin* 20 of^s] S *deleted* Sicocelle] Sicocelle *outer margin (cross-reference indicated with the astronomical sign of Piscis (♓) in the body of text, over the preceding deletion)* 23 herbes] root*es*. *outer margin (cross-reference indicated with the astronomical sign of Mars (♂) in the body of text)*

Glasgow, GUL, Hunter MS 513, ff. 2r–37r

Basel, Ö.B.U., MS D.II.11, ff. 172r–177v

¶ And ther for this is the Cure for |
soche maladies ¶ First it behouethe
to purgen | the stomake and the
brayne of suche humour · ℞ |
20   reubarbari the lesse esule rede
saundres mirabol*anum* cit*r*ini | an*a*
ʒ.j. of agarik q*uarter* ·ʒ*e*· of fenell
sp*e*racle p*e*rsili Sma||llache
Sicatelle cicorye capill venerys
an*a*·M·j· & | sethe these herbes by
hem selfe in water till the ||
19v   haluendele of the water be at
consumed than clense | it and in
that colature putte ye two pounde
of zucc*ar* e | and make of these
thinges a·Sirup laxatyf ¶ But |
vnderstonde that whan ye putten

---

18 soche] C *added in outer margin*

Oxford, Bodleian Library, Ashmole MS 1468, pp. 1–6

Biblio.-Médiathèques de Metz, MS 176, ff. 1r–16r

    res supra|dictas bene puluerizatas
et libras ij boni | zucari, et faciatis
10 inde sirupum laxa|tiuum, sed
quando ponetis res supradictas |
cum zucaro non debent bullire
nisi | parum, quia amitteret vim
eorum et | virtutes suas. Et iterum
coletur et de | illo sirupo bibat bis
15 in ebdomada, | et iterum custo-
diat se a contrarijs a calidis | et
siccis et a cibis grossis et fumosis |
et ab eis que sunt dure digestionis,
ex | alia parte faciatis ei cauteria in
tim |poribus prope auriculas sicut
20 uidetis | designatum in cauterijs
nostris. |

Glasgow, GUL, Hunter MS 503, pp. 1–135

make þerof a syrup lax|atyff. but
when ȝe put the spycys | and   10
suger. be ware þat yt boylle not |
after but lytle. for þan shal the
spy|cys lese theyr wertu & her
myght. | And when it ys redy.
clense yt a|geyn. And of thys
syrup. lete the | pacyent drynk   15
twyes yn the weke || And yn the   [69]
mene tyme. lete hym | abstene
hym from contr*aryous* metys. |
And from such as byth of harde
dy|gestyon. And also lete hym be
caute|ryzed on the templys   5
besydys the erys | as ȝe q*uo*d he
shall se assygned in my |
cauteryes,

London, British Library, Sloane MS 661, ff. 32r–46r

water till halfe be consumed. | then clarifye it, after take the aforesayd spi|ces finelye   25
powdred. and put them vnto the | sayd liquo*r*. and w*ith* ij ℔. of Suga*r* make | there of a
Syrupe laxatiue, but when yo*w* | put in the spices & suga*r* beware that yt boyle | but little
after, for then theye ˪   spices ˩ shall lose there | force & vertew. then clense yt againe   30

---

24 then] Here as I thincke | ether my Author | or he that first | translated the | Booke, have
mis|taken the trew | meaninge of the | first Author. | for that as yt | appeareth, by | Him, yt
shoulde | be made an Elec|tuarye, and not | a syrupe, as well | maye appeare, | both by the
manner of makinge the medicine and allso he na|meth yt an Electuarye in the begininge And
therefore I | woulde counsell, first after the decoctinge of the root*es* of | fenell, Asperagus,
Bruscus, Parsleye, Smaledge, Sircocella Cicorye | Polipodye Capillis veneris &c. the*n* to straine
yt, & to put vnto yt | the Suga*r*, & boyle yt to a consistence for an Electuarye After | put vnto yt
the other ingrediencie finely powdred & make an | Elect: *outer margin*

Glasgow, GUL, Hunter MS 513, ff. 2r–37r   *Basel, Ö.B.U., MS D.II.11, ff. 172r–177v*

5   yn the forsaide | spices w*ith* the zucr*e* · it shall sethe but alitell for yif | they seithe moche they lesen her myght*es* and her stre|ngthe ¶ And yet lete the pacient be kepte fro hote | And drie and from Drynkes Also and from alle | grete metes and fumose and from all
10   met*es* that | ben of harde digestiou*n* ¶ And on the tothir side | make hym cauterijs in the templis ny3e the eres | as ye shull see in our cauterijs and so we haue | delyu*e*rid many and so doo ye ·/·

Oxford, Bodleian Library, Ashmole MS 1468, pp. 1–6

Biblio.-Médiathèques de Metz, MS 176, ff. 1r–16r	Glasgow, GUL, Hunter MS 503, pp. 1–135
49. Habetis de prima infirmitate que pro|cedit in oculis ex habundancia co|lere, nunc docebimus vos de secunda. | Dicimus ergo quod secunda infirmitas est illa | que apparet super tunicam oculorum | aut lucem quasi nebula sparsa in aere | claro, sed non accidit nisi in illis in | quibus colera magis dominatur scilicet cum | febricitant. Vnde cessante febre rema|net eis istud vicium, ideo quia non fue|runt bene purgati a principio et non | custodierunt se a cibis contrarijs. Dicto | de signis, hec est cura: ℞ saphirum | et tere in mortario et inde fac puluerem | subtilissimum et in uase deaurato re|seruetur, et in oculis pacientis semel | in die ponatis et liberabitur ad plenum. | Et adhuc recipiatis fel taxonis et sic|cetis et reducatis in puluerem et po|natis in oculum, et liberabitur. Item | ℞ gummam	¶ The secunde sekenes | causyd of color. ys whan þer aperyth | vpon the tonycle of the eye before the | syght. as yt were athyn clowde yn | a clere eyre. and vnneth yt may be | seyn. And thys sekenesse fallyth not | but to þem. to whom. and yn whom | coler reygnyth. And when þei be yn | an accesse. And when the acces ys || goon thys dysease remayneth for | lak of due cure be tyme. And for þat | absteyne not from contrarious metys | But for thys sekenes thys ys the | cure. ¶ Take a saphyr and breke | yt yn a morter yn to sotyl powder. | and the powder to be kept yn a vessyl | of golde. And onys on the day put | of þat yn the pacyent eye. and he | shall be hoole yn schort tyme. The | same

10 yn] a thin cloud *added in outer moargin in an Elizabethan hand*

London, British Library, Sloane MS 661, ff. 32r–46r

And \| of this syrupe let the patient drincke twise \| a weeke. And let him abstaine from sutch \| meates as of hard digestion, And let him \| be cauterized on the temples, as I have \| will assigne in my booke of Cauteries. \|\|

[49] The second syckenes caused of Choller is when \| there appeareth vppon the tunicles of the \| Eye before the sighte as yt wer a thyn clowde \| in a clere ayre. and yt can Scarselye be \| seene And this syckenes faulleth not but to \| them in whom choller reyneth, and when \| theye be in an accesse And when the accesse \| is goone this disease remayneth for lacke \| of due cuer be tyme ffor this yow shall take \| a Saphyre and breake

---

1 when] The second \| syckenes cau\|sed of Coller. *outer margin* 2 tunicles] befor *deleted*
4 Scarselye] Barrowe is \| verye faultye. \| in lettinge pass \| all the errors \| as he founde \| them. *outer margin* 6 choller] it *deleted*

Glasgow, GUL, Hunter MS 513, ff. 2r–37r   Basel, Ö.B.U., MS D.II.11, ff. 172r–177v

Of þe secunde | maner of coler & the cure of it. |

15   SEcunde infirmite of colre ys that appereth | on the tonicle of the ey3en before the sight | of the ey3e / as it were a·cloude in the | clere eyre disperpled ¶ wherfor knowe that this | ne fallethe nou3t but
20   hem in whom that colre | hathe dominion vpon ¶ whan they ben feue*r*ous | and whan the feuer ys y cessed · than leuyth | hym this vice of maladie For they were nought | well y cured first at begynnyng · neyther they | were nought wele y kepte at begynnyng from ||
20r contrarious met*es* ¶ The gloriouse cure of this ma|ladie that is right well y preuyd after the moste | y preued crafte of ey3en ys this of poudres // | ¶ TAke a·stone that is

---

14 maner] **15** *added in outer margin*

Oxford, Bodleian Library, Ashmole MS 1468, pp. 1–6

Biblio.-Médiathèques de Metz, MS 176, ff. 1r–16r

  feniculi ʒ iiij et tres partes | de
puluere nabetis – primo pulueri-
zetis | gummam et ponatur cum
puluere nabetis | et ducatur
45 adinuicem et in oculis mitta|tis.
Hec tria facit: corrodit pannum,
mun|dificat oculum, et clarificat
9rb eius lumen || vsque in finem vite
sue. Vnde karissimi dicimus |
vobis uere quia super gummam |
feniculi Ypocrates et Galenus et
omnes alij philosophi | concordati
sunt simul et habent ipsam pro
5 summa | medicina oculorum. Et
non mirantur | tamen intrat oculos
si oculi vident, | sed dicunt etiam
quod cum est in manibus manus |
deberent videre, tamen non
nominabant ipsam | gummam sed
10 feniculum, quia nole|bant expo-
nere virtutem veram. Et nos |
explanauimus vobis illud quod
occul|tauerunt, quia laudabant
solummodo | herbam et non

Glasgow, GUL, Hunter MS 503, pp. 1–135

doth the galle of a bawson yf | yt
be dryed. & powder red. And put |
yn the eye. |

London, British Library, Sloane MS 661, ff. 32r–46r

yt in a mortar into very | fine powder, and kepe the powder in a vessell | of goulde, | and
put there of once a daye | into the patientes Eye, and yt will cuer him | in short tyme. The
same doth the galle | of a Bawson if yt be dryed & powdred. | 15

---

15 Bawson] Bawson, doth | Barrow calle | a Hare. *outer margin (cross-reference indicated with the astronomical sign of the Sun (☉) in the body of text)*

Glasgow, GUL, Hunter MS 513, ff. 2r–37r   *Basel, Ö.B.U., MS D.II.11, ff. 172r–177v*

5   cleped a saffir stone and gry|nde
hym in a brasyn morter Also
diligentliche | and Also sotillich as
it may till it be most sotill | poudre
that may be and kepe this poudre
in a· | vessell of golde and doo it
in to the ey3en of the | pac*ient*
onys a·day and he shall be de-
10 liu*er*ed at the Full | and this for
lordis ¶ Also take the galle of the |
best that is clepid a·grey or brocke
and drie it & | make pouder of it
and putte that poudre in to | the
pacientes ey3e onys aday and he
shall be | deliu*er*ed at full thorugh
15 this medicyne ¶ Also take | fenell
sede ·ʒ· iiij on the tother side &
thre p*ar*ties | of poudre nabat*is* on
the tone side and in a brasyn |
morter make poudre of the forsaide
gu*m*me and | medle it and after-

---

4 grynde] 1. *added in outer margin*
10 the²] 2. *added in outer margin*
14 take] ℞ 3. *added in outer margin*

Oxford, Bodleian Library, Ashmole MS 1468, pp. 1–6

Biblio.-Médiathèques de Metz, MS 176, ff. 1r–16r

    gummam illis scientibus | ubi erat
    virtus vera. Vnde postquam Deo |
15 placuit ut cognoscerem suam
    virtutem, | cum ipsa sanctissima
    gumma innumerabiles | homines
    liberauimus et curauimus | et quod
    fuit in multis occultum exper|tum
    et declaratum est vobis a nobis, |
20 operamini ergo ipsam cum
    salute. |

Glasgow, GUL, Hunter MS 503, pp. 1–135

London, British Library, Sloane MS 661, ff. 32r–46r

Glasgow, GUL, Hunter MS 513, ff. 2r–37r   *Basel, Ö.B.U., MS D.II.11, ff. 172r–177v*

```
        warde do hem bothe in to the |
        morter to giders till bothe be right
20      sotill and | Do  this poudre in to
        the ey3e and / For sothe it | dothe
        thre thinges first it freteth the
        webbe 2ᵉ· | and it softethe and
        clerethe the ey3e and it
        con|seruethe light till is lyues ende
20v     / wherfor on þe ‖ gumme of fenell
        ypocras and galien and all the |
        olde leches were accorded to
        geders and helde | it for a high
        medecyn ¶ And wete ye well that |
        they nemenyd it none gumme but
5       fenell for þey | nould   naught
        shewe where in his vertue | was /
        and for certayne we wole shewen
        For | they praysed the herbe and
        the sede but no|ught the gumme
        though they couthe hit / but | they
        hidden where that the verray
10      trewth | was  · wherfor with that
        holy herbe we haue | delyuerd
```

Oxford, Bodleian Library, Ashmole MS 1468, pp. 1–6

Biblio.-Médiathèques de Metz, MS 176, ff. 1r–16r

50. Dicimus ergo uobis quod propter humorem melancolicum | in multis generantur multe diuerse et | varie infirmitates in oculis, et dice|mus de prima. Aliquando propter nimiam |habundanciam melancolie perturbatur cerebrum | ita quod nerui optici conturbantur et opi|lantur tali modo quod spiritus visibilis | non recto modo valet pertransire, et post | opilacionem apparent ante oculos pacien|tis in die quasi musce volare per | aerem ante oculos suos, et quando respicit | lucernam videtur ei de vna 4 esse, | scilicet et de vna luna 4, et quando respicit | in facie hominis videtur sibi simile | sicut et superius et sic de singulis. | Istud magis

25

30

35

---

34 sibi] M esse *expunged*

Glasgow, GUL, Hunter MS 503, pp. 1–135

Off the Infymytees of Malen|colye, || 15 [72]
For the humor malenco|ly ys gendyrd y myche | peple many dyuerse | dysease yn eyon come þerof. wherof | oon ys thys. Sum   5
tyme for the | habundance of malencolye. the | brayn ys so troublyd. þat the nerfe | obtyk ys so opylate and stoppide. | þat the vysyble spyryt may not | passe   10
the ryght wey. And when | thys nerfe. ys opylate and ouerleid. | þen aperen a fore the pacyentis eyon. | as yt were fleyng flyes yn the | ayre on the day lyght. And of

---

10 when] Gutta Serena *added in outer margin in an Italic hand* 12 eyon] vide pag, 26 *added in outer margin in an Italic hand* 13 the[1]] flying flies | & doble seinge *added in outer margin in an Elizabethan hand*

London, British Library, Sloane MS 661, ff. 32r–46r

[50] The 7º. Chap. of the infirmities | of the Eye caused of Melancholye. | ffor that the Humor of melancholye is bredd | in manye People It is an occation to cause | manye and divers diseases in the Eyes. Some | tymes through this humor there is caused   20
sutch | troble in the braine that the Opticke synowe | is so stopped that the visible sperit can not | passe And when this opilation hapneth. there | appeareth as yt wer flyinge fyes,   25
before the | patientes Eyes, and obiectes presented to there | sighte doe seme to be quadrible, as the moone | or a candell semeth 4. moones or 4. candells. | This kinde of disease doth rather happen to | oulde melancholye men, Then to men | of any other   30
complexion And to sutch patientes | yow maye not put any medicins into the Eye | but

---

20 Some] The first | disease of Me|lancholye is | as though they did see flyes | flyinge before | there Eyes. *outer margin* 30 men[1]] where *deleted*

Glasgow, GUL, Hunter MS 513, ff. 2r–37r   *Basel, Ö.B.U., MS D.II.11, ff. 172r–177v*

    many and that þ*at* was hidde
    nowe | it is open and proued
    Of ·6· infirmi|tees of malencoly &
    the cure of þe first. |
    Nowe of the infirmitees that
15   comyn | thorowe the accasion of
    emlancoly in |to A mannes sight
    and in to his ey3en | wherfor we
    sayne that for the melanco|lious
    humour in many engendreþ
    dyiu*er*se | infirmitees in the ey3en
20   and we wolle tell | you of the first
    ¶ Su*m*me tyme for of ouer | to
    moche habundaunce of mel*ancol*ie
    the brayne is | disturbled · So that
    the holwe synewes ben | y stopped
21r in that maner that the visible spi||rit
    may nought wende in the right
    maner ¶ And | after that stoppyng
    ther appereth a fore the | pacientes
    sight as it were fleyng flyes in þe |

---

12 infirmitees] 16 *added   in   outer margin*

Oxford, Bodleian Library, Ashmole MS 1468, pp. 1–6

Biblio.-Médiathèques de Metz, MS 176, ff. 1r–16r

accidit illis qui naturaliter | sunt melancolici quando senescunt quam alijs com|plexionibus. Et cum videtis aliquem | pacientem cum istis signis nullam | medi-
40 cinam ponere in oculis presu-matis, | sed faciatis ei istud electuarium restau|ratiuum et mitigatiuum, ut nerui concaui | opilati possint aperiri, ita ut spiritus visi|bilis possit libere pertransire.
45 ℞ suci | liqueritie ℔ ß, seminis rute, basiliconis, vrtice trans|marine uel Siciliane, seminis feniculi,
9va alexandrini, || apii, carui ana ʒ ij, masticis, gariofili, | nucis muscati, cinamomi, cubebe, gumme | amigdale, cerase, pomi, gumme ara|bici, dragontee, croci ana ʒ ß,
5 grana | citoniorum pomorum ana ʒ 1. Omnia hec | terantur et in subtilissimum pul|uerem redigantur et cum bono | zucaro conficiantur et fiat inde | electuarium, et

Glasgow, GUL, Hunter MS 503, pp. 1–135

a lan|terne of ly3te. or of the 15
moone. yt || semyth þat yt were [73]
iiij. And yf he | loke yn the face of
a man. yt semyth | to hym the
same. ¶ Thys maner of | sekenes
yt happenyth to them raþer | þat 5
be naturally malycolyus. when |
þei vexen aged. raþer than to
menn | of oþer complexion.
wherfor the prac|tysers when 3e se
such a pacyent. | put no medycyne
yn hys eye. but | make hym a 10
lectuarye my tyg a | tyff and
aperytyff. whych schall | swage
the peyn and open the opy|lacion
of the hole neruys þat the | spyryt
of syght may passe esely | by 15
them. And þus it shalbe made || ¶ [74]

---

15 yt¹] you shall finde this disease | in the 26. page: reconed | amongst the vncurable | Cataractes. *added in outer margin in an Italic hand*

London, British Library, Sloane MS 661, ff. 32r–46r

make them an Electuarye mitigatiue & || and aperatiue, whitch must swage the paine, 43v
and open | the stoppinge of the opticke synowe, and yt shalbe | made after this sorte.
Take of Sugar of lyco|rise of Euphrase of Siler montaine & hylwort ana | halfe a pound. 5
Of the seedes of Rewe, of the seedes | of Basilicon of Nettles that come from be yond
the | seaes of ffenell of Alexander of Smallage of Car|uy. ana ij owncees Of masticke of
Cloves. of Nutmegges | of Synamonde of Cubibes Gumme of Almondes, Cerase | Pyonie 10
Gummarum Arabici, Draganti Safforne | ana ʒ ß. the Kyrnells of Quinces Pioniorum

---

33 &] aperitiue *lower margin* **4 &**] This compositi|on diffareth | mutch from that | whitch Barrowe | hath published. *outer margin (cross-reference indicated with an asterisk in the body of text—see next lemma).* **7 Caruy**] *an asterisk over this word, apparently indicating the end of the recipe that 'diffareth mutch from that whitch Barrowe hath published'*

Glasgow, GUL, Hunter MS 513, ff. 2r–37r

eyre in the day light ¶ And whan
he lokeþ | alanterne with light he
wenythe that ther is two | lanternes
or foure / and of one mone he
wenythe | that ther is foure monys
And whan he lokethe | in aman his
face he wenithe that ther is two |
faces or moo and so hym semythe
Also of all oþer | thing*es* ¶
wherfor knowe ye well that this
falleth | more to hem that ben
naturallich melancoliouse after |
that they wexen olde than any
other folke // And | whan ye se
any pacientes of this infirmite be
þes | signes afore saide ¶ Than be
ware that ye putte no*n*e |
medecyne in to the ey3en nought
so hardy but mAkeþ | this letuarie
restauratif and moysting to this
mala|die that the holwe senewis
that ben y stoppid mowe | be vndo
her stoppyng and be opened and
that the | visible spirite mowe

Basel, Ö.B.U., MS D.II.11, ff. 172r–177v

Oxford, Bodleian Library, Ashmole MS 1468, pp. 1–6

Biblio.-Médiathèques de Metz, MS 176, ff. 1r–16r

10 paciens recipiat de eo | mane et sero cum iuerit dormitum, | et recuperabit lumen suum sicut desi|derat. Et dicimus vobis quod non tantum | ad istam infirmitatem valet sed eciam | illis qui non clare
15 vident et qui | habent quasi caliginem in oculis, et | simile valet illis omnibus qui propter | magnam tristiciam et planctum lacri|marum, vigilias, ieiunium, et fatiga|ciones corporis et alia
20 similia illis la|borant. Et vocamus illud electua|rium declaracio oculorum, ideo quia | clarificat lumen oculorum et spiritum | viuificat.

Glasgow, GUL, Hunter MS 503, pp. 1–135

Take suger. lycoryse. eufrasie. | siler mownten. i. hylwort an*a* halfe | a pounde. Off the seedys of rewe | basylycon. vrtice vltra marine. | fenel alexand*er*.   5
smalege. Caruy. | an*a* ij vnc*er*. Mastic*is*. clowys. not|myggi*s*. Cynomo*n*. Cubib*is*. Gu*m*me | of almandys. Cerase. pyonie. gu*m*|mar*um* arabici. dragaganti. safron. | halfe an vnc*er* gra*n*a   10
cytemor*um*. pio|nior*um*. an vnc*er*. All thyes muste | be betyn to gyddyr to smal poud*er* | and wele sarsed. and þan confect | wyth goode sug*er*. and make a lectu|arye. And of thys lete the   15
pacy||ent ete. fyrst at morn*n*. and   [75]
laste | at yeven. and he shalbe hoole, ¶ | Thys sayd lectuarye ys not oonly | good for thys sekenes.

---

1 eufrasie] Clarifica|cio Occu|lorum *added in outer margin in an Italic hand*

London, British Library, Sloane MS 661, ff. 32r–46r

ana ℥ j. | All th[e]se must be beaten into fine powd*er*. & well sear|sed, and make there of an Electuarye. w*ith* suffitient | good sugar. And of this let the patient eate mor|ninge and   15
Eveninge first and last. This Elec|tuarye is not onlye good for this syckenes, but | allso for all thos[e] w*hi*tch see not clerelye, but have | in manne*r* a miste before there Eyes. caused ether | of thoughte and great heavines, or of weepinge, | or of watchinge or of fastinge,   20
and therefore yt | is called Clarificatio Oculoru*m*.

---

12 these] *First* e *is blotted* 17 those] *Final* e *is blotted* 21 is] Clarificatio Occulorum *outer margin*

Glasgow, GUL, Hunter MS 513, ff. 2r–37r

   freliche passyn ¶ Take Inde |
20 liquorice ·℔·ß rewe sed
   basilicoun nettils of beyonde | see
   or of cicile fenell sede stanmarche
   smaleach carui | ana ·ʒ·ij mastike
   gariofil cucubys note mowges
   gumme | of Almoundes gum of
   cheritre gingiuer p$_t$i$_j$onie gum
   arabie | Dragaganti saffroun ana
   ·ʒ j· kirnelles of quynys & of ||
21v apples ana ·ʒ·j grynde all these
   right sotilliche in to pou|dre and
   confice hem with good hony or
   withe zucre in a· | pewtre vessell
   and make of hem a letuarie and
   the | pacient shall vsen therof
   erlich and late and he shall |
5 receyue his sight aʒeen ¶ And we
   saye that þis le|tuarye is nought
   only to this infirmite it profethe |
   but also to all hem that mewe not
   so clerelich but | they haue hete in

Basel, Ö.B.U., MS D.II.11, ff. 172r–177v

---

19 Inde] ℞ *added in outer margin*

Oxford, Bodleian Library, Ashmole MS 1468, pp. 1–6

Biblio.-Médiathèques de Metz, MS 176, ff. 1r–16r

51. Et dicimus adhuc quod aliquando | ascendit dolor ad oculos propter | humorem melancolicum sic subito quod exci|tat oculos pacientis extra conca|uitatem uel fontem oculorum, et ap|parent oculi inflati ultra modum, | et multi de illis sunt qui propter | occasionem illam amittunt lumen ex | toto, et alij sunt de talibus qui | vident sed male. Vnde scias quod omnes | possunt liberari si a principio egritudi|nis sunt curati cum istis curis: primo | purgare debemus cerebrum et stoma|cum

Glasgow, GUL, Hunter MS 503, pp. 1–135

but also for | all tho whych see no clerely. but | haue yn maner a myste yn þer eyon. | causyd eiþer of thou3te and grete he|uynes of a grete weepyng or of | wacche. or of fastyng. or of such | oþer. And þerfor thys lectuarye ys | clepyd. Clarificacio oculorum, This | ys the clarifyers of eyon.

¶ Ther | ys also a noþer sekenes causyd of | malyncolye. & yt ys when the | payne sodonly ascendyth yn to || the eyon. and so greuouly þat it | semyth the eyon wolde stert oute | of theyr places. And þei aperyn | passyngly bollen. and of thys ma|ner of pacyentis. som lese holy þer | syght. And som seen but feblye. | And not for than all thyes may | be holpe yf

12 ys] Swelling of the | eie, and paine | that they be re|die to starte out *added in outer margin in an Elizabethan hand*

London, British Library, Sloane MS 661, ff. 32r–46r

[51] There is | allso an other syckenes caused of Melancholye | and that is when the paine sodainelye ascendeth | into the Eyes, and that so grevouslye that yt see|meth to the patient the Eyes will breake out of | there places, and the Eyes be verye mutch | swollen, and manye of this disease doe wholye | lose there sighte. And yet these maye be holpen | if theye be taken in the Bigininge by these remo|dyes that I will sett yow downe. Take of Aloes He|paticke. of Myrabolanes citrine of Turbith Saunders | citrine Rhabarbe ana ʒ ß. Scamonie, Suffron, Bal|samum, Myrh, Masticke, Lignum Aloes. Olibanum album | Agaricke. Nux Indica Succum Liquoritiæ, the seedes | of Smalledges, lettuce, Cicherye, Basilicon and ʒ j. | Beate the all into fine powder, and make them | into a masse of Pills

24 into] Paine and swel|linge of the Eyes, | so vehement that | theye be readye | to start owt | of there places. *outer margin* 29 remodyes] Pills of Comfort *outer margin*

Glasgow, GUL, Hunter MS 513, ff. 2r–37r

    her ey3en ¶ Also it is good to
hem | that for grete sorwe and for
10 moch wepyng of teris | and for
wakyng and fastyng and for
traueillyng of | her body ben nygh
blynde and we clepe þis elec-
*tuariu*m | the cleryng of ey3en for
why the light of the ey3en | it
clerithe and quyketh the spirites
**Of the | secunde cure of malen-
coly & þe cure of it |**
15 SEcunde infirmite that comethe
thorwe the | accasiou*n* of melan-
colie ¶ And we sayne that | su*m*
tyme they Ariseth an vnsuffrable
pen*a*nce | and ache in the ey3e for
that melancolie humour so |
sodaynlich that it sterethe the
20 ey3en of the pacient | oute of her
holwenesse And oute from the
wellis of | ey3en and that the

Basel, Ö.B.U., MS D.II.11, ff. 172r–177v

---

14 secunde] 17 *added in outer margin*

Oxford, Bodleian Library, Ashmole MS 1468, pp. 1–6

Biblio.-Médiathèques de Metz, MS 176, ff. 1r–16r

 cum pillulis nostris consolacionis
ad quas: | ℞ aloe epatici, mirabo-
lani citrini, turbith, | sandali
citrini, reubarbi ana ʒ ß, sca-
mo|nee, croci, balsa, mirre, mas-
40 ticis, ligni | aloes, olibani albi,
agarici, nucis Indie, | suci lique-
ritie, seminis apii, lactuce, cicoree,
ba|siliconis ana ʒ 1. Hec omnia
pulueri|zentur et cum suco rosarum
recenti | conficiantur, et detur de
45 eo secundum | vires pacientis.
Purgato cerebro | super oculum
ponatis de emplastro lau|dabili,
quod de istis rebus componitur: ||
9vb ℞ poma acerba et coque sub
cinere calido | ita quod
mollificentur, et mundentur a |
cortice et in mortario [eneo]
pistentur, | et cum 4 pomis
5 iungatur clara oui | et simul

Glasgow, GUL, Hunter MS 503, pp. 1–135

they be cured yn the be|gynnyng
of theyr sekenes. wyth | thyes 10
medycynes that I shal sey | yow. ¶
Fyrst the stomake and | the brayn
must be porged wyth oure | pelat*is*
of comforth. whych are ma|de on
thys wyse. ¶ Take aloes | epatyk. 15
mirabolys. cytryne. tur||byt. [77]
saunde*r*s. cit*r*ine. rubarbe. an*a*. |
halfe an vnc*er* scamony. safrone. |
balsami. mirre. mastyci. lygnu*m* |
aloes. olibanu*m* album. agaricus. |
nuces Indie. succu*m* liqueryce. 5
the | seed of smalache. letuce.
cicorie. | basylicon. an*a* of eche a
drame, | bet all yn to powder and
confecte | þem wyth the Jows of
roses. & | make pelatys. And yif 10
yt the pa|cyent after hys power.
And when | the stomake & the
brayn ben powr|ged. ley on the ey

---

3 eneo] M ereo, VP2 (f. 302v), VR
(f. 48v) eneo

14 aloes] pills of | Comfort *added in outer margin in an Italic hand*

London, British Library, Sloane MS 661, ff. 32r–46r

w*ith* the Juyce of Roses | w*h*itch I call pills of comfort, And when the | stomacke and
braine is purged. laye vnto the || Eye my plaist*er* called. Emplastru*m* Laudabile | w*h*itch 44r
is thus made. Take of Sower Apples called | crabbes and roste them in the Embars till
theye be | softe. then take from them the paringe, and the Coore. | and beate them well in 5
a morta*r*. and vnto the pulpe | of 4. Crabbes put the white of an egg and beate | them
togethe*r* till theye be well incorporate, & | be in manne*r* of an Oyntme*n*t. And of this |
plaister, let be applyed vnto the Eye, vppon | pledgette*s* of towe twise in the daye, 10
morninge | and Eveninge. And after this manner yo*w* shall | cue*r* this kinde of disease
The vertewes | of this plaister are these ffirst yt doth | asswage the swelling. there of.

---

39 the] Eye *lower margin* 1 Laudabile] Emplastrum | Laudabile *outer margin*

Glasgow, GUL, Hunter MS 513, ff. 2r–37r *Basel, Ö.B.U., MS D.II.11, ff. 172r–177v*

    ey3en semyn all for swolle oute |
of mesure and ther ben many of
thoo that thorowe | that occasiou*n*
that lesyn all the sight of her
22r ey3en || ¶ And yef ther be any of
suche that sein full euyll | they
seyn ¶ And knowith well that all
tho mowe | be y cured fro the
begynnyng of her maladies wiþ |
these medecynes / First thowe
5 moste purgen the sto|make withe
these pil*u*llis of oure consaille ¶ ℞
aloe | epatic*a* mirabol*anum* cit*r*i
turbithe sandas cit*r*ini reubi*um*
croci bal|sami mirre mastike ligni
nuc*es* indice succi liquericie |
seme*n* apij lactuce acorie basili-
conis ana ·ʒ·1· alle þe|se shull be y
made in to right sotill poudre and
10 w*ith* | the iuse of Ros*arum*
freysshe they shullen be confited |
and thou shalte yeue her of after

---

5 aloe] ℞ *added in outer margin*

Oxford, Bodleian Library, Ashmole MS 1468, pp. 1–6

Biblio.-Médiathèques de Metz, MS 176, ff. 1r–16r

  ducatur in mortario donec fiat |
emplastrum ad modum vnguenti.
Et de isto lau|dabili emplastro, cum
stuppa, oculo clauso, |
superponatis bis in die scilicet
mane et sero, | et cum istis curis
10 liberabitis pacien|tes a principio
de ista infirmitate quia | nos
innumerabiles homines cum ipsis
curis | curauimus et liberauimus.
Dicimus | etiam uobis quantas
habet virtutes illud pre|dictum
emplastrum: primo detumescit
15 oculum, | secundario collocat
oculum in loco suo, tercio |
mitigat dolorem et recipit lumen |
pacientis, id est recuperat.

Glasgow, GUL, Hunter MS 503, pp. 1–135

my plaster cle|pyd. Emplastru*m*
laudabile. whych | ys made on 15
thys wyse. ¶ Take ‖ sowre apples [78]
þat ys Crabbes. and | roost þem
hoote yn the embrys tyll | they
soft. than voyde away the parow |
and the core. And bruse þem
wele | yn a mort*er*. And to iiij. 5
Crabbys. | put the whyte of an egg
glayre. & | bray þem to geddyr. tyl
þei be In|corp*er*atte yn man*er* of an
oynement. | And of thys lawdable
plaster. ley | on flexen herdys. 10
and plaster yt on | on the eye.
twyes on the daye. morn | &
yeuen. And yn thys wyse ye shal |
cure thys man*er* of disease. yf it be
a|plied. & vsed. At the be-
gynnyng. | Of thys plaster thyes 15

---

1 and] Emplast. | Laudabile *added in outer margin in an Italic hand*
6 egg] *The drawing of the brevigraph for* er *at the end of this word appears to have stopped midway*

London, British Library, Sloane MS 661, ff. 32r–46r

and kepeth | the Eye in his place. yt easeth *the* paine | and comforteth the sighte and for 15
these cau|ses I call yt Laudable.

---

15 yt] are *deleted*

De Probatissima Arte Oculorum 369

Glasgow, GUL, Hunter MS 513, ff. 2r–37r   *Basel, Ö.B.U., MS D.II.11, ff. 172r–177v*

    the strengthe is | of the pacient ¶
    And whan that the brayne is | thus
    y purged layeth ouer the ey3e of þe
    worship|full plastre that is y made
15 of these thinges take | sour applis
    and roste hem vnder hote emery
    and | whan they ben well neysshe
    and from her parell | y mundefyed
    than bete hem in a·brasyn morter
    & | putte ther to the glayre of
    a·nay and well distemper | hem to
    gidres in the morter till they be in
20 maner | of aplaster or of an
    o y n e m e n t / A n d o f t h i s
    worship|full plaister with stupis ley
    it on the ey3e twies a· | day ·i· erly
    and late and so with this cure at
    beginnyng | of this maladie ye
    shull deliuere pacientes as we ||
22v haue y prouyd ofte tyme ¶ wherfor
    of this emp|lastre we saye firste for
    it swagethe that maladie | ·2$^{e·}$ for it
    setteth in his stede 3$^{e·}$ for it dothe
    a w a y e | t h e a k t h e A n d i t

Oxford, Bodleian Library, Ashmole MS 1468, pp. 1–6

Biblio.-Médiathèques de Metz, MS 176, ff. 1r–16r

52. Dicimus | adhuc uobis quod propter humorem melancolicum | generantur vngule in oculis, et incipiunt | crescere a parte lacrimalis minoris et com|plexantur adinuicem – cursus earum semper | est versus pupillam et si postquam super | tunicas oculorum ueniunt, non inciduntur | antequam occupent pupillam et pro|hibeant lumen. Non postea de facili | curantur sicut a principio. Et aliquando | nascitur alia vngula a parte lacrimalis | [maioris] et complexatur adinuicem | et

28 maioris] M minoris, VP3 (f. 104v), Bo (f. 76v) maioris

Glasgow, GUL, Hunter MS 503, pp. 1–135

be vertues. || Fyrst yt swagyth the [79] bolnyng. It | settyth the eye fyxe yn hys place. It | lesseth the payn. and refreshyth the | syght. And for thies causes I cal it | laudable. that ys worthy to be *pray*|sed.
Also sup*er*habundance of the hu|mor of malencolye is often gendryd | yn the ey a dysease callyd. vngula. | a nayle. for it ys muche lyke a fyng*er* | nayle. and begynnyth comonly to | growe. In lacrimabili minore, þat | ys to sey. yn the corner of the eye. | to the ereward. And the course of | the growyng ys towarde the pupil | þat ys to sey to the sy3te. And yf it || be not cut a way or it ocupye the | [80] pupil and let the sy3ght. Afterwarde | it wyll not be easely curyd. Also | sum tyme þ*er*e

9 a] vngula *added in outer margin in an Elizabethan hand*

London, British Library, Sloane MS 661, ff. 32r–46r

[52] Allso ⌊ of ⌋ superabundance | of Melancholye is ingendred in the Eye a | disease called Vngula. so called for that yt | is like to the Nayle of our finga*r*, and begin|neth most com*m*onlye in that corne*r* of the Eye | nexte to the Eare, and yt spredeth yt selfe & | groweth towar*d*es the Pupill. and if yt be not | cutt a waye before yt coue*r* the Pupill, & | hinde*r* the sighte, after yt will not be easelye | cured. Allso some tymes there groweth an | other vngula in that corner of the Eye next | to the nose: and if these 2. happen to knytt | to gether and to coue*r* all the Eye, and to hinde*r* | all the sighte, then yt is more harde to Cuer | yet bey hedefull workinge w*ith* the hand yt | maye be cured after this manner. Take a | twytch of siluer & there w*ith* | subtillye lifte vpp the vngula from the |

19 Vngula] be *deleted* yt] Vngula *outer margin* 28 happen] *Final* n *crossed with a slant line* 31 yt] m *deleted* 33 of] sill *deleted* with] suttlelye *deleted*

De Probatissima Arte Oculorum

Glasgow, GUL, Hunter MS 513, ff. 2r–37r

comfortethe the sight of þe pacient |

Basel, Ö.B.U., MS D.II.11, ff. 172r–177v

5 **Of þe ·3· cure of malencoli & þe cure of it** |
Nowe the thirdde infirmite thorugh occasion | of mel*anco*lie ¶ we sayne for the melancolie hu|mour in the ey3en ben engendred vngule | ·i· the horne of a·nayle and it begynnethe to wexe*n* |
10 toward the lasse tery place and his cours is toward | the ey3e appull and it couereþ it ¶ And sum*m*e tyme | ther wexethe a nother vngula toward the more te|ry place & they rynnen to giders and helyn all the | ey3e and fornemethe the pacient all his

---

5 Of] 18 *added in outer margin*

Oxford, Bodleian Library, Ashmole MS 1468, pp. 1–6

Biblio.-Médiathèques de Metz, MS 176, ff. 1r–16r

    occupat totum oculum et prohibet
30 lumen | pacientis. Et dicimus
quod omnes sunt cura|biles, sed
cum magna discrecione et o|pera-
cione manuum. Cura eorum hec
est: | accipiatis vncinum de
argento et | cum ipso suspendetis
35 ipsam vngulam | a tunica oculi,
et cum rasorio ipsam in|cidatis ita
diuidendo uadas usque ad | lacri-
male ubi ipsa habet originem
suam | et incidatis eam ex toto.
Hoc facto bom|bacem intinctum in
40 albumine oui, clau|so oculo,
superponatis usque ad x dies. |
Finito numero x dierum abluat se
aqua | calida, et abluto oculo
mittatis intus | de puluere nabetis
mane et sero do|nec oculus sit
45 clarificatus et rehabe|at lumen
suum sicut desiderat. Et iterum |
custodiat se a contrarijs, et ||

---

45 iterum] M desiderat *expunged*

Glasgow, GUL, Hunter MS 503, pp. 1–135

growyth a noþer | vngyll jn the   5
corner of the eye. | nexte the
noose. and yf thies ij. | happyn to
be knyt to gydd*er*. and | to
occupye all the eye. and to let | all
the sy3th. þan it ys more hard | to   10
cure. But nat for than. boyth | be
curable but by grete dyscrec*i*on |
& sotyl workyng or wrythyng | of
the honde. And þis must be | the
cure. ¶ Take a twych of | sylu*er*   15
and þerwyth sotylly lyftvpe || the   [81]
vngle from the tonycle p*ro*cedyng |
forthe to the lacrymal where he
toke | hys growyng. And when it
is all | cut awey wyth a rasour
sotilly. lete | the pacyent spere yn   5
hys eye. and lay | þe*r*to a plaster
of the whyte of an egg | x. dayes
folowyng. twyes on the day |
renewed. whych so past. lete hym
wash | hym w*ith* hote water. and
þan put yn | hys ey. at morn and   10
euyn. of my | powd*er*. callyd.

London, British Library, Sloane MS 661, ff. 32r–46r

tunicle procedinge forth to the lacrimall | where he first looke his begininge. and when || 35
yt is all cutt awaye w*ith* a raso*r*, let the pati|ent close his Eyes, and laye for the space | of   44v
.x. dayes followinge, pledgett*es* wet in | the whites of egg*es*, renuige them everye | daye   5
twise morninge and Eveninge. and at | the end of x. dayes, let him wash his Eyes | w*ith*
warme wate*r*. and after put into his | Eyes of the powder called pulvis Nabe|tus. before
described & so continew till the | Eye be suffitientlye clered. and in the | meane tyme let   10
him avoyde all meates *that* | maye brede any offence to the Eye. |

---

36 when] yt is *lower margin*   8 Nabetus] fol. 17 *outer margin*

Glasgow, GUL, Hunter MS 513, ff. 2r–37r

15   sight | And we sayne that all ben curable · But withe | grete Discrecioun and worchyng of handes ¶ And this | is the Cure Take and hoke of siluer and w*ith* that | hoke take that vngula · and lifte vp the nedill & | so w*ith* a Rasour kutte her dyuiding · go to
20   the lacri|mall where that vngula wexeth and than kutte | her A waye / And whan ye haue so y donn on þe | ey3e lay a·sponge y wette in the glayre of a·nay | whan the ey3e is y shitte and do it a nowarde | till the ferthe day ¶ And
23r   whan the ferthe daye || is ended wasshe the ey3e w*ith* hote water ¶ And whan | the ey3en is so wasshen than do ther ynne þe poudre | nabat*is* erliche and late / till the ey3e be y clered and | that it haue his sight ¶ And ayeneward
5   that the pa|cient kepe hym well from malancolious metes & |

Basel, Ö.B.U., MS D.II.11, ff. 172r–177v

Oxford, Bodleian Library, Ashmole MS 1468, pp. 1–6

Biblio.-Médiathèques de Metz, MS 176, ff. 1r–16r

10ra nullam medicinam ponatis in oculum, | quia probata improbatis non de|betis relinquere – ex improviso multi fal|luntur.

Glasgow, GUL, Hunter MS 503, pp. 1–135

Puluis nabetus. tyl | the eye be clere sufficyently. And yn | the mene tyme lete hym absteyne | hym from cont*r*aryo*us* metys. And | noon*n* o*þ*er medycyne yn the eye. ‖   15

53. Et dicimus quod aliquando
5   habun|dat in cerebro sanguis melancolicus et | incipit habere cursum suum per oculos | propter nimiam habundanciam et facit de|siccare palpebras. Et illa desiccicacio ver|titur postea in
10   ardorem et pruritum, | ideo quia non sumit purgationem et non | custodiuit se a contrarijs in principio in|firmitatis. Docuimus vobis signa | et hec est cura: si est juuenis facia|tis eum minuere de
15   vena que est in | medio frontis,

¶ It happyth sum tyme *þ*at the   [82]
ma|lencolyo*us* humor habunda*n*t
yn the | brayn begynnyth to haue
hys course | by the eyon. And for
the supe*r*habun|dance *þer*eof. it   5
makyth the ey ledys | to wexe
drye. And *þ*at drynes tor|nyth afte*r*
to an ycche. and to brynny*n*g | and
the cause of thys bry*n*nyng and |
ycche. ys. for that he tooke no   10
purga|c*i*on yn the begynnyng of

———————————

15 eye] it happyth *added in lower margin*   **6** tornyth] drines of the | ey lid*es* and | ytch. and | burninge. *added in outer margin in an Elizabethan hand*

———————————

2 probata] M impro *expunged*

London, British Library, Sloane MS 661, ff. 32r–46r

[53] It hapneth oftentymes that this melancholye | humor, abundant in the braine begineth to have | the corse by the Eyes, and can seth a great | drynes in the Eye lidd*es*,   15
and that drynes | turneth to an ytch and borninge, and the | cause there of is, for that he was nether pur|get not did abstaine from hurtfull meates | at the begininge of his disease.   20
In the Cuer | of this disease it is good if the patient be | younge. to let him blood on the vaine in | the middest of the forehead. w*h*itch beinge done | let him be cured w*i*th a remodye called Col|lerium Rubrum made after this manne*r*. | Take 40. tender croppes of   25
Bramble. and stampe | them so small as greene sawce, and the*n* put | them into a new earthen pott, and put to them | a quarte of good white wyne, and boyle them | vppon a   30

———————————

16 drynes] Drynes. | Itch and | Borninge of |the Eyes lidd*es*. *outer margin*   **22** blood] or *deleted*
24 Collerium] Collerium | Rubrum *outer margin*

Glasgow, GUL, Hunter MS 513, ff. 2r–37r

    contrarious to the pacient ¶ And
loke that ye do | none othir
medicyne in to the ey3en but this
that | we haue y prouyd and y
taught it to you as for | well y
proued and for vnprouyd
10 medecyns we shall | nought leue
./.

**Of the ·4· maladie of | malyncoly
& the cure of it.** |

Of the 4ᵉ infirmite thorugh
accasiou*n* of melan|colie we sayne
that su*m*me melancolious blode |
habundeþ in the brayne and it
15 begynneþ | to haue his cours by
the ey3en for his ouer moch |
habundaunce and it makeþ that the
ey3e liddes ben | to drye and that
drying turnethe to moche sore |
woo and ache as of moche peple ·
For defaute of | purgacions and for
they kepte not hem selfe from |

Basel, Ö.B.U., MS D.II.11, ff. 172r–177v

---

10 of] 19 *added in outer margin*

Oxford, Bodleian Library, Ashmole MS 1468, pp. 1–6

Biblio.-Médiathèques de Metz, MS 176, ff. 1r–16r

facta minucione medice|tis eum
cum collirio [ruborum], ad quod |
℞ xl tallos [ruborum] teneres et
pis|tetis eos ad modum salse, et
cum hoc | misceatis ij ℔ boni vini
20 albi, et in | noua olla simul
bulliantur donec vi|num illud
reuertatur ad medietatem. | Postea
coletur et de isto collirio intus
ocu|lis bis in die ponatis et sic
liberabitur | paciens usque ad
25 plenum. Et scias quod | magis
inuenimus de istam infirmita|tem
habentibus in Roma quam in alijs
pro|uincijs. Et dicimus quod hoc
collirirum valet | ad omnes
scaldaturas et rubedinem | palpebrarum et vocamus ipsum colli-

---

16 ruborum] M rumborum
17 tallos...teneres] M tallos
rumborum teneres, N (f. 67r) talos
teneros rubrorum, VP2 (f.303r) calos
ruborum teneros

Glasgow, GUL, Hunter MS 503, pp. 1–135

the sekenesse | nor absteyned from
contraryous metys. | ¶ Off thys
dysease thus ys the | cure. yf the
pacyent be yong. lete | hym blode
on the veyne yn the myd|dys of   15
the forhede. whych so doon. | cure   [83]
hym with a colerie clepid.
Cole|rium ruborum. thus made. ¶
Take | xl^{ti}. tendyr croppys of the
bremyl | and stampe them as
smale as sauce. | and put it yn a   5
new erthen pot with | a quarte of
goode whyte wyne. and | boyle it
wyth an esy fyre tyl halfe | be
consumede. Than clense yt. and |
kepe it yn a glasse. wherof twyes
yn | the day put yn the pacyentis   10
eye. and | noon oþer thyng tyl he
be hole. And | thys colerie ys
goode a geyne al skal|dyng and

---

1 cure] Colerium | Ruborum *added in outer margin in an Italic hand* 3 xlti] Sc *added in outer margin in an Elizabethan hand*

London, British Library, Sloane MS 661, ff. 32r–46r

softe fyer till halfe be consumed. | Then clense yt, and kepe yt in a glasse And | twise
everye daye put some there of into | the patientes Eyes. and vse nothinge Ellse | vntill he
be cured. And this medicine | is good against all scaldinge & reddnes of || the Eyes   35 | 45r
caused by the aforesayde syckenes. | I found more in Rome (sayth my Author) | then in
any other province.

---

33 Ellse] in *deleted* 35 of] the Eyes *lower margin* 2 Rome] Trobled with | this disease. *outer margin (cross-reference indicated with a cross over* Rome *in the body of text)*

Glasgow, GUL, Hunter MS 513, ff. 2r–37r *Basel, Ö.B.U., MS D.II.11, ff. 172r–177v*

20   contrarijs dietyng*es* in the be
gynnyng of that in |firmite ¶
wherfore when ye see suche
maladies | thus ye shull Cure hem
yif he be yong First ma|ke that he
be y lete blode on the veyne that is
in | the myddell of the frount and
25   afterward ye shull | hele hem
w*ith* this collerie of breres ¶ TAke
23v   ·xl· || braunches or croppes of
breres and grynde hem right |
small as any sauce and withe hem
menge ·℔·ij of | gode white wyne
in a newe erthin potte and lete |
hem sethe in the forsaid wyne till
5   the haluende|le be y soden a waye
· and whan it is comen sode*n* | in
to the haluendele than clense it ¶
And of this | colerye doithe twies
on a day into the ey3e till | the
pacient be deliu*er*ed atte full as we
exp*er*te & | well prouid // And we

---

25 ·xl·] ℞ *added in outer margin*

Oxford, Bodleian Library, Ashmole MS 1468, pp. 1–6

Biblio.-Médiathèques de Metz, MS 176, ff. 1r–16r

30   rium | ruborum   quia fit de tallis
     ruborum. |

Glasgow, GUL, Hunter MS 503, pp. 1–135

rednesse of the maladies | of the
forseyd sekenes. Qu*o*d the autor | I   15
fonde mo yn Rome than yn any ||
othir pr*o*uince.   [84]

54. Nascitur quidam humor extra
oculum | inter cilium et palpebram
et tumescit, | ob hoc palpebra et
totus oculus circum|circa ipsum
35   cum medietate palpebre | faciei,
sed non offendit oculum. Et Tus|ci
vocant ipsum humorem bene-
dictum, Ro|mani uaximam, Cici-
liani et Creci | papulam, ultrama-
rini et Francigene | vocant ipsam
maledictam – et certe bene |
40   dicunt   ideo quia est nimio magno
do|lore et terrore nata. Et hec sunt
sig|na cognoscendi eam, quia ex
ista tota palpebra | est dura, rubea,

Moreoure of such sup*er*|fluyte of
malencolie. su*m* tyme þ*ere*
grou|yth a corupte humor wythout
the | eye betwyxte the place.
where the he|re growyth. and the   5
eye lydde. whych | bolnyth not
oonly the eye lydde. but | all the
eye. wyth halfe the face. but | it
hurtyth not the eye. And men | of
tuskan calle it. Humeris
b*e*n*edictum*. | Them of Rome call   10
it. Nexionam. | And men of Cicile.

4 here] a swelling a|bout the eie |
lede. *added in outer margin in an
Elizabethan hand*

London, British Library, Sloane MS 661, ff. 32r–46r

[54]   More ou*er* of sutch | superfluitye of melancholye some tymes | there groweth a   5
corrupte humo*r* wi*th*out the | Eye betwixte the place where the heares | groweth and the
Eye lidd, w*h*itch swelleth not | onlye the Eye lidd, but all the Eye, and | halfe the face but
yt hurteth not the Eye. | and this disease (sayth my Autho*r*) in diuers | cuntryes hath   10
diuers names. In Tuskan | yt is called Humoris b*e*n*edictu*m In Rome | theye call yt
Noxionam. In Cicili and Grece | they call yt Papulam But the vltra|mountaines &   15
ffrentchme*n* call yt Male|dictam and no wondar for yt groweth | w*i*th great sorenes. and
great paine. | and thus yow shall knowe yt It maketh | the Eye lidd*es* harde, redd, &

6 betwixte] I thincke he | meaneth only | vppon the lower | Eye lidd. *outer   margin
(cross-reference indicated with the astronomical sign of Piscis (♓) in the body of text).*
14 vltramountaines] A swellinge | in the Eye | lidd*es outer margin*

Glasgow, GUL, Hunter MS 513, ff. 2r–37r

10 sayne that this collerie | is gode for iij thinges that is it is gode ayenst | all scaldinges and for the rednes of the ey3e lid|des ¶ And we clepe this collerio of breres / and | of these maladies we fonde moste At Rome & | that pro*u*ince of Rome cou*n*tre more than aure ellz |

15 **Of the ·5· maladie of malencoly & þe cure | of it. |**

ALso we saye that a nother diu*er*se infirmite | that is the fifthe that wexethe of this | humour bitwene the ey3e and the ey3e |lidde and it swellethe w*ith* halfe the visage of |

20 the face ¶ And it is an horrible maladie and it | hathe dyu*er*se namys / For sum*m*e clepen it y cur|sid and sum*m*e y blissed

24r maladie · For it comeþ || withe moche sorowe and ache and w*ith*

Basel, Ö.B.U., MS D.II.11, ff. 172r–177v

---

15 Of] 20 *added in outer margin*

Oxford, Bodleian Library, Ashmole MS 1468, pp. 1–6

Biblio.-Médiathèques de Metz, MS 176, ff. 1r–16r

    et tumefacta, | et tenet oculum ita
45 clausum quod paciens | nullo
    modo potest aperire eum. Audi-
    uistis | istius supradicte infirmitatis
    signa, | nunc docebimus vos pro
10rb i p s a m o p tim a m || e t
    probatissimam curam ad quam: ℞ |
    medullam frumenti ueteris, vi|tella
    ouorum ana ʒ 1, croci ʒ 1. Hec in
    simul | incorpora et pistentur et
5 cum lacte mulieris | mollificentur
    ut fiant sicut vnguentum, | et de
    isto emplastro ponatis super illam |
    benedictam, sed inter vnam
    palpebram | et aliam ponatis
    licinium de panno | ut retineat
10 emplastrum ad hoc ut non | intret
    oculum. Sciatis quod tria facit |
    emplastrum istud: primum quia
    totum humorem | [coadunat] in
    vno loco, secundario quia |

---

12 coadunat] M coadiuuat, VV (f. 178v) quoadunat, VP2 (f. 303v), VR (f. 50r) coadunat

Glasgow, GUL, Hunter MS 503, pp. 1–135

and Grekys cal | it Papulam, But
the citramown|tayns and frenshe-
men and oþer cal | it. Maledictam.
A no wonder for | yt growyth   15
with grette sorones and || grete   [85]
peyn. and thies ben the know|yng
þerof. It makyth the ey ledys al |
harde red & bolnyn. and kepyth
the ey | so shyt. þat the pacyent
may not | open it. Off whych   5
disease thys | is the cure. ¶ Take
fyne pure | flowre of olde whete.
and ʒelkys | of eggis as much. of
eche an vncer. | of safron a drame.
and stampe | them wele to geddyr   10
wyth wo|mans mylke. mollifi yt.
tyl yt | be as an oynement. wherof
make | a plaster and lay it to the
sore. and | be tweyne the ij. ey
lyddys ley a | smayl lyst of lynnen   15
cloyth to kepe || that on. þat noon   [86]
of the plaster entre | yn to the ey.
And iij tymes doo þis | plaster. It
gederyth too gheder all the |

London, British Library, Sloane MS 661, ff. 32r–46r

swelled, & | kepeth the Eye so shutt that patient can | not open yt And yow are to cuer   20
yt | after this sorte. Take fine puer flo|wer, of oulde wheate, and as mutch yelkes | of
egges, of etch an ownce of Safforne ʒj. | and beate them well together with so mutch | 25
womans mylke as will make yt into the | forme of a softe Oyntment (or as I thincke |
rather ₍a₎ Cataplasme) and applye this | vppon pledgettes to the sore Eye providinge | by   30
some fine pece of Sylke or lyninge cloth | to kepe yt from enteringe into the Eye be|twixte
the Eye liddes It gathereth to gether | all the humors & ripeneth them, & yt doth | ease
the paine, & many have bene cured there | with. || 35

---

28 rather]) deleted a] c deleted, a added over the deletion

Glasgow, GUL, Hunter MS 513, ff. 2r–37r

    grete fernesse | and horrible drede
it wexeth ¶ And the signis of | it in
knowyng is this all the ey3e liddes
ys hard | and for swollen and the
5 pacient haldeth his ey3e | closed
and y shitte that he maye nought
opyn his | ey3es ¶ Nowe y shall
teche the this cure moste | prouyd
take the floure of eldest whete þe
white | of eyren and the þe*nn*e of
saffron ana ·2·q· and | all these
grynde to giders withe womans
10 milke | make it neysshe in maner
of a noynement but | make it
nought moche neysshe w*ith* this
emplas*tr*e | on that benedicta leye
it but bytwene one ey3e | lyd and
that other laye ye a·pece of lynnen
cloþe | that it may holden the
15 emplastre that it goo | nought in
to the ey3e ¶ And we sayne that
þis | emph*astr*e dothe iij thing*es* ¶
First for it bryngeth | to geder all
the humour in to o place secunde

Basel, Ö.B.U., MS D.II.11, ff. 172r–177v

Oxford, Bodleian Library, Ashmole MS 1468, pp. 1–6

Biblio.-Médiathèques de Metz, MS 176, ff. 1r–16r

[maturat], tertio uero quia attrahit et | mitigat dolorem. Cum isto
15 emplastro | innumerabiles homines curauimus et libe|rauimus de ista infirmitate, et ma|gis regnat in iuuenibus quam in senibus | et plus inuenimus de istis in Tuscia | quam in alijs prouincijs.
20 **55.** Item aliam | medicinam pro ista infirmitate: Accipe | radicem lilij et ponatis eam sub ci|neribus calidis ut bene coquantur, postea | habeatis poma acerba et sub cineribus | simile coquantur donec
25 mollificentur et | a cortice mundari possint. Hoc facto | mundificentur et cum predicta radice pis|tentur et tantum sit de vno quantum de | alio, et cum albumine oui distemperentur | ita quod fiat bene liquidum. Et de isto

---

13 maturat] M muturat, VP2 (f. 303v), VR (f. 50r) maturat

Glasgow, GUL, Hunter MS 503, pp. 1–135

humors into oonn place. than after | rypeth it. and for the þryd 5
yt swa|gyth the payn. and wyth þis. ma|ny haue ben holpen. of thys disea|se.

¶ A noþer medicyne also for the | same. Take a lilie roote and roost | yt yn hoot embers. Take also 10
crab|bys & rooste hem yn the hoote fyre | or embrys is better tyll þei be roost. | þan a voyde the parrowr & the core. | and stampe þem and the root to | to gydder 15
asmych by weyght of the || toon [87]
as of the tooþer. tyl þei be welle | incorperate. and temper þem with the | whitte of eggis tyll þei be wele liquyde | And plaster the sore wyth this ony|ment tyl all the humor be consumyd. | and that the 5
ey may open & shytte. | And on

London, British Library, Sloane MS 661, ff. 32r–46r

[55] An other medicine allso for the same Take a | lyllye roote and roste yt in hoate 45v
Imbers Take | allso of crabbes, and rost them, in hoate imbers | the take of the pills & the cores, and stampe | them, and the lillye roote together, as mutch | by wayghte of the on, 5
as of the other, till | theye be well incorporate & temper them with | the whites of egges as mutch as will suffire | and applye yt to the Eye till all the humors, | be consumed, and 10
that the Eye can open | and shutt againe. But to the sore where the | swellinge did breake & the matter issu forth | yow shall applye this oyntment called vng: | Subtile. made after this sorte. Take of Aloes | Hepaticke. of Hennes grece oyle of bitter | allmons and white 15

---

3 allso] An other | Cataplasme | to the same | intent. *outer margin*   14 Subtile] vnguentum | Subtile. *outer margin*

Glasgow, GUL, Hunter MS 513, ff. 2r–37r   *Basel, Ö.B.U., MS D.II.11, ff. 172r–177v*

    for | it maturethe The ·iije· for it
draweth and swa|gethe the akthe /
And withe this emplastre we |
20 haue delyue*r*id fele and moste of
this maladie we | founde in
tuskene than aure elles

    ¶ Also we | shull teche a nother
medycyne for this infirmite | ¶
Take lilie rotis and Do hem in hote
24v emery || and lete hem roste well
and after that haue wode crab|bes
and w*ith* the forsaid lylie rotis in
a·brasyn morter | bruse hem an*a*
of hem bothe w*ith* the white of a
naye | temp*er* hem so that it be
5 nought moche neysshe ne | moche
harde and doo it on this infirmite
till all | the humour and all the
swellyng ben don awaye | and that
the ey3e mowe opyn and shitte and

---

23 emery] ℞ *added in outer margin*

Oxford, Bodleian Library, Ashmole MS 1468, pp. 1–6

Biblio.-Médiathèques de Metz, MS 176, ff. 1r–16r

30 em|plastro super istam infirmitatem pona|tis quousque totus ille humor con|sumatur et oculus possit claudi et | aperiri, et semper cicatricem ponatis de vn|guento
35 subtili quod fit de aloe epatico | et anxugia gallina et oleo amigdalarum | amarum et cera alba ana ʒ 1, et sic con|solidabitur et subtiliabitur cicatrix | cum isto vnguento taliter et tali modo | ac si
40 non fuisset ibi vlla macula, | et paciens liberabitur sine dolore | et cum gaudio laudans Deum et bene|dicens studio nostro.

56. Sed recorda|mur uobis ut semper habeatis uobiscum | de vnguento alabastro in omnibus
45 curis | vestris oculorum, et ponatis semel in | die, scilicet in
10va sero vngatur de eo ‖ timpora

Glasgow, GUL, Hunter MS 503, pp. 1–135

the stepe of the wonde there | the sore was. ley on an oynement | callyd. Vnguentum subtile. whych | ys made thus. ¶ Take aloe epa|tik. hennys grece. oyle of bitter | almandys. & white waxe. ana of | ycche. j ʒ. and Incorperate them to|gheder in to an oynement. and þis | shal consowdyn & subtilizen. so the ‖ skyn of the wonde. þat þer shal no | stepe apperynn yn the wonde.

10

15
[88]

Also | I counsel yow þat ye haue wythyou | Vnguentum alabastrum. and yn euery | cure of the eyon. 5 onys yn the day | þat is at even. anoynte the pacy|entis forhede. templys. and browis | þer wyth.

42 Sed...habuisset] Final paragraph of shorter recension

9 callyd] vng: Sub|tile added in outer margin in an Italic hand

London, British Library, Sloane MS 661, ff. 32r–46r

waxe of ether ʒ j. & incor|porate them together into the forme of an | oyntment. and this will consound & heale | the wounde perfectlye.
[56] I councell yow | (sayth my Author) that yow neuer be withowt | vng Alabastrinum, 20 and in everye Cuer of | the Eyes once in the daye annoynt the | Patientes forehead, temples, and browes | there with for that helpeth yor medicines | and asswageth the 25 paine & suffereth not | the humors to discend to the parte affected |

21 vng] fol. 14. outer margin 23 forehead] foreho before correction

Glasgow, GUL, Hunter MS 513, ff. 2r–37r

on | the wounde laye theron of the sotill poudre that is | y made of aloes epatik w*ith* hennes grece and
10   w*ith* the | oyle of bitter almoundes and white wexe an*a* to | the wheyght of an vnce for eu*er*yche and it shall | be y consouded and it shall sotill the skynne w*ith* | this sotill oynement in this maner as though he | hadde none wemme ne spot and the
15   pacient | w*ith*outen woo shall be delyu*er*d and they praisy*n*g | and worschippyng oure studye

¶ But we telle | you that he haue w*ith* oure vnguentu*m* de Alabastro | nostro in almaner of cures of eʒen as in cate|ractis as in othir maladies that comyn as
20   emy|grayne and other that fallen to hem eu*er*more | erlyich and late anoynte the temples and the | forhede and the browes of the eyʒe

Basel, Ö.B.U., MS D.II.11, ff. 172r–177v

¶ Deuetz saber senhors que en | totas las emfermetatz dels | uelhs   10
quals que sian niquals | q*ue* no. uos deuetz auer del en|guent alabaustro lo calh uos | auem dith de sobre que se fay | am las   15

---

10 dels] u *expunged*

Oxford, Bodleian Library, Ashmole MS 1468, pp. 1–6

386   *De Probatissima Arte Oculorum*

Biblio.-Médiathèques de Metz, MS 176, ff. 1r–16r

    frontem et supercilia pa|cientis, quia multa facit: primo | adiuuat omnem medicinam nostram | oculorum, secundo mitigat do-
5   lorem, | tercio non permittit ad locum dolen|tem descendere spiritus et humores, | quarto uero facit pacientem requi|escere die noctuque ac si nullam | maculam habuisset.

Glasgow, GUL, Hunter MS 503, pp. 1–135

For þat helpyth your me|dicyns and swagyth the peyne. & | suffryth not the humers to   10
descend | to the hurt place. And it makyth | the pacyent to haue rest.

10   **57**. Multi de illis | qui fuerunt passi talem infirmi|tatem uenerunt coram nobis cum | palpebris reuersatis, ad hoc ut | possent curari et liberari. Et nos in|terro-gauimus eos qualiter accidit eis, |
15   et ipsi dixerunt nobis: "domine habu|imus quoddam apostema quod bene|dicta vocatur et non fuimus bene | curati, vnde a conseruacione illius | cicatricis
20   remanserunt nobis pal|pebre

More|oure quod. Benemicius. I wyl þat | 3e practysers that many of þem | þat suffre this seid   15
sekenes to cum ‖ to me with þeir   [89]
ey lydys reuersed foule | for lak of sufficyent cure as þei sey | to me. and so yt was yn whos | cure yt procedid. For wyth a rasor | I   5
deuyed it suttilly and discretely | the ey lyd from the cycatryes of | the wonde. so þat the eye lede my|ght turne vp and downn.

London, British Library, Sloane MS 661, ff. 32r–46r

[57] There hath come vnto me sayth Beneuenutus | many that after the cuer of this sayd sycke|nes, have had there Eye liddes reuersed, for | lacke of suffitient care in there cuer.   30
And | to those with a Rasor I did subtillye devide | the Eye lidd from the Cicatrizes of the | wound so that the Eye lidd might torne ‖ vpp and downe. and then I made a little   46r
boul|ster of lynninge cloth, in the manner of a little | childes fingar and wett yt in the white of an | egg & layed ʟ yt ⌐ there vppon, and bound yt vpp till | the nexte dressinge   5
& I continued yt for the | space of xv. dayes. and then I made an | oyntment of Hennes grece & white wax and | there with I annoynted the boulster as I did | before. & layed yt to the wounde. as before | till yt was perfectlye cured. And sometyme | I made my   10

---

27 There] The reuersion | of the Eye | liddes. [caused   *deleted*] *outer margin*   33 torne] vpp & downe. *lower margin*

Glasgow, GUL, Hunter MS 513, ff. 2r–37r

    liddes / For | it Dothe moche gode
25r for it helpethe and after || warde it
    dothe A way ache the thridde it
    suffreth | nought to falle downe
    spirit*es* and humours to the | place
    of ache ¶ The Firste it makethe the
    pacient | to resten nyght and day
5 from ache As though | he hadde
    none spot neither webbe ne
    penaunce in | his ey3e ·/·

**Of the turnyng of ey3e liddis |
and of þe same infirmite & of the
cure.** |
    MAny that were suche infirmiteis
    comen | afore vs with her ey3e
10 liddes ouer turned | Saynige we
    hauethe apostome that is | clepid

---

23 after] warde *added in outer margin* **1** dothe] Francis Sleighe *added in upper margin in an Italic hand* **6** liddis] 21 *added in outer margin*

Oxford, Bodleian Library, Ashmole MS 1468, pp. 1–6

Basel, Ö.B.U., MS D.II.11, ff. 172r–177v

cimas d*e* las ronze e la pei|ra ques
anom alabaustro ede|uetz onchar
las templas elas silas.|
¶ Quant alcun es feritz per | colp
pres deluelh et aparlosa*n*c | pres   20
del uelh. aias .i^a. teula ro|ssa
efaylan escalfar alfoc ben | epueis
met sobre lateula sobre | ditha de
melh elayssa bolir ben | epueis etu
aias de coton mu|lath am baquel   25
melh e met | de sobrel colp ecera
gueritz

---

15 las…ronze] *added in a different hand*

Biblio.-Médiathèques de Metz, MS 176, ff. 1r–16r

reuersate." Et ipsi faciebant | pactum nobiscum ad hoc ut pos|sent per me curari et liberari. | Facto pacto accipiebamus raso|rium et diuidebamus palpe-
25 bram | a cicatrice ita subiliter et discrete | quod palpebra reuertebatur sursum. | Facta illa incisione ponebamus | postea desuper puluillum de panno | lineo ad
30 modum digiti factum et in|tinctum in albumine oui, et dimit|tebamus ita usque ad alium diem | cum fascia ligatum. Et de illo die | inantea imitabamur curam et oper|acionem istam, et faciebamus
35 vn|guentum de anxungia galline et | cera alba, et vngebamus puluillos | sicut primo faciebamus de albumine | oui, et ponebamus super illam cy|catricem illos
40 puluillos donec ci|catrix illa erat consolidata et eci|am remanebat palpebra in bono | statu. Tamen ter

Glasgow, GUL, Hunter MS 503, pp. 1–135

which | so doon. I made a lytyl pylowe of | ly*n*nen cloth yn the   10
mane*r* of a ly|tyl chyldys fynge*r* and wett it in | the whyte of an egg. and layd | þ*er* vpon. and bonde it to wyth a | lynnen bande to the nexte reme|uyng aȝen. and   15
so contynue þis || medycyne   [90]
daylly. to the xv. daye | and than I made an oynement | of hennys grece and of whyte | wexe. And þerwyth I anoynted | the pelowe   5
lyke as I dyd before. | wyth the whyte of an egg. and | leyd it on the cicatryce. or on the | wonde. like as I haue doon before | tyl it was p*er*fiȝtly sensowdid. and | the   10
ey lyde hole and yn good asta|te. Or els sum tyme I made a pe|lowe of a sponge and leyd it on | the wounde. for the p*ro*purte of the | sponge is to distroye waste flech |

---

7 cicatryce] *over erasure*

London, British Library, Sloane MS 661, ff. 32r–46r

boulste*r* of Spunge & kepte | that vppon the wounde, for the propertye | of the spunge is to kep downe proude flesh. | Never the lesse of the torninge vpp of the Eye | lydd*es*   15
caused through the abundance of sup*er*flu|ous bloode, and not beinge cured, wi*th*in a yeare. | Beware that yo*w* enter not the vttar p*ar*te of the | Eye lidd, but wi*th* a hooke lifte vpp the corne*r* | where the flesh is vnder the Eye lidd, and | then wi*th* yo*r* rasor cut yt so   20
directelye that that | yo*w* toutch not that part of the Eye lidd | where in the heare groweth. And havinge so | done applye pledget*es* as before is taughte in | the forme*r* cuer. and dresse yt twise in the | daye.   25

Glasgow, GUL, Hunter MS 513, ff. 2r–37r

    benedicta and we were not well y
cured | ther of wherfor the keping
of that heled wound | tho ey3e
liddes were so ouer turned outward
¶ In | this cause we token a ¶
15 Rasour and we kutte | and
deuided the ey3e lydde from the
heled wound | so sotillich and so
curiousliche that the ey3e lydde |
turned vp / And whan that the
kutty*n*g was y done | than we
layden alitell pelwe y made in the
shap | of a fynger of lynnen clothe
20 & we watte it in | the white of
a·naye and we leide it on the
wou*n*d | tille that other day y
bounde w*ith* a · bounde And |
from inforward we chaunged that
25v pilwis doy*n*g || so as it is saide till
xv dayes ¶ And than we chaun|gid
this cure And we made an-
oynement of hennes | grece and of
white wexe and we anoynted ther
|w*ith* the litill pilwe as we did first

Basel, Ö.B.U., MS D.II.11, ff. 172r–177v

Oxford, Bodleian Library, Ashmole MS 1468, pp. 1–6

Biblio.-Médiathèques de Metz, MS 176, ff. 1r–16r

      in ebdomada pone|bamus de
spongia marina ad | modum
45   puluilli ad hoc ut illa super|fluitas
quam cicatrix facit consu|meretur,
quia spongia marina tria | facit:
10vb primo quia destruit carnosi|||tatem
et pulmonositatem quam cicatrix |
facit ad consolidacionem, secundo
quia at|trahit et viuificat spiritum et
sanguinem, | tercio uero quia facit
5   plagam consolidari | tali modo
quod remanet in bono statu. | Et
taliter curabimus omnes qui
habebat | palpebras reuersatas de
quocumque | modo uenerat causa,
preter illos quorum pal|pebre erant
10   versate occasione ponderis | multe
carnositatis et simili occasione, |
scilicet habundancia sanguinis et
pruri|tu palpebrarum (sicut habetis
in primo | tractatu nostro de
pruritu oculorum | qui fit ex
habundancia sanguinis) quando |
15   per annum vnum stant quod non

Glasgow, GUL, Hunter MS 503, pp. 1–135

to drawe & to quyken the spiryt || 15
of the blode. & to consowdyn &   [91]
knit | the wounde. and to bryng yt
to | good astate. And on thys wyse
quod | he. I cured all that hade
þere eylydys. | turnyd by the   5
same cause. Neþer the | lees of
thys turnyng of the eyleddis | of
superhabundance of superfluite
of | blode not curid wythyn a
yere. | be ware the practisers that
3e enter | not the vtter parte of the   10
eye lydde. | but wyth a twycche
sotilly liftevp | the corner. where
the wast fleche | ys vnder the eye
lyd. And wyth a | rasur cutt it so
discretly þat 3e tou|che not. the   15
parte of the eylede that || the here   [92]
growyth. whych so doon. | ley
þerto such smale peletis as it | ys
said yn the cure before. And
chan|ge it twyes on the day till it be
ful | hoole. And of thys maner of   5
seke fol|kys. I found moyst yn

London, British Library, Sloane MS 661, ff. 32r–46r

Glasgow, GUL, Hunter MS 513, ff. 2r–37r

  5 w*ith* the white | of   anay and we
layde on the wounde thoo litill |
pilwes as it is saide till that the
wounde was | y heled / and
afterward that ey3e lidde lefte in |
good state ¶ And afterward neuer
the lesse we | dide to that wounde
10 of a·sponge y made in the | maner
of alitill pilwe for it shuld kepen
the | wounde and Do away the
supe*r*fluyte that the | wounde
hadde y made For the see sponge
is | gode for iij·skeles / First for it
distroiethe þe Fles|shi hede and the
lunge that the drie wounde hade |
15 y made thorugh his consowdyng ·
Se*cun*de for draweþ | and
quckethe the spirite and blode /
The iij^{de} for it | makethe the
wounde to conseuden in soche
maner | as it may fayrist stonde ¶
And so we heled | all thoo that
hadden her ey3eliddes ouer
20 turned | of   what eu*ere* cause it

Oxford, Bodleian Library, Ashmole MS 1468, pp. 1–6

Basel, Ö.B.U., MS D.II.11, ff. 172r–177v

Biblio.-Médiathèques de Metz, MS 176, ff. 1r–16r

    sunt curati, | palpebre oculorum
reuersantur. Vnde | karissimi istos
tales non debetis incidere | in
extrinseca parte [sed] in intrinseca
– to|tam illam carnositatem cum
20   vncino | et rasorio ita sagaciter et
discrete quod | palpebras ubi
nascuntur pili non | incidatis. Hoc
facto habeatis puluillos | sicut in
alijs curis de reuersatis, in |
extrinseca parte ponatis et mit-
25   tetis | bis in die puluillos pre-
dictos mane | et sero. Et sic
liberabuntur pacientes | usque ad
plenum, laudantes et bene|dicebant
Deum nostrum Ihesum Christum.
Et | sciatis quod magis inuenimus
30   de istis in | Tuscia et in Bononia
quam in alijs pro|uincijs.

Glasgow, GUL, Hunter MS 503, pp. 1–135

tuskeyn. | than yn any oþer
prouince.

---

18 sed] M nisi, VP2 (f. 304v), VR (f. 51v) sed

London, British Library, Sloane MS 661, ff. 32r–46r

Glasgow, GUL, Hunter MS 513, ff. 2r–37r

    come outtake thoo of whom | the ey3e liddes were ouer turned thorugh occasioun | of berthen of moche flesshe or liche to hem ¶ And | Also thorugh occasioun of ouer habundaunce of blod | and of 3eiche of the ey3eliddes as ye haue
26r in the ‖ First tretise of ye3che of ey3en the whiche is tho|rugh the habundaunce of blode whan they ben | nought in A yere y cured than the ey3elyddes | ben ouer turned wherfor my Dere Frendes |
5   ye shull nought kutt in the outeside but on the | inwarde par*t*ie all that Flesshe mater that is more | than y nowe w*ith* ahoke and with a· Rasour doyng | it away neuertheles wysolich that vndre that | ey3e lid where the here wexethe that ye kutte hym |
10   nought whan that is don hauethe litill pilwes | as in other cures of the ouer turnynges of ey3elid|des ·i·

Basel, Ö.B.U., MS D.II.11, ff. 172r–177v

Oxford, Bodleian Library, Ashmole MS 1468, pp. 1–6

Biblio.-Médiathèques de Metz, MS 176, ff. 1r–16r   Glasgow, GUL, Hunter MS 503, pp. 1–135

58. Item de humore melancolico generaļtur in multis hominibus quedam infirļmitas inter nasum et oculum et est | quasi carnositas, et in multis locis | vocatur muru, id est vulgariter corsu, | et in multis vocatur fungus. Vnde | cum videritis talem infirmitatem taļliter procedatis in curacione: Accipit rasoļrium et cum illo [rasorio] illum morbum | incidatis et excipietis a radicibus | suis, postea habeatis ferrum calidum et | cauterizate locum vnde habet originem, | ita tamen sagaciter et

¶ And | also of the malencoly*us* humor q*uo*d | the autor ther is gendrid yn many | men a sekenes that growyth betwe|ne the nose and the ey. and it appe|ryth lyke the pece of a long. and it | gr*au*elo*us* and voydyth allway fylth. | and co*mmu*nly it towchyth w*ith*yn the | ou*er*eye lede. and also the neþ*er*. And ‖ in many placis thys sore is clepyd. | Muri or wulgalpus. Off whych | thys ys the cure. wyth a twych so|tylly lyftvp the sore. and wyth the | poynt of a rasour cut yt vp by the | roote. and then wyth a

39 cum…rasorio] M cum illo rasario, VR (f. 51v) cum illo, VP2 (f. 303r) cum rasorio

8 quod] wolgaspus | Muri in | the corner | of the eye *added in outer margin in an Elizabethan hand*

London, British Library, Sloane MS 661, ff. 32r–46r

[58] There allso is caused of this melan|cholye humo*r* a disease growinge betwene *the* nose | and the Eye and yt appeareth like a pece of the | langes and yt is g*r*evelous & voydeth all waye | fylth & com*m*onlye yt towcheth w*ith*in the ou*er* | Eye lidd, and allso the nether. And in manye | places this sore is called Muri or wulgal|pus, and yt is thus cured ffirst w*ith* a hooke | lifte vpp the sore and w*ith* the poynt of a rasor | cutt yt vpp by the roote: and then w*ith* a whoate | Iron cauterize yt in the place where the sore | first tooke his begininge so warylye that yo*w* | hurt not the Eye: and annoynt yt w*ith* vng|uentu*m* subtile till yt be whole.

25 melancholye] Muri or wul|galpus a pece | of flesh gro|winge betwixt | the Eye & the | nose. *outer margin* 31 or] wol *deleted* 38 vnguentum] pag. 28 *outer margin*

Glasgow, GUL, Hunter MS 513, ff. 2r–37r　　*Basel, Ö.B.U., MS D.II.11, ff. 172r–177v*

    we haue saide aboue And doo thoo
litill pilwes | w*ith*in twies in a
daye that erlyche and late and we |
haue cured so many at the full in
15 Tusken and abou|ten boleyne we
founden moo than aure elles ·/· |
<O>f þe ·6· i*n*firmite of malyn-
coly & þe cure of it |
The sixte infirmite that wexeth of
malanco|lye humour in many and
that is a·infirmite | wexing a twene
20 the ey3e and the nose and | it is
as it were in the maner of Flesshy
mater and | of many it is cleped
mauri // The Cure of it is this |
Take a·Rasour and ku tte the
maladie and kutte hym | vp w*ith*
all hit Rotis and afterward hauethe
26v an hote || yren and cauterize it
where that is that the maladie | had
his begynnyg So wisely that ye
offonde nought | the ey3e · For

---

16 it] 22 *added in outer margin*

Oxford, Bodleian Library, Ashmole MS 1468, pp. 1–6

Biblio.-Médiathèques de Metz, MS 176, ff. 1r–16r

    discrete ut non | offendetis
oculum, quia muru illud semper |
45 nascitur inter nasum et lacri-
male. | Postea ponatis desuper
11ra stuppam intinc||tam in albumine
oui bis in die donec de|siccetur et
constringatur et consolidetur |
vsque ad plenum. Sic faciebamus
et sic | facietis cum benediccione
Ihesu Christi et mea. |
5 **59.** Adhuc dicimus vobis alia
signa de | predicto muru. Dicimus
ergo uobis quod ap|paret quasi
pulmo et est granellosus | et
semper emittat putredinem. Et
appre|hendit palpebram superiorem
10 ab illa | parte ubi oritur, id est
inter nasum et lacri|male. Quando
homo vult apprehendere ipsum |
cum vncino et rasorio non tenetur |
nec teneri potest propter suam
teneritatem, quia | tenerum est
propter suam gummositatem, et
15 gra|nellosus est propter suam

Glasgow, GUL, Hunter MS 503, pp. 1–135

hoote yron | cauteryse it yn the
place where the | sore tooke hys
orygynal begynny*ng*. | so weryly
that ʒe hurt not the eye. | And an*n*   10
noynt it w*ith* the oyneme*nt* |
callyd. Vnguentu*m* subtile. tyll it |
be hoole. |

London, British Library, Sloane MS 661, ff. 32r–46r

Glasgow, GUL, Hunter MS 513, ff. 2r–37r   *Basel, Ö.B.U., MS D.II.11, ff. 172r–177v*

    why this mury wexethe at twene |
    the nose and the lacrimal place and
5   afterward a·stupe | y wette in to
    the white of a ney twies a day till |
    it be y Dryed vp and y constrayned
    and y helyd vp | at the Full

    ¶ A nothir token ther ys of the
    forsaid | mury is this · we saye that
    it is liche a lunge & | it is kernelly
    and euer more it castethe oute
10 rothed | and   it strecchethe right
    in to the ouer ey3elid and | to the
    nether ey3e lid ¶ And ther as he
    hathe his be|gyn*n*ynyng and
    wexethe atwene the nose and the |
    tery place ¶ And whan eny body
    take it with an | hoke and w*ith* a
    Rasour it holdethe nought · For it |
15 is   right neysshe and roten and for
    his tendrenes|se it is tendre for his

Oxford, Bodleian Library, Ashmole MS 1468, pp. 1–6

Biblio.-Médiathèques de Metz, MS 176, ff. 1r–16r

frigiditatem, quia | semper
habundat de humoribus frigidis
superfluis et corruptis. |

60. Expleuimus uobis tractatum 4
humorum, | scilicet sanguinis,
flegmatis, colerice, melancolie. |
20 Docuimus uos curas et signa
infir|mitatum que procedunt ex eis,
et Artem | a nobis Beneuenuto de
Iherusalem compositam, | quia
expertum et probatissimum reddit |
artificem, et quia est sapientum
25 semper | dare, et audientium
conseruare. Et au|diendo et conser-
uando a primis dantibus | et
secundis operantibus exit nostra
Ars.

───────────────

17 corruptis] M expliciunt morbi
oculorum ab initio *added in margin
in another contemporary hand*

London, British Library, Sloane MS 661, ff. 32r–46r

Glasgow, GUL, Hunter MS 503, pp. 1–135

IN the fyrst partye of thys | tretys.
ȝe practysers quod my | autor. I   15
declared to yow || what ann eye is.   [94]
And how it ys | maid after myn
opynyon and oþer | menys also.
and what is a cater|acte. and how
many spycys be þere|of curable.   5
and how many vncu|rable. and
how the cure of the cu|rable ys.
And how the cure of | the vn-
curable ys by ann easy de-
ly|uerance of honde by a craft   10
callyd. | Ars acuaria. that is the
crafte | of the nedyl. And after yn
the | secunde partye I tauȝt yow of
the | infirmitees of eyon that be
cau|sed Inwarde. by occasyon of
dis|temperance of the iiij humers.   15
þat || ys to wyt. blode. color.   [95]

Glasgow, GUL, Hunter MS 513, ff. 2r–37r   *Basel, Ö.B.U., MS D.II.11, ff. 172r–177v*

gu*m*mosite and it is of gray|nes for his coldenesse · For allway it habundithe | and wexeth of roten humours ·/·
Of smy|tyng & hurtyng of þ*e*
20 **ey3e & brekyng of the | tunicle and the cure ther of.** |
For why it is of wise men to yeue alwey | audiens and to kepen that that is taken | of wysdom and so in hering and in keping | from firste yeuyng and from the secunde y
25 wrought | connyng commethe therof

---

18 smytyng] **23** *added in outer margin*

Oxford, Bodleian Library, Ashmole MS 1468, pp. 1–6

400   *De Probatissima Arte Oculorum*

Biblio.-Médiathèques de Metz, MS 176, ff. 1r–16r

Glasgow, GUL, Hunter MS 503, pp. 1–135

61. Am|modo docebimus uos de illis infirmi|tatibus que ueniunt in
30   oculis ex parte | extrinseca et ex vi cause percussionis, | scilicet quando oculi sunt percussi baculo uel | lapide, virga, alapa, pugillo, uel | pugno – aut cum paruuncula sagitta si|cut pueri faciunt quando
35   ludunt, aut cum | manu aut canna, aut aliquo alio sti|pite duro et alijs similibus. Dicimus | ergo quod quando videbitis aliquem percussum, | succurratis ei cum albumine oui quam | cicius pote-
40   ritis antequam humores con|currant et dissoluantur, scilicet vitreus | cristallinus et albugineus, ne forte, | propter nimium dolorem quem sustinuit in | oculo propter percussionem, humores oculorum | destruantur. Et nullam medi-
45   cinam | ponatis in oculis istam

flewme. & | malyncolye. and þeir cures. ¶ |
And now yn thys thyrde pαrtye and | last of my tretys. I wyll tel yow | of þies hurtis and diseases   5
causyd | yn eyon from wythouteward. as | wyth smytyng of stekkys and stonys | & staues. or ony such oþer. wherfore | here ere that I pρocede to any specyall | cure. I generally counseyl yow.   10
that | when ʒe se any suche come to yow | socowre them wyth the whyte of | ann egg. And as sone as ʒe mowe | leying to the ey a plaster made of | flexen hurdys.   15
and the whyte of || an egg. And   [96]
yff it happen for the grete | payn the humurs of the eye. be distro|yd and dyssoluyd. and thys plaster | renewith. iiij. sythes on the day &

---

13 ann] supe or out|ward quick in the eyes. *added in outer margin in an Elizabethan hand*

London, British Library, Sloane MS 661, ff. 32r–46r

Glasgow, GUL, Hunter MS 513, ff. 2r–37r   *Basel, Ö.B.U., MS D.II.11, ff. 172r–177v*

¶ Nowe hens forward | we shull
teche you of the maladies of ey3en
27r   that || comyn of cause of
w*ith*outen forthe as is smytyng
w*ith* staf | or w*ith* stone or suche
other ¶ And whan ye se any |
suche helpe hem w*ith* the glayre of
a·nay as sone as | ye mowe / or
that the humours of the ey3en ben
5   dis|solued and that by happe ne
falle nought for moche | payne of
the stroke the humours of the
ey3en wer | distroyed and that ye
done none medecyn but the |
glayre of an ey well y swugen and
w*ith* cotoun y |layde on that ey3e
10   iiij· tymes on a·day and twyes | a
nyght ¶ do thus xv· dayes / And
yef the tonicle | be to broke putte
in the ey3e the medicyn that is |
clepen de virtute a·deo data ¶ And
that is y made | of the streynes of

Oxford, Bodleian Library, Ashmole MS 1468, pp. 1–6

Biblio.-Médiathèques de Metz, MS 176, ff. 1r–16r

	infirmita|tem pacientibus nisi
	albumen oui bene ductum et
11rb	verberatum cum subtili ‖ stipite
	uel virga donec totum reuer|tatur in
	spumam. Et habeatis bombacem │
	et intingatis in illa clara et oculo │
	clauso superponatis quater in die
5	bis │ in nocte usque ad xv dies sic
	faciendo. │ Sed tamen si tunica est
	fracta ponatis │ in oculo de virtute
	a Deo data inuen|ta a nobis et ita
	vocamus ipsam │ quia virtutibus
10	magnis est plena, da|tis a Deo
	– que facta est de graminibus
	ouo|rum sicut in subscriptis ratio-
	nibus, │ ascendemus bis in die
	semel in nocte, │ et propter hoc
	non dimittatis quando pona|tis
	bombacem intinctum in albumine
15	oui │ super oculum clausum
	usque ad predictum │ terminum.
	Sed dum medicabitis infir|mos
	vestros vngatis eis timpora │
	frontem et supercilia vngento

London, British Library, Sloane MS 661, ff. 32r–46r

Glasgow, GUL, Hunter MS 503, pp. 1–135

twys │ on the ny3te. xv. days to 5
gydd*er*. And │ yf it happyn by the
hurte takyn the │ tonycle to be
hurte or brokyn. put │ twyes on the
day & oonys of the nyght │ of a
medycyne founde be p*ra*ctyffe
callyd. │ Virtus a deo data. whos 10
makyng │ shal be tau3t a noon
after. but not │ for þan ley not the
forseyd plast*er*. │ tyl the forseyd
tyme be past. and │ also foryetyth
not a noyntyng the │ pacyentys 15
templys. hys forhede ‖ and hys [97]
browes w*ith* the p*re*scyous
oy|nement of Alabastru*m*,

---

11 not¹] pag. 98 *added in outer margin in an Italic hand*

Glasgow, GUL, Hunter MS 513, ff. 2r–37r   *Basel, Ö.B.U., MS D.II.11, ff. 172r–177v*

eyryn and we shull shewe | you of
that medicyn do it in the ey3en
15   twyes | a   day and ones at nyght ¶
Nought for that | leue ye nought to
ley cotoun y wette in the glayre |
of a·nay y beten to water till fiftene
daies ben | fulfilled ¶ And anoynte
ye the browes & þe for|hede and
the templis w*ith* the oynement
Alabaustri |

Oxford, Bodleian Library, Ashmole MS 1468, pp. 1–6

Biblio.-Médiathèques de Metz, MS 176, ff. 1r–16r

ala|bastro quod confortat cerebrum
20 et vi|uificat spiritum et dolorem
expellit. |
62. Et sciatis karissimi quod si a
principio | cum sunt percussi non
sunt cum istis | curis nostris curati,
scilicet cum albumine | oui et
virtute a Deo data antequam |
25 oculi incipiant tumescere uel
pu|tresceri, raro enim postea aut
nunquam | curantur cum clara oui
et virtute | a Deo data. Vnde
narrabimus uo|bis virtutem et
30 potenciam diuinam | que est in
clara oui specialiter pro istis |
percussionibus oculorum. Dicimus
ergo | quod tria facit ad oculum
percussum: primo | quia mitigat
dolorem, secundo quia | con-
stringit humores oculorum, tercio |
35 quia purificat oculum – et nullam
su|perfluitatem aliorum humorum
neque | spirituum permittit ad
oculos peruenire. | Ergo digne

London, British Library, Sloane MS 661, ff. 32r–46r

Glasgow, GUL, Hunter MS 503, pp. 1–135

and yf þei | that be hurte. or
smyten wyth thys | be not curyd
on the seid wyse bety|mes at the 5
begynnyng ere that the | ey
begynne to bolne or to roote. þei |
shal neuer be cured nor helyd
wyth | any oþer medycyne. ¶ For I
wyll | ȝe knowe. iij grete vertuous
of the white | of an egg. and 10
specyally for suche | smytyng. ¶
The fyrst it swagith | the sorow
and the payn. the secunde | it
constrenyth the humers of the
eyon | and purifyeth the eyon. the
thyrd | it suffryth no superfluyte 15
of humers || to come in to the [98]
eyon. and as for the | medycyne
callyd. Virtus a deo data. | that

---

15 humers] to come *added in lower margin*

Glasgow, GUL, Hunter MS 513, ff. 2r–37r   *Basel, Ö.B.U., MS D.II.11, ff. 172r–177v*

20   ¶ yif they fro the begynnyng were
y smyte ben | nought y heled ne
Cured w*ith* these medecyns | or
that they begynne to swelle and to
27v wexe rote*n* ‖ selden after or neuer
shull they be y cured oneliche |
withe these medicyns ¶ wherfor
the white of anay | that specialich
for smytyng*es* is good and wete
ye | for why · For it first for-
5   nemythe the ache · 2ᵉ after|ward
constraynethe the humours of the
eyen and | it clensethe the ey3e· 3ᵉ
it suffrethe nought that none |
superflue humours neyther of
spirite to come to the | ey3e · 4ᵉ·
and it confortethe the ey3e liche to
hym in | kynde ¶ The Cure of the
10 tonicle y broken ys w*ith* | the

---

9 kynde] cure *added in outer margin*

Oxford, Bodleian Library, Ashmole MS 1468, pp. 1–6

[62] do we did nedill it after þe maner of agul|lyng as it is y taught aboue in doctrine of   1a
ca|taract*es* and so he was clenelich y heled and | clerely he toke and recouered his si3t /
And þus | we haue serued many worshiping be to god // | And so do 3e and dothe none   5
oþer cure

Biblio.-Médiathèques de Metz, MS 176, ff. 1r–16r

```
          nominata est clara oui,  | quia cum
 40    intrat oculos clarificat,  | purificat
          oculum, eius dolorem mitigat  | qui
          fit ex percussionibus, et hoc facit  |
          cum suauitate sue dulcedinis,
          quia  | suauis est et dulcis et
          percussionem  | sanat. Et dicitur
 45    clara quia clari|ficat  oculum et
          confortat suum similem.  | Et hec
          est cura tunice fracte cum  ||
 11va  medicina   que vocatur virtus a
          Deo data  | que sic fit: Recipiatis
          oua recencia  | que nascuntur de
          gallinis albis, extra|hatis inde
 5      germina pullorum usque ad xii  | et
          ponatis ipsa in mortario pulchro et
          mundo et ducatis ea ad modum
          vnguenti. Hoc facto in vase vitreo
          seruetur, et paulatim in oculo seu
          oculis pacientis bis in die ponatis
 10    donec  | tunica  saluatrix
          consolidetur, quam  | Iohannicius
          vocat coniunctiuam. Et di|cimus
          uobis karissimi sicut vnguenta
```

London, British Library, Sloane MS 661, ff. 32r–46r

Glasgow, GUL, Hunter MS 503, pp. 1–135

knyttyth and sowdeth the tony|cle a
geyn yf it be brokyn. and it | is   5
made on thys wyse. ¶ Take | xij.
stren*us* of new freshe leyd egg*is*. |
of white hennys. and put them i*n* |
a mort*er*. and labur them wele
w*ith* | a pestel. tyl thei be wele
yncorp*er*ate | to gydder yn man*er*   10
of a oynement. | And þan put it yn
a vessel of glase | and put it yn the
eye. as it ys se|yd. be fore twyes on
the daye. and | oonys on the nyght.
For lyke as | othyr consolydatyfe   15
oynementys || consowdyn and   [99]
purifye othir won|dys. so thys vertu
youen of god co*n*|sowdyth the
tonycle of the eye. yf | it be hurte
and purified the eye. & | w*ith* thys   5
ryght v*er*tuo*us* medycyne ma|ny
one haue I cured and hopen. me*n*. |

---

5 Take] virtus a deo | data *[quid deleted]* added in outer margin in an Elizabethan hand **13** fore] *a comma, written in a darker ink, follows.*

Glasgow, GUL, Hunter MS 513, ff. 2r–37r

    vertue y yeuen fro god and that is this | ¶ Take newe y leide henne eyren and take out her | streynes ·24· and grynde hem in aclene morter in | maner of a noyntement and kepe it in a glasyn ves|sell and doo therof a litell in to the ey3e of
15 the pa|cient twies a·Day till that tunicle saluatrix | be hole and Cured ¶ And Right as oynement*es* that | ben soden helyn and clensyn woundes Right so | this medicyne y yeuen of god consowdeth the | tunicle and purifiethe the ey3e ¶
20 And yit withe | this vertuouse cure we haue delyu*er*de many ¶ But | take good hede that after that the ey3e is y con|souded of the tonicle so broken the ey3e leuethe | clere but the pacient ne seithe nought w*ith* his ey3e | for ther in the ey3e ys y woxe
28r a·cataract ¶ And || ther knowe ye well that of suche smytyng*es* howe

Basel, Ö.B.U., MS D.II.11, ff. 172r–177v

Oxford, Bodleian Library, Ashmole MS 1468, pp. 1–6

Biblio.-Médiathèques de Metz, MS 176, ff. 1r–16r

con|solidativa consolidant et
purificant | vulnera, ita ista
15 medicina virtus | a Deo data
consolidat tunicam illam | et
purificat oculum a macula, id est |
de percussione illa quam oculus
sus|tinuit. Et ideo vocamus ipsam
vir|tutem a Deo datam quia
20 habuimus | ipsam ex virtute Dei
et cum ista | virtuosissima cura
multos homines | de istis percus-
sionibus sic faciendo | liberauimus
et curauimus. Inter | quos autem
25 inuenimus quendam puerum | in
Messana qui habebat oculum
inci|sum per medium et erat tunica
sal|uatrix incisa sic quod tres
humores | oculorum videbantur, et
pater suus et | consanguinei sui
30 [duxerunt] eum | coram nobis et
nos incepimus ipsum | curare sicut

22 faciendo] M de *expunged*
29 duxerunt] M dixerunt, *emended in a different hand*

London, British Library, Sloane MS 661, ff. 32r–46r

Glasgow, GUL, Hunter MS 503, pp. 1–135

women. and chyldren. yn dyuers |
placys. Amonge whych yn a
cetee | callyd. Messana. was
brought to | me a chylde whos   10
eye was oute yn | the myddys. so
that I myght se. iij. | humers. And
wyth thys forseyde | medycyne. I
saued hys eye hoole. | but he
myght not see. for hys ey | was   15
cateracte of the vyolence of the ||
stroke. as it ys declaryd be forn [100]
yn | the fyrst spice of the curable
cateracter. | wherfore I lete hym
be so. iiij mo|nethys after. tyll. the
cateracter was | confermed. and
þan I cured hym | as I haue tauȝt   5
beforn yn the cu|rable cateracter.

Glasgow, GUL, Hunter MS 513, ff. 2r–37r   *Basel, Ö.B.U., MS D.II.11, ff. 172r–177v*

|eu*er* that the ey3e be y hurte it
wexethe therin | cataract*es* right as
ye haue in the first spice of
cata|ract*es* of smytyng in the first
5 tretise of cataract*es* | ¶ And ther
for do ye as y did to a childe In
mas|sana whos ey3e was cloven a
two in the myd|des w*ith* a stroke
and saluatrix tonicle was kutte |
And the 3^(e.) humours were y sey /
And we did after | the forsaid cure
and heled hym vp and that Child |
10 receyued his ey3e ¶ But neuer the
lesse he say | nought ther w*ith* for
the lyght was y cataracted | ¶ But
y lete hym be so foure monthes to
fulfilly*ng* | of that cataract*es* / And
whan this was y do | we did nedill
15 it after the maner of agulyng as | it
is y taught aboue in doctrine of
cataract*es* and | so he was clene-
lich y heled and clerely he toke |
and recouered his sight / And thus
we haue ser|ued many worshiping

Oxford, Bodleian Library, Ashmole MS 1468, pp. 1–6

Biblio.-Médiathèques de Metz, MS 176, ff. 1r–16r   *Glasgow, GUL, Hunter MS 503, pp. 1–135*

      docuimus uos in presen|ti cura:
      intus oculum ponebamus | de
      virtute a Deo data, et oculo clau|so
      superponebamus bombacem
35   intinc|tum in clara oui usque ad
      xv di|es, et bis in die ponebamus
      intus | oculum de virtute a Deo
      data et | semel in nocte. Et puer sic
      recupera|uit oculum suum, sed
40   tamen nichil vide|bat quia lux erat
      catharactata | sicut habetis in
      tractatu catharac|tarum curabilium,
      de prima specie que | accidit extra
      oculum ex vi cause per|cussionis.
      Vnde sciatis karissimi quod de |
45   istis percussionibus quocumque
      modo | oculi fuerint percussi, ipsi
11vb oculi || catharactantur, sed post-
      quam erunt cu|rati cum predictis
      curis nostris de percussi|onibus
      quibuscumque remanent clari sed |
      nichil vident. Non timeatis ergo si
5   non | vident. Dimittatis post
      pacientem stare | sic per 4 menses

London, British Library, Sloane MS 661, ff. 32r–46r

Glasgow, GUL, Hunter MS 513, ff. 2r–37r   *Basel, Ö.B.U., MS D.II.11, ff. 172r–177v*
   be god and so do ye and | dothe
none other cure

Oxford, Bodleian Library, Ashmole MS 1468, pp. 1–6

Biblio.-Médiathèques de Metz, MS 176, ff. 1r–16r

    et plures, completo | hoc termino
acuate eum sicut docui|mus uos in
curis nostris catharactarum |
curabilium, quia et nos siquidem |
10   fecimus de illo puero et de
pluribus alijs. |
    63. Ita debetis curare pacientes de
per|cussionibus, scilicet cum clara
oui et virtute | a Deo data, et non
sicut faciunt stoli|di medici qui
15   ignorant Artem et curam, | quia
quando vident aliquem percussum
acci|piunt ceram et ciminum
puluerizatum et com|miscent
insimul et faciunt de istis duo|bus
emplastrum et calefaciunt ipsum et
po|nunt super oculum percussum.
20   Et vultis | audire quanta mala
facit? Si tunica | est fracta illud
emplastrum attrahit to|tam sub-
stantiam oculi et consumit omnes
hu|mores oculorum. Cera duo facit:
attra|hit et consumit, et ciminum
25   dissoluit et | liquefacit propter

Glasgow, GUL, Hunter MS 503, pp. 1–135

On thys wyse shall | ȝe cure all tho
þat arnn hurte in the | ey wyth
stroke or smytyng. and | not os   10
lewde leches arnn wont to | doo.
wyth a plaster made of waxe | and
powder of comyn. whych they |
leyd hoot to the ey hurte and
bro|ken. for yf the tonycle of the
eye | be hurte or brokyn. a noon it   15
draw||yth all the substance of the   [101]
eye and | consumyt the humers.
for wex of his | propurtee drawyth
and consumyth. | And commyn
dyssoluyth & meltyth. | And thus   5
by drawyng. dyssoluyng | &
consumyng. the eye ys distroyed. |
and ys foule dysfigured. And the |
ey be smytyn and hurte wythoute |

London, British Library, Sloane MS 661, ff. 32r–46r

Glasgow, GUL, Hunter MS 513, ff. 2r–37r   *Basel, Ö.B.U., MS D.II.11, ff. 172r–177v*

20   ¶ And be ware that ye do | nought
as summe vnwise and foly leches
vnknow|yng the cure & the
connyng Done for why whan |
they sein a body y hurte or y smyte
in the ey3e | they taken wexe that
28v is actractifi and ¶ the ey3e || that is
y hurte drawethe humours to hym
and | comyn y poudred the whiche
dissoluethe vndothe and | meltethe
for hete and moystenes that is in
hem two | and of hem they make
5   emplastre and all warme | they
ley it to the ey3e and so hem that
they shuld | hele they fornem hem
her sight · For why se howe |
contrarie they don that leyn an
emplastre that vn|doyng dissoluyn

Oxford, Bodleian Library, Ashmole MS 1468, pp. 1–6

[63] ¶ And | beware þat 3e do nou3t as summe vnwise and | foly leches vnknowyng þe cure and þe connyng | done ffor why whan þey sein a body y hurte | or y smyte in þe   10
ey3e þey taken wex þat is | attractyf and to þe ey3e þat is y hurte draweþ | humours to hym and comyn y poudred þe which | dissolueth vndoth and melteth for hete and |
moystenes þat is in hem two and of hem þey | make emplastre and all warme þey ley it   15
to þe | ey3e and so hem þat þey shulde hele þey forneme | hemm her si3t · ffor why se howe contrarie þey | don þat leyn an emplastre þat vndoyng diss|oluyng drawyng
wastyng þat distroieth þe | ey3e and leuith it defouled ¶ And yif it were | so þat þe ey3e   20
were nou3t to broke / yit þis | emplastre noyeþ · ffor it draweth to hym spirites | and
humours and woo and akþe on ayþer side | fi3tyng on euery side of þe ey3e and so þey
beten | till þe ey3e be wasted / and we haue say many | þat haue loste all þe substaunce   25
of þe ey3e by þat | emplastre · wherfore we amoneste 3ow þat in | what euer wey þat þe
ey3e ys y smete with yn or | with owt / hele it with þe glaire of a ney / ffor euer | y lich   30

Biblio.-Médiathèques de Metz, MS 176, ff. 1r–16r

    suam caliditatem et sicci|tatem. Et ecce tria contraria, quia at-tra|hendo, dissoluendo, et consumendo dis|currit tota substantia oculi, et sic discurren|do destruitur oculus tali modo quod oculus |
30 remanet postea deturpatus. Et si tuni|ca non est fracta attrahit ibi spiritus | et humores, vndique pungentes circum|circa oculum, et tantum pulsant donec oculus | deuastatur cum tota sua substantia.
35 Et | nos vidimus quam plures homines qui fu|erunt percussi et amiserunt totam substantiam | oculi, et nos interrogauimus quomodo ami|serant lumen oculorum et ipsi dixerunt | nobis: "Domine, fuimus percussi in oculis
40 sed | tamen videbamus aliquantulum. Postea fu|imus curati cum cera et cimino, | et ab illa hora amisimus lumen oculorum | ex toto ex illa medicina, quia

London, British Library, Sloane MS 661, ff. 32r–46r

Glasgow, GUL, Hunter MS 503, pp. 1–135

brekyn of the tonycle. than this | plast*er* drawyth þereto the spyrit | 10
and the hum*ers*. and causyth grete | sorowe rounde a bowte the eye. and | so betyth boyth the ey and the tem|plys. that often the ey ys wasted | & dystroyed þerby. as   15
I haue often || founde yn dyu*ers*   [102]
placys. ¶ Also | sum haue lost þeir sy3te wyth pla|sters made of wormewode & oliba|nu*m* and of such hote and dyssoua|tyfe   5
thyng*is*. wherfore I counsel you | to be ware of all suche plast*ers*.

Glasgow, GUL, Hunter MS 513, ff. 2r–37r   *Basel, Ö.B.U., MS D.II.11, ff. 172r–177v*

    drawyng wastyng that distroyethe |
    the ey3e and leuethe it defouled ¶
10 And yif it were | so that the ey3e
    were nought to broke yit this
    em|plastre noyethe · For it
    Drawethe to hym spiritus | And
    and woo & akthe on ayther side
    fi3tyng on eu*er*y | side of the ey3e
    and the beten till the ey3e be
    was|ted And we haue say many
15 that haue loste all the | substaunce
    of ey3e by that emplastre wherfor
    we | amoneste you that in whAt
    euer wey that the ey3e | ys y smete
    w*ith*in or w*ith*owte hele it with the
    glay|re of a ney For euer y liche
    conforteth and nurshe|the his liche
    And the ey ys of colde kynde and
20 so | is   the ey3e And many
    pacient*es* were that haue | loste he
    ey3en And her syght namelyche
    p*ro* empla|stris y made of
    wormode & olybano and suche
    oþ*er* | hote thing*es* dissolutiuis ·/·

Oxford, Bodleian Library, Ashmole MS 1468, pp. 1–6

conforteth and nursheth his lyche / And þe | ey ys of a colde kynde and so is þe ey3e /
And | many pacient*es* were þat haue loste her ey3en*n* | and her si3t namely p*ro* emplastris
y made of wor|mode & olibano and suche other hote þinges | dissolutiuis ·/·| 35

Biblio.-Médiathèques de Metz, MS 176, ff. 1r–16r

    lacri|mando exiuit paulatim tota
45 substantia | oculi cum maximis
    doloribus et | angustijs." Vnde
12ra monemus vos || quod quocumque
    modo oculus fuerit percussus |
    extra uel intus, medicetis eum
    cum | clara oui qui simile nutrit et
    gubernat | suum similem. Post-
    quam oculus est frigide com|ple-
5 xionis, oportet ut cum percutitur
    et le|ditur quod et gubernetur et
    medicetur | cum rebus frigidis, ut
    humores oculorum | non dissol-
    uantur a suis nutrimentis | propter
    percussionem quam sustinuerunt.
10 Et | multi alij fuerunt qui amise-
    runt lu|men pro emplastris factis ex
    absinthio | et olibano et cum alijs
    rebus calidis | et dissolutiuis.
    64. Audiuistis contraria que |
    stolidi medici faciebant in oculis |
15 percussis, et eciam docuimus uos
    pro ipsis | probatissimam curam
    nostram. Ammodo | docebimus

London, British Library, Sloane MS 661, ff. 32r–46r

Glasgow, GUL, Hunter MS 503, pp. 1–135

And | haue all weye yn all hurtys
of eyon | caused of owtwardys by
stroke or | smytyng to the
gr*a*cy*ou*s medycyne of | the   10

Glasgow, GUL, Hunter MS 513, ff. 2r–37r   *Basel, Ö.B.U., MS D.II.11, ff. 172r–177v*

29r **Of smytyng of || þe ey3e liddis &
in þe temples & þe lacrimal
place & þe cure | þerof. |**

---

1 temples] 24 *added in outer margin*

Oxford, Bodleian Library, Ashmole MS 1468, pp. 1–6

[64] Of smytyng in þe ey3e liddes & in þe temples | & þe lacrimal place and þe cure þerof ·/·|
Nowe we shull teche yow of þe smytynges | þe whiche benn ayenst þe ey3e as in þe |
ey3e liddis and in þe templis and of þe | lasse lacrimale place and in bene þat ys vnder | 40
þe neþer ey3e lyd // And we say 3if a man be || y smete in þe ey3e liddes and þat 1b
smytyng be | moche and it touche þe bone þat is aboute þe | ey3e þou3 it touche not þe
ey3e ¶ The ey3e | appereth clere and neuer þe lesse hit hath losten | his li3t · ffor þat 5
smytyng neruus opticus ys | stopped in so moche þat þe visible spirit may no3t | come to
þe ey3e ¶ Also þe smytyng in þe temples | it distourbleþ þe humours of þe ey3enn / for
why | þe pacient may nou3t clerelich se summe tyme | And 3if it be it is vnder þe ey3e 10
lid in þe neþer | partie / So þat it toucheth þe bone þat is vnder | þe nether eye lid / And
also he seyþ nou3t þo3 | he haue a clere ey3e wherfore whan 3e se | any suche beholdeth
in to þat ey3e and yif þe | balle of þe ey3e be brode or yif þat he be more | þan his 15

Biblio.-Médiathèques de Metz, MS 176, ff. 1r–16r

vos de illis percussionibus | que
fiunt circumcirca oculum, scilicet
in super|cilijs, in timporibus, et a
20 parte lacrimalis | minoris, et in
osse quod subtus uel super |
palpebras oculorum est, scilicet
inferiorem. | Et primo dicimus
vobis de prima et de | supercilijs.
Si homo est percussus cum |
gladio et tangit os quod est circum-
25 circa | oculum, id est subtus
palpebram et supra, | et est magna
percussio uel punctura | quamuis
non tangat oculum, oculus ap|paret
clarus tamen amittit lumen quia |
propter percussionem neruus
30 opticus est | ita opilatus quod
spiritus uisibilis per|transire non
potest usque ad oculum. Item |
percussio que fit in timporibus
con|turbat sic humores oculorum

Glasgow, GUL, Hunter MS 503, pp. 1–135

whyte of egg*er*. that I haue tolde |
yf ȝe wyll not erre. |

---

32 conturbat] M confirturbat *before correction*

London, British Library, Sloane MS 661, ff. 32r–46r

Glasgow, GUL, Hunter MS 513, ff. 2r–37r *Basel, Ö.B.U., MS D.II.11, ff. 172r–177v*

NOwe we shull teche of the
smytynge*s* the | whiche ben ayenst
the ey3e as in the ey3eliddis | and
in the templis and of the lasse
5 lacrima|le place and in bone that
is vndre the nether ey3e |lid // And
we say yif aman be y smete in the
ey3e |liddes and that smytyng be
moche and it towche þe | bone that
is a bought the ey3e though it
towch not | the ey3e ¶ The ey3e
apperethe clere and neuer the |
10 lesse hit hathe losten his lyght ·
For that smytyng | neruus opticus
is stoppid in so moch that the
visi|ble spirite may nought come to
the ey3e ¶ Also þe | smytyng of
the templis it distourblethe the
hu|mours of the ey3en For why the
15 pacyent may no|ught clerelich se
su*m*me tyme and yef it so be it is |
vndre the ey3e lid in the nether
p*ar*tie So that it | towchethe the
bone that is vndre nether ey3elid |

Oxford, Bodleian Library, Ashmole MS 1468, pp. 1–6

felawe knowe ye well þat he seiþ nou3t | ¶ And yif þe pacient sey þat he seith · loke yif |
þe appill of þe ey3e · 3if it is made brode and con|streyned ׃ it is to leue þat he seyþ · for
why þe | visible spirit comyng by þe holwe synewe to his | out passage makeþ þe ey3e   20
appill to wexe | abrode and to constrayne ¶ And yif it be no3t | y gone abrode and to
constrayne as it doiþ in | an hole ey3e / And þou3 me semeth þat he haue | a clere ey3e   25
as þe toþer ey3e ey3e is clere · whan | he hath þese signes as we haue y said doþe | none
cure / ffor þe holwe nerffe is so stopped þat | þe visible spirite by none wey may nou3t
co*m*me | to þe ey3e / And knoweþ well þat þe senewe | holwe moste is stopped in hem   30
þat bene y smete | all about þe ey3e þan in oþer causes as it | fareth w*ith* men þat vsen
moche swevyng and | ben y plesed w*ith* suche doing laboure or be|tyngg*es* or for
fastynge*s* or for teres or for me|lancolye humours / and soch oþer doynge*s* ·/·| 35

Biblio.-Médiathèques de Metz, MS 176, ff. 1r–16r

      quod paciens | non potest clare
35 videre, et si est in inferiori | parte
      subter palpebram ita quod tangat
      os | quod est subtus inferiorem
      palpebram, | similiter non videt
      quamuis habeat oculum | clarum.
      Vnde dicimus vobis quod illi qui |
      sunt in tali loco percussi, de illo
40 oculo | in quo sunt percussi nichil
      vident. Vnde | cum videritis
      aliquem [talem] et uos | vultis
      certificari an videat an non, |
      respiciatis ei in oculum et videatis
      si | pupilla est dilatata, et si est
45 maior | alia   sciatis quia nichil
12rb vident. Et si || dixit   uobis quod
      non videat, respicia|tis pupillam si
      dilatatur et con|stringitur sicut facit
      in alio sano | oculo, credendum est
5   quia videt, quia | spiritus visibilis
      ueniendo per neruum | concauum

---

41 talem] M talium, VP2 (f. 307r),
VR (f. 54r) talem

London, British Library, Sloane MS 661, ff. 32r–46r

De Probatissima Arte Oculorum 421

Glasgow, GUL, Hunter MS 513, ff. 2r–37r *Basel, Ö.B.U., MS D.II.11, ff. 172r–177v*

¶ Also he seythe nought though he
hAue a clere ey3e | wherfor whan
ye see any such beholdethe in to
20 þat | ey3e and yef the balle of the
ey3e be brode or yif | it be more
than his felawe knowe ye well that
he | seithe nought ¶ And yif the
pacient sey that he | seith loke yif
the appill of the ey3e yef it is ||
29v made brode and constreyned it is
to leue that he seiþ | for why the
visible spirit comyng by the
holwe | synewe to his oute passage
makethe the ey3e appill | to wexe
abrode and to constrayne ¶ And
5 yef it be | nought y gone A brode
and to constrayne as it doþe | in an
hole ey3e / And though me semeth
that he haue | a clere ey3e as the
tother ey3e ey3e is clere whan | he
hathe these signes as we haue y
saide dothe no | cure For the
holowe nerffe is so stoppid that the
10 vi|sible spirite by none wey may

Oxford, Bodleian Library, Ashmole MS 1468, pp. 1–6

Biblio.-Médiathèques de Metz, MS 176, ff. 1r–16r   ***Glasgow, GUL, Hunter MS 503, pp. 1–135***

    ad exitum suum facit pupil|lam
dilatare et constringere, et si non |
dilatatur et constringitur sicut |
facit in oculo sano, quamuis
10 videatur | habere oculum sanum
et clarum sicut | alium, nichil videt
et habet ante lucem | ista signa
sicut prediximus in quo | nullam
curam facere presumatis, | quia
neruus concauus est ita opilatus |
15 quod spiritus uisibilis nullo modo
potest ad | oculum peruenire. Et
dicimus uobis | karissimi quot
modis nerui [optici] opi|lantur et
possunt opilari: primo possunt |
opilari per multa ieiunia et ui|gi-
20 lias, secundo per multas angus-
tias | et planctum lacrimarum,
tercio per | multas verberaciones
capitis et fa|tigaciones corporis, et
similiter accidit mul|tis hominibus

---

17 optici] M conticij, VP2 (f. 307r),
VR (f. 54v) optici

London, British Library, Sloane MS 661, ff. 32r–46r

Glasgow, GUL, Hunter MS 513, ff. 2r–37r　　**Basel, Ö.B.U., MS D.II.11, ff. 172r–177v**

  nowght come to the | ey3e / And
knowithe well that the senewe
holwe most | is stopped in hem
that ben y smete all a boute the |
ey3e than in other causes as it
farethe w*ith* men þ*at* | vsen
swevyng and ben y pleased w*ith*
15 such doing labo*ur* | or betyngg*es*
or for fastyng*es* or for teres or for
melan|colye humours / and such
othir doyng*es* ·/·

Oxford, Bodleian Library, Ashmole MS 1468, pp. 1–6

Biblio.-Médiathèques de Metz, MS 176, ff. 1r–16r

25   per nimium coitum | – accidit
     etiam per multum legere et |
     multum scribere, opilantur etiam |
     per nimiam melancoliam, et magis
     opi|lantur in illis et cicius qui sunt
     per|cussi circumcirca oculum
30   quam in aliqui|bus istorum, sicut
     superius diximus. |
     65. Nunc dicimus vobis quandam
     infir|mitatem que uenit in oculis
     oc|casione percussionis. Accidit
     enim in | multis qui sunt percussi
35   inter super|cilia et nasum quod
     oritur ibi quidam | humor cor-
     ruptus exiendo per | puncturas
     palpebrarum iuxta na|sum ad
     modum lacrime, et medici | vocant
     ipsum humorem fistulam. Et |
40   apparet iste humor quasi pu-
     tredo | mixta cum lacrimis, et
     semper ha|bundat cursum suum et
     intrat ocu|los et apparent oculi
     semper lacrimosi. | Vnde dicimus
     uobis cum videritis oculos |

London, British Library, Sloane MS 661, ff. 32r–46r

Glasgow, GUL, Hunter MS 503, pp. 1–135

BUt here it ys to be noted | and
vnderstonde that yn | my latenn
apy lacked an | hoole Chapytere.   15
In whych tretys of || hurtys taken   [103]
a boute the eyon as by | strokys of
the forhede and the brow|ys the ey
lyddes. the boyth lacrymall. | the
temples. and such oþer of their |
cures.   5

Glasgow, GUL, Hunter MS 513, ff. 2r–37r

Basel, Ö.B.U., MS D.II.11, ff. 172r–177v

Of | smytyng i*n* þe forheued atwix the browes or | on þe nose side & þe cure þerof. |
Smete in the forhede atwene the
20 two browez and the | nose on the
to side or on that other side And it
fal||lethe other while ther wexethe
a·maner of corrupte | humour
goyng oute by the poyntes of the
ey3e liddes bi|side the nose as it
were teres and leches clepen þa*t* |
humour fistule for it wexeth as it
25 were rothed y meynte   w*ith* teres

---

17 smytyng] 25 *added   in   outer margin*

Oxford, Bodleian Library, Ashmole MS 1468, pp. 1–6

[65] Of smyting in þe forheued atwix þe browez | or on þe nose side & þe cure þerof ·/·|
Ismete in þe forehede atwene þe two browez | and þe nose on þe to side or on þat oþer |
side   And it falleþ otherwhile þer wexeþ | a maner of corrupte humour goyng oute by | 40
þe poyntes of þe ey3e liddes beside þe nose as it | were teres and leches clepen þat
humou*re* fist|ule for it wexeth as it were rothed y meynte w*ith* || teres   and his cours   2a
alwey it habundeth and wex|eþ more and more and it entreth in to þe ey3en*n* | and þan
þey appere alwey terifull ¶ wherfore | whan ye sein þe ey3en terifull / and yif ye will be |
certayne   whether it be corrupt humour or fistula | or clere teres ⸱ putte yo*ur* shewyng   5
fynger .i. lyk|potte bitwene þe nose and þe lacrimale fro þe | neiþer ey3e lidd and þer
afterward lokeþ into | þe ey3e ⸱ and in þe hyrne of þe ey3e ye shull see | rothed   come   10
oute by þe poynt*es* of þe ey3e liddes | beside þe nose ¶ wherfore vnkunnyng leches and |
foles þat knowen nou3t þat place where þat | rothed comeþ out and wenen þat it comeþ

Biblio.-Médiathèques de Metz, MS 176, ff. 1r–16r

45 |	lacrimosos et vultis certificari || si
12va	est humor corruptus qui dicitur |
	fistula sicut supradiximus an | sint
	lacrime naturales et clare, | ponatis
5	digitum uestrum indicem | inter
	nasum et lacrimalem palpebram |
	inferiorem. Postea respiciatis
	intus | oculum et in illo angulo
	videbitis | putredinem iuxta nasum
	exire | per punctas palpebrarum si
10	in | eam est predictus humor.
	Vnde | multi stolidi medici igno-
	rantes | proprium locum vnde exit
	humor ille | siue putredo illa
	credunt quod ue|niat per medium
15	lacrimale iuxta | nasum inter
	vnam palpebram et | aliam et
	faciunt istam pessimam | curam:
	Habent ferrum candentem | et cum
	ipso perforant nasum per |
	medium lacrimale inter palpe-
20	bram | superiorem et inferiorem
	et detur|pant locum illum et
	credunt | humorem illum desiccare

Glasgow, GUL, Hunter MS 503, pp. 1–135

London, British Library, Sloane MS 661, ff. 32r–46r

Glasgow, GUL, Hunter MS 513, ff. 2r–37r

  and his cours allwey it habundeþ ‖
30r and wexethe more and more and it
  entrethe in to the | ey3en and than
  they appere alwey teryfull ¶
  wher|for whan ye sein the ey3en
  terifull / And yif ye will | certayne
  whether it be corruppte humour or
5 fistula | or clere teres putte your
  shewyng fyngre ·i· lykpotte |
  bitwene the nose and the lacrimall
  for the neyther | ey3e lidde and
  ther after lokethe in to the ey3e
  And | in the herne of the eye ye
  shull see rothed come oute | by the
  poyntes of the ey3e liddes beside
10 the nose // | ¶ wherfor vn-
  kunnyng leches and foles that
  knowen | nought that place where
  that rothed cometh out | and
  wenen that it comethe oute by the
  myddill lacri|male beside the nose
  beside that ey3e lidde and that |
  other / and they do this cure worste
15 / they hauen a· | glowyng yren

Basel, Ö.B.U., MS D.II.11, ff. 172r–177v

Oxford, Bodleian Library, Ashmole MS 1468, pp. 1–6

out | by þe myddill lacrimale beside þe nose beside þat | ey3e lidde and þat oþer / and 15
þey do þis cure | worste ׃ þey hauen a glowyng yren and þey | persen þorwe þe nose by
þe mydde of þe lacrimal | atwene þe ouer ey3e lid and þe nether and þei | defoulen þat
place and þey wenen to drie | vp so þat place and þey do nou3t / But þey | corrumpen 20
þat place but þey maken a cauterie | and þur3 þat many lesyn her si3t þur3 suche |
cauteryng / and also for þe neruis of ey3en ha|ven her way besiden and þe fellyng fyre
þey | be made drie 25

---

25 be] C *added in outer margin*

Biblio.-Médiathèques de Metz, MS 176, ff. 1r–16r

sic et | nichil faciunt sed corrum-
punt | locum in quo faciunt
25 cauterium. | Et multis pacientibus
accidit quod | pro illa occasione
amittunt lumen | oculorum quia
nerui oculorum habent | viam
[iuxta siue prope nasum], vnde
ac|cidit quod nerui illi desic-
30 cantur | sencientes calorem et
ardorem | cauterij quod illi stolidi
medici faci|unt.

66. Nos autem diximus uobis |
quod primo debetis purgare
pacien|tis stomacum cum pillulis
35 nostris ihero|solimitanis. Facta
purgacione | faciatis eis incisio-
nem cum | puncta rasorij inter
palpebram | inferiorem et nasum,
ita discrete | quod non tangatis

Glasgow, GUL, Hunter MS 503, pp. 1–135

---

28 iuxta...nasum] M iuxta ita siue
prope, VP2 (f. 308r) iuxta nasum

London, British Library, Sloane MS 661, ff. 32r–46r

Glasgow, GUL, Hunter MS 513, ff. 2r–37r *Basel, Ö.B.U., MS D.II.11, ff. 172r–177v*

  and they persen thorowe the nose |
by the mydde of the lacrimal
atwene the ouer | eyelid and the
nether and they Defoulen that
place | and they wenen to drie vp
so that place and þey | do nought ¶
Butt they corrumpen that place
20 but | they maken a cautarie and
though that lesyn her | syght
thorough suche cauteryng Also for
the neruis | of ey3en hauen her
waye bysiden and they fellyng |
fyre they be made drie
  ¶ And ye shull cure these | thus
first purge her stomak w*ith* oure
25 pill of Jer*usa*lem | and they ben
purged ye shull make a kuttyng
30v w*ith* || w*ith* a·poynte of a ¶
Rasour atwene the nether ey3e |lid
and the nose so wyselich and
discretelich that | ye towche
nought the ey3e nether the ey3elid
// | ¶ But make a·kerffe beside the
5 nose alete that kut|tyng be full

Oxford, Bodleian Library, Ashmole MS 1468, pp. 1–6

[66] ¶ And ye shull cure these þus | first purge her stomak w*ith* oure pill of Jer*usa*lem |
And þey ben*n* y purged ye shull make a kutt|yng wiþ a poynte of a · Rasour atwene þe |
nether ey3e lid and þe nose so wyseliche & | discretelich þat 3e touche nou3t þe ey3e 30
neþer | þe ey3elid ¶ But make a · kerffe beside þe | nose a longe in kuttyng þe hide onely
⁚ and | lete þat kuttyng be full litell / and whan þou | hast made þat kuttyng putte in þat
wounde | a grayne of pesen þat is cleped chichis & | after þat ye shull putte þeron a litill 35
pilwe of | lynnen cloth and binde it well w*ith* a clothe | So þat chiche goo nat ou3t till
anoþer day | .i. on þe morwe / and on þe morwe in þe hole | þat þe chiche hath y made 40
3e putte þerin of our*e* | poudre corrosiue and mortificatiue as we shull | shewe yow in þe
ende of þis book for almaner | fistulys where euer þey ben in þe body and || whan ye put 2b
in þat poudre make þe pacient | to shitte his ey3e and ley on þe ey3e coton y|watte in þe
glaire of a neye ⁚ So þat þis pou|dre by no way come in to þe ey3e and bynde it | to w*ith* 5
a · lynnen clothe and binde it to a nother | morwe ⁚ In þe morwe putte þer*e* þe poudre

Biblio.-Médiathèques de Metz, MS 176, ff. 1r–16r

40 palpebram neque | substantiam
oculi. Et fiat incisura iuxta | nasum
per longum, et sit paruun|cula et
non incidatis nisi corium tan|tum.
Facta incisione ponatis intus | in
illa cicatrice 1 granum ciceris, |
45 postea ponatis puluillum panni |
linei desuper et bene ligetis cum ||
12vb fascia ita quod cicer non possit
exire usque | ad alium diem. In
alio die in fora|mine quod cicer
fecerit ponatis de pul|uere nostro
5 corrosiuo et mortificativo, | sicut
demonstrauimus uobis in fine |
nostri libri pro omnibus fistulis
ubi|cumque fuerint in corpore, et
posueri|tis intus de puluere nostro,
faciatis ei | claudere oculum et
10 superponatis | oculo clauso
bombacem intinctum | in clara oui
ita quod puluis nullo modo | possit
intrare oculum, et cum fascia |
linea ligetis usque in alium diem.
In | alia die uero desuper ponatis

London, British Library, Sloane MS 661, ff. 32r–46r

Glasgow, GUL, Hunter MS 513, ff. 2r–37r *Basel, Ö.B.U., MS D.II.11, ff. 172r–177v*

    litell / and whan thowe haste |
made that kuttyng putt in that
wound a·gray|ne of pesen that is
cleped chichis and after that | ye
shull putte theron a·litill pilwe of
lynnen | clothe and bynde it well
10 withe a·clothe So þat | chiche
goo nat oute till anothir day .i· on
the | morwe / and on the morowe
in the hole that þe | chiche hathe y
made ye putte therin of oure
po|udre corrosyue and mortifi-
catiue as we shuld | shewe you in
the of this booke for almaner
15 fistu|lis where euer they ben in
the body and whan | ye putte in
that poudre make the pacynet to
shi|tte ys ey3en and ley on the ey3e
cotoun y watte in | the glayre of a
neye / So that this poudre by | no
way come in to the ey3e and bynde
20 it to a | nother morwe / In the
morwe putte ther the | poudre lay
grece of a·yonge souwe alwel till

Oxford, Bodleian Library, Ashmole MS 1468, pp. 1–6

lay | grece of a · yonge souwe alwell till þat þe dede | flesshe be y rered vp wiþ þe
poudre and þat | place leuen open and þan afterward ye shull | see afterward þe place y   10
putrified where þat | þe well was of rothed and þat cours þat was | in þe lacrimal shall be
dried vp · and afterward | a see sponge þe mountaunce of a · chiche in þat | hole shall be
done þat þe poudre made till it | be ri3t well y purged · ffor þe see sponge openeþ | and   15
wasteth wycked humours · also longe | as þe wounde ys corrupte // And afterward |
whan þat place ys well y dried as well by | þe puncte of þe lacrimal as by þe wounde so |
þat neiþer quitour neiþer humour ne none | rothed comeþ out in to þe ey3e as it did   20
be|fore neiþer by olde wounde leue ther y made | of þe corrosyue and þat drie flesshe and
quicke | appere þer ׃ þan with lynet of lynnen cloþ | þou shalt consoude it vp withouten   25
any oþer | fathede / and þan is þe pacient deliuered withouten | any drede or perill or any
difformite .i. vn|shappynes ׃ But euery euenyng þe whiles | ye leche hem 3if hym of oure
maruelous electuarie | whan he goth to bedde as moche as a chestaynn ·| 30

Biblio.-Médiathèques de Metz, MS 176, ff. 1r–16r

15 de anx|ugia suellina, semper donec caro morti|ficata eleuetur cum puluere, et re|maneat locus apertus et uidebitis | postea videbitis locum putrefactum | ubi
20 erat origo putredinis, et ille cur|sus qui erat in lacrimali desiccatur. Postea | de spongia marina in foramine quod | puluis fecerit ponatis ad modum | ciceris quousque bene purgetur et de|siccetur locus ille, quia spongia
25 ma|rina duo facit: aperit et consumit malos | humores dum vulnus est corruptum, | postquam locus erit desiccatus tam | per puncta lacrimalis quam per cica|tricem, dimittatis spongiam et
30 cum | fimbrijs panni linei consolidabitis sine | aliqua vnctione – et paciens erit libe|ratus sine periculo. Sed dum medica|ueritis tales pacientes et quolibet, | sero detis
35 eis de nostro mirabili elec|tuario

Glasgow, GUL, Hunter MS 503, pp. 1–135

London, British Library, Sloane MS 661, ff. 32r–46r

Glasgow, GUL, Hunter MS 513, ff. 2r–37r   *Basel, Ö.B.U., MS D.II.11, ff. 172r–177v*

     þ*at* | the dede flesshe be y rered vp
     w*ith* the poudre | and that place
     leuen open and than afterward | ye
     shull see afterward the place y
31r putryfied || wher that the well was
     of rothed and that cours | that was
     in the lacrimall shall be dryed vp
     and | afterward a·see sponge the
     mountaunce of a chich in | that
     hole shall be done that the poudre
5   made till it | be right well y
     purged For the see sponge
     openethe | and wasteth wycked
     humours · Also longe as the
     wo|unde ys corrupte ¶ And after-
     ward whan that place | ys well y
     dryed as well by the puncte of the
     lacri|mall as by the wounde so that
10 neither quitour neither | humour
     ne none rothed comethe oute in to
     the ey3e | as it did be fore neither

---

1 well] *spelling unsure as there is an ink blot over the word*

Oxford, Bodleian Library, Ashmole MS 1468, pp. 1–6

Biblio.-Médiathèques de Metz, MS 176, ff. 1r–16r

cum iuerit dormitum ad modum |
et ad quantitatem unius castanee. |

Glasgow, GUL, Hunter MS 503, pp. 1–135

London, British Library, Sloane MS 661, ff. 32r–46r

67. Docuimus uos probatissimam curam | pro lacrimis oculorum corruptis secundum | nos, nam secundum alios fistule dicuntur. | Ammodo demonstrauimus vobis de na|turalibus lacrimis vnde habeant exitum, | ideo quia multi credunt quod lacrime | habeant exitum et exeant de oculis | sed decipiuntur. Alij putant quod

And more ou*e*re the nexte cha|py*tre* folowyng in the be-gynnyng | lakked sum what. but not muche | as I suppose. wher he tretyth of wa|try eyon. and of teres. of corrupte | hum*ers* lyke teres. whych leches cal|len festeles. wherfore q*uo*d Benny|micius, of them oure lorde ih*esu* yaue | knowlege and exp*e*riens of the

Glasgow, GUL, Hunter MS 513, ff. 2r–37r

by olde wounde leue ther | y made
of the corrosyue and that drie
flesshe and | quicke appere there /
than w*ith* lynet of lynnen clothe |
thou shalt consoude it vp
15 w*ith*outen any other fathede | and
than is the pacient deliu*er*d
w*ith*outen any drede | or p*er*ill or
any difformite ·i· vnshappynes ¶
But eue|ry euenyng the whyles ye
leche hem yif hym of | our*e*
meruelous electuare whan he goth
to bedde as | moche as a·Chestayn
·/·
20 **Of natural teres | & of fistule of**
the wherof they come |
BUt there as the naturall teres gone
oute | sum*m*e wenen that from the
ey3en of hem | and sum*m*e wenen
from the lacrimal they | comyn
oute ¶ But we Beneuenutus of
31v Jerusalem || say that they comen

Basel, Ö.B.U., MS D.II.11, ff. 172r–177v

---

19 teres] **23** *added in outer margin*

Oxford, Bodleian Library, Ashmole MS 1468, pp. 1–6

[67] Of naturall teres & of fistule of þe ey3e | wherof þey come ·/· |
But þere as þe naturall teres gone | out su*m*me wenen þat from þe ey3en | of hem and   35
su*m*me wenen from þe | lacrimal þey comen out / But we Beneue|mitus of Jerusalem say
þat þei comen out by | þe poynt*es* palpebrar*um* · que stant iuxta nasum | wherof þe
lacrimal ys y saide / and þey comen | oute   as well of þe ouer lacrimal as of the nedyr | 40
lacrimal / and þer ben two holes in bothe ey3e | liddes from wham þe teres comyn oute
the | whiche 3e mowe see hem þer yif he will ouer|turne þe ey3e liddes // And from þe
ouer ey3e || lidde hole þer come oute teres su*m*me tyme roten | of þe whiche we speke of   3a
in fistula abouesaid | þe whiche ben y cleped fistula oculi

Biblio.-Médiathèques de Metz, MS 176, ff. 1r–16r

45 ueni|ant de cerebro et habeant
13ra meatum et viam || similiter intus
per oculos, qui similiter | deci-
piuntur – sed non ex toto quia |
bene sunt quedam que veniunt a
cere|bro sed non per oculos. Alij
5 credunt | quod exeant per
medium lacrimale maius, | qui
similiter decipiuntur. Alij credunt
quod ue|niant per medium oculi
intus super | pupillam oculi, qui
omnes falluntur nec | sunt in
cognicione ueritatis. Nos uero |
10 Beneuenutus de Iherusalem cui
Dominus noster | Ihesus Christus,
de quo omnia bona procedunt, |
dedit ueram experienciam et
agnicionem | de omnibus infirmi-
tatibus que super|ueniunt et
possunt accidere in oculis et de |
15 substancijs, humoribus, et
complexionibus eorum, | et quis
eorum melius uideat et possit |
videre, et qua de causa et in quo

London, British Library, Sloane MS 661, ff. 32r–46r

Glasgow, GUL, Hunter MS 503, pp. 1–135

infir|mytees of eyon. humers and
complex|yons. and the cures yf   15
practysers wyll || verely be   [104]
certyfyed wheþer the humor be | a.
Fistula. or a clere tere. do þus.
put|tyth your secunde fyngers ende.
whych | ys callyd. Index. the
shewyng fynger. | betwene the   5
nose and the lacrimall | besyde the
neþer eye lede. and þere shall | ȝe
se the corrupte humor. that is the |
mater of the fystyl. goyng oute by
the | poyntys of the eye leddys
betwene the | nose and the eye.   10
But many boystus | leches and
ignorant not knowyng | the very
place of yssuyng of the cor|rupte.
whych ys the mater of the fys|tyll.
but weenyng that the goyng | out   15

1 certyfyed] Fistula *added in upper margin in a late hand* 3 whych] To knowe wher | it be a fistula | in the ey. *added in outer margin in an Elizabethan hand*

Glasgow, GUL, Hunter MS 513, ff. 2r–37r   *Basel, Ö.B.U., MS D.II.11, ff. 172r–177v*

    oute by the poynt*es* palpebra*rum* |
    que stant iuxta nasum / where of
    the lacrimal ys | y saide and they
    comen oute as well of the ouer |
    lacrimal / and ther ben to holes in
5   bothe eyӡe liddes | from wham
    the teres comyn oute the whiche |
    ye mowe see hem ther yif he will
    ouer turne the | eyӡe liddes // And
    from the ouer eyӡe lidde hole |
    ther come oute teres su*m*me tyme
    roten of the whi|che we speke of in
    fistula abouesaid the whiche ben |
10 y cleped fistula oculi

Oxford, Bodleian Library, Ashmole MS 1468, pp. 1–6

Biblio.-Médiathèques de Metz, MS 176, ff. 1r–16r

spiritus | uisibilis magis operatur,
et potest ope|rari qua de causa
20   similiter. Dicimus | ergo quod
lacrime exeunt per punctas |
palpebrarum que stant et sunt
iuxta | nasum ubi dicitur 'lacri-
male' et exeunt | tam de superio-
ribus quam de inferioribus |
punctis palpebrarum ubi sunt duo
25   fo|ramina: uidelicet in ambabus
pal|pebris vnde exeunt lacrime. Et
si vul|tis certificari et dimittere
errorem | antiquum, reuersetis
palpebram et | prospiciatis in
30   lacrimale maiori, si|cut diximus in
capite palpebre ubi | finiuntur pili,
et ibi inuenietis vnum | foramen de
quo exeunt lacrime, et | similiter
est foramen in simili loco supe-
rioris | palpebre de quo eodem
35   loco exeunt | lacrime et habent
cursum suum. Et eciam | lacrime
putrefacte de quibus supra|di-
ximus.

London, British Library, Sloane MS 661, ff. 32r–46r

Glasgow, GUL, Hunter MS 503, pp. 1–135

of the corrupc*i*on were yn the ||
myddys of the lacrymal. besydys   [105]
the | nose betwyxt boyth the eye
ledys. & | þei vsen for to cure a
craft that ys | a cause of lesyng of
manny mans | sy3thtys. And it ys   5
thus. ¶ They | taken an hoote yron
and make a | cauterye vpon the
nose yn the myd|dys of the
lacrymall betwyx the ou*e*re|ylede
and the neþerlyd weenyng for | to   10
dry vp the place where the cor|rupt
mat*er* of the fystyl ys gendryd |
but þei do not curee but deforme
fou|le the face yn the place. whych
þei | cauteryse. and many as I haue
se|yd defo*ur*rem and dystreyen the   15
sy3th || of the vysyble synews that   [106]
arn*n* clepyd. | Nerui optici. goyng
be twyxt besyde | the nose by the
Cautaryzac*i*on ben dri|ed. and the
sy3te destroyed. wherfore | yf 3e
wyll not dysteyne your name | nor   5
hurt your pacyent*is* in cure of |

Glasgow, GUL, Hunter MS 513, ff. 2r–37r   *Basel, Ö.B.U., MS D.II.11, ff. 172r–177v*

Oxford, Bodleian Library, Ashmole MS 1468, pp. 1–6

Biblio.-Médiathèques de Metz, MS 176, ff. 1r–16r

Glasgow, GUL, Hunter MS 503, pp. 1–135

thys man*er* of fystyl. leue thys
fore|seyd lewde craft. and do as I
schall | teche yow. ¶ Fyrst clense
the pa|cyentys stomake wyth the   10
peletys | of ier*usa*lem. wherof the
makyng ys | tau3t before. whych
purgac*i*on made. | þen 3e shall
make a lytle Insysyon*n* | wyth the
poynt of a rasor. betwyxt | the   15
neþ*er*eylyd and the nose. so
dyscre|||tly that 3e touchnot the eye [107]
lede and | the nose. neþ*er* the
substance of the eye. | And thys
Incysion*n* or kuttyng shal | be but
oonly þorugh the skyn in len|ght   5
wyse. In whych yncysion. put | the
grane of a fecche. and lay þ*er*on |
a lytle pylowe made of lynnen |
cloth. and bynd it wyth a lynnen |
bende. that the fecche remoue not |
from the place where it is leyd.   10

---

9 pacyentys] festula *added in outer margin in a late hand*

London, British Library, Sloane MS 661, ff. 32r–46r

Glasgow, GUL, Hunter MS 513, ff. 2r–37r   *Basel, Ö.B.U., MS D.II.11, ff. 172r–177v*

Oxford, Bodleian Library, Ashmole MS 1468, pp. 1–6

Biblio.-Médiathèques de Metz, MS 176, ff. 1r–16r   *Glasgow, GUL, Hunter MS 503, pp. 1–135*

                                            & | so lete it lye tyl the nexte day.
than | remoue the fecche. and yn
the hole | that it hath made. ley of
the coresey | and the mortificat
powder. whych I | shall teche yn   15
the ende of the tretis. || ageyne all   [108]
man*er* of fystyll*is*. wherso|eu*ere*
they be. whych powd*er* put yn. |
do the pacyens shyt hys eye. that
the | powder may not entre. Or
vpon the | eyelyd lay a plast*er* of   5
coton. or flex|en hardys. I wet yn
the whyte of | an egg. and bynd it
þ*er*to wyth a lyn|nen bande tyl the
nexte day. and þan | anoynte yt. or
ley þ*er*to clene freshe | swynes   10
grece. tyl the mortifyed fleshe | be
reysed vp wyth the powd*er*. and
the | place remayne opyn. And
than shal | 3e se the place
putrifyed wher the | begynnyng of
the corrupte mat*er* of | the fystyl   15
was. and how the cowrs || þ*er*eof   [109]
yn the lacrymall shalbe dryed. |

London, British Library, Sloane MS 661, ff. 32r–46r

Glasgow, GUL, Hunter MS 513, ff. 2r–37r *Basel, Ö.B.U., MS D.II.11, ff. 172r–177v*

Oxford, Bodleian Library, Ashmole MS 1468, pp. 1–6

Biblio.-Médiathèques de Metz, MS 176, ff. 1r–16r   *Glasgow, GUL, Hunter MS 503, pp. 1–135*

and aft*er* thys take a lytle pece of a
spon|ge the q*ua*ntyte of a fecche.
and ley yt | yn the hoole. that the
powd*er* mayd tyl | it be pourgyd   5
and dryed. For the p*ropar*|te of the
spounge ys to opyn. to con|sume
wykkyd hum*er*s. And when | the
place ys dryed boyth be the poynt |
of the lacrymall and the
Cicatryce | made by the fyrst   10
Incysyon. Than | leue the sponge.
and ley þereto nat els. | but fayre
lynet of feyr lynnen cloth. |
wythoute ony man*er* of
oynyment | tyl yt be p*er*fy3tly
consowded. and so | shall the be   15
delyu*er*d wythout perell. ||
Neu*er*thelees eu*er*y ny3te whyle   [110]
he ys | yn curyng. when he goth to
bedde. | yeue hym of oure
electuarie callyd. | Electuariu*m*
mirabile. the q*ua*ntite | of a
chasteyn.   5

London, British Library, Sloane MS 661, ff. 32r–46r

Glasgow, GUL, Hunter MS 513, ff. 2r–37r   **Basel, Ö.B.U., MS D.II.11, ff. 172r–177v**

Oxford, Bodleian Library, Ashmole MS 1468, pp. 1–6

Biblio.-Médiathèques de Metz, MS 176, ff. 1r–16r

68. Iam docuimus uos vnde | lacrime oculorum habent cursum et vnde | semper exeant. Ammodo
40 docebimus vos | differentiam inter eas que exeunt ex pal|pebris superioribus et eas que exeunt | ex inferioribus. Dicimus ergo quod lacri|me que exeunt per palpebras inferi|ores procedunt a corde, scilicet quando aliquis | constrin-
45 gitur pro aliquo dolore ad | plorandum, quia ueniunt ex vi et ||
13rb iste non sunt durabiles, quia mitigato dolore et cessante cessant et lacrime. Ille uero lacrime que ueniunt et exeunt per palpebras
5 superiores | veniunt a cerebro, scilicet pro aliqua cor|rupcione uel habundancia super|fluitatum humorum, et cursus aquarum | non cessat nec potest cessare nisi materia | purgetur. Adiuuetur et
10 detineatur | cum electuarijs nostris et cauterijs, secundum |

London, British Library, Sloane MS 661, ff. 32r–46r

Glasgow, GUL, Hunter MS 503, pp. 1–135

¶ Now I haue | shewed q*uo*d he the knowlege of cor|rupt terys. wherof ben*n* caused fys|tyllys. and the cures of them. ¶ | Now I teche yow the v*e*rry knowlege | of 10
v*er*ry terys. and yn what place | they v*e*ryly spryng. many mene we|ne that wepyng terys come out | of the eyon. but yt is not so. for | theyr yssue ys oute of the eye ledys. | boyth the ou*er* and the 15
neþ*er* at the ho|||les yn the lacrimal [111]
be syde the nose | at the ende of the grounde of the | herys as ʒe shall euydently aspye | yf ʒe wyll reu*er*se and turne the ey|ledys. But 5
nat forthan. þere is | different causes of teres. whych | spyrng out of the ou*e*rey lede. And | whych spryng oute of the nether. | For tho whych come out of the ne|ther eye lyde. pr*o*ceden from 10
the hert. | eyther for sorow. drede. or smart. | and be caused by

Glasgow, GUL, Hunter MS 513, ff. 2r–37r   *Basel, Ö.B.U., MS D.II.11, ff. 172r–177v*

¶ The difference of these teres | as
to hir cause is this for tho teres that
comen | oute by the neyther ey3e
liddes fro the herte of | su*m*me
grete sorowe but they be nought
durable | for whan the grete sorwe
15 is passed than sesen | thoo teres ¶
But thoo teris that comyn from |
the ouer ey3e liddes they comyn
from the brayne and | comyn of
plentenes of humours of fleume
·/· |

Oxford, Bodleian Library, Ashmole MS 1468, pp. 1–6

[68] ¶ The difference of þese teres as to hir cause is þis for þo | teres þat comen oute by 5
þe neither ey3e liddes | fro þe herte of su*m*me grete sorwe but þey be no3t | durable for
whan þe grete sorwe is passed | þan sesen þoo teres ¶ But þoo teres þat | comen from þe
ouer ey3e liddes þey co*m*myn | from þe brayne and comyn of plentenes of | humours 10
and of fleume ·/· |

Biblio.-Médiathèques de Metz, MS 176, ff. 1r–16r

quod Ars Nostra Probatissima Oculorum | demonstrat.

69. Audiuistis differentiam que | est inter vnam lacrimam et aliam. Am|modo docebimus uobis de
15 alijs | infirmitatibus que accidunt in | oculis ex percussionibus in multis ho|minibus, et magis in illis qui fran|gunt lapides, id est lathomis et molen|dinarijs et similiter in
20 fabris, quia aliquando | resultat aliquid de ferramento in ocu|lis et incarnatur super pupillam | uel

London, British Library, Sloane MS 661, ff. 32r–46r

Glasgow, GUL, Hunter MS 503, pp. 1–135

amane*r* of vyole*n*|ce. but they be
not durable nor | a bydyng. for
when the cause | þ*er*of cesyth. þei   15
sesyn. But the te||res whych cu*m*   [112]
oute of the hoole of | the oue*r*lyd
of the ey. p*r*ocede*nn* from the |
brayn and be causid of sum
corrup|c*i*on of habundans of
sup*er*fluytee | of hume*r*s. and her   5
cours ceceth not. | but yf the mat*er*
be po*ur*gyd and hol|pen wyth oure
electuaryes and | cautaryes lyke as
we haue tauȝth | be forne. |
Now aft*er* that I haue | tauȝth   10
yow q*uo*d he of | the hurtys that
co*m*me | to the eyon outwarde. as
by stro|kys yn the forhede templys
or | browys. and naturally of   15
cor||rupte and naturale terys. ¶   [113]
Now | wyll I speke of the hurtys.

---

2 wyll] when ani duste | or other thinge | falleth into the | eyes. or chips | or durst &c. *added in outer margin in an Elizabethan hand*

Glasgow, GUL, Hunter MS 513, ff. 2r–37r   *Basel, Ö.B.U., MS D.II.11, ff. 172r–177v*

<O>f smytyng in þe ey3e as
fallethe to ma|sons and smythes
& the cure therof. |
20 Nowe we shull sey of smytynges
that hap|peþe many and more
comonly hem that | breken stones
as masons and mylwardes & |
smethes / For why somme smale
peces smyght in |to the ey3e and

---

19 Of] 27 *added in outer margin*

Oxford, Bodleian Library, Ashmole MS 1468, pp. 1–6

[69] **Of smyting in þe ey3e as falleþ to ma|sons & smethes & þe cure þerof** ·/·|
Now we shull sey of smytynges þat happ|eth   many and more comonly hem þat | breken   15
stones / as masons and mylwardes | and smethes ¶ ffor why somme smale peces smyte |
in to þe ey3e and þey ben entred on þe tonicle | of þe ey3e and for þat akþe þe ey3en
alway te|ren and watrin in so moche þat þe pacient | may nou3t open his ey3en ¶ And we   20
mowe | fynde many þat hauen þat litell pece of þat | ston stille in her ey3en an hey3 or þat
þei ben | y entred in to þe si3t and ben faste // And othere | hauyn   ayenst sy3t and many   25
atwene þe white | and þe blaknes of þe ey3e ¶ This is þe cure / make | þe pacient sitten
afore þe vpri3t and put his | hede bitwene thy kneys and make hym to shitte | his hole
ey3e and to open his other ey3e and | with   a siluerem nedill remeue þou þat pece | of   30
stone fro þat place þere it is on softely and | wisely þat none maner touche þou nou3t þe |

---

26 and] C *added in outer margin*

Biblio.-Médiathèques de Metz, MS 176, ff. 1r–16r

super tunicam oculi. Vnde accidit
quod | propter illum dolorem
quem facit illum | tantillum, siue
25 sit de ferramento | siue de
batitura lapidis, oculi semper |
lacrimantur, ita quod paciens non
potest | aperire oculos propter
illud tantillum fer|ramentum. Et
multis inuenietis de | illis qui
habent illud ferramentum uel
30 la|pidem uel aliquid aliud simile
istis | incarnatum super lucem,
alios circa | lucem, et multi sunt
qui habent illud | ferramentum
inter nigredinem et | albedinem
35 oculi. Diximus uobis | causam et
cetera sed hec est cura: fa|ciatis
sedere pacientem coram uobis |
supinum et ponatis caput suum
inter | crura uestra et genua, et
faciatis ei | claudere oculum
40 sanum et aperire alium | (scilicet

Glasgow, GUL, Hunter MS 503, pp. 1–135

whych ca|sually falle vnto dyue*r*se
artifycers. | as to masons. myllers.
wryghtys. | smythes. and oþe*r*. 5
For yt happyth þat | sum of here
fragmentys sterte ynto | there eyes.
vnwysyli and rechelesly | be left
þe*r*yn. tyll þei be incarnate. vpon |
the tonycles. of the ey. and the
payn | causeth contynually þe*r* 10
eyon to water. | so that the pacyent
may no wele opon | hys eye. and
of thyes ȝe schal fynde | som þat
haue the fragment of ston | or of
styke opon the lyght Incarnat. |
Som be syde the lyght. and som be 15
twe|ne the blak and the white. [114]
And of all | thyes þe*r* ys but oon*n*
mane*r* of cure. and | yt ys thus.
Make the pacyent to sytt | downe

---

6 sum] strok*is added in outer margin in a late hand* **15** twene] ne the blak. *added in lower margin*

London, British Library, Sloane MS 661, ff. 32r–46r

Glasgow, GUL, Hunter MS 513, ff. 2r–37r   *Basel, Ö.B.U., MS D.II.11, ff. 172r–177v*

      they ben entred on the tonicle of
32r   þe ‖ ey3e and for that akthe the
      ey3en alway teren and | wateren in
      so moche that the pacient may
      nought open | his ey3en ¶ And we
      mowe fynde many that hauen |
      that litill pece of that ston stille in
5   her ey3en an hey3 | or that they
      ben y entred in to the syght and
      many | atwene the white and the
      blaknes of the ey3e // This | is the
      Cure / make the pacient sitten
      afore the vpri|ght and put his hede
      bitwene thy kneys and make | hym
      to shitte his hole ey3e and to open
10   his other ey3e | and w*ith* a
      silueren nedill remeue thou that
      pece of | stone fro that place ther it
      is on softely and whisely | that
      none maner touch thou nought the
      tonicle w*ith* | the forsaid nedill
      that it prike nought the ey3e w*ith* |
      the nedeles poynte but lede the
15   nedill on the tonicle | as me

Oxford, Bodleian Library, Ashmole MS 1468, pp. 1–6

tonicle wiþ þe forsaid nedill / þat it prike | nou3t þe ey3e with þe nedeles poynte but |
lede þe nedill on*n* þe tonicle as me wolde shaue | as barbours done wiþ a · Rasour / and   35
yif þ*ou* | Doist þus · þou shalte departe þat pece | of stone fro þe tonicle / And yif þat
hole be moch | putte therin þan of vertu of god y 3eue and | on þe ey3e lay cotun · y   40
wette in þe white of | aney twies a · day and onys a · ny3t / and he | shall be deliu*e*red
in thre Dayes / and yif suche | be nou3t y cured / And yif þat pece abide þere ‖ any   3b
while on þat tonicle of þe ey3e till þe | tonicle wexeþ white and lesith his li3t ·/· |

---

37 departe] of *deleted*

De Probatissima Arte Oculorum

Biblio.-Médiathèques de Metz, MS 176, ff. 1r–16r

[pacientis] in quo est illud ferra|mentum). Et cum acu argenti divi|datis illud ferramentum uel illud tan|tillum a tunica oculi uel a loco ubi | manet et se tenet, tamen
45 ita suauiter et | discrete quod nullo modo tangatis tunicam ||
13va oculi cum predicta acu – maxime cum | puncta – sed ducatis eam acum super | tunicam, radendo sicut faciunt barba|rij siue barbi-
5 tonsores barbam et | super barbam cum rasorio. Et sic fa|ciendo separabitis ipsum a tunica illa | et a loco illo, et si foramen est magnum | mittatis intus oculum de virtute | a Deo data, et super oculum ponatis |
10 exterius bombacem intinctum in al|bumine oui bis in die et semel | in nocte. Et sic erit liberatus

---

40 pacientis] M pacientem, VR (f. 56v) patientis

London, British Library, Sloane MS 661, ff. 32r–46r

Glasgow, GUL, Hunter MS 503, pp. 1–135

and bakwarde to ley hys hede. | betwene your legges. and þen doo   5
hy*m* | shyt hys hoole eye. and af*ter* open the | sore eye. and wyth a nedyll of syluer | deuyde the fragment from the place | þat it ys on so sotelly and so discre|tely   10
that yn nowyse 3e hurt not the | tonycle. but lede it so softly and so so|tylly yn the ma*ner* of a barbor vpon a | mans berde. And so ledyng forth the | nedyll by ma*ner* of shauyng. 3e shall | remoue it   15
from the place where it lay || and   [115]
þat doon. 3e shall easely haue it | out. and yit yn the place wher yt | lay. be made a grete pyt. put into | the eye of the oynement callyd. The | vertu youen of god. whych I   5
tau|gte be fore. and on the eye

---

4 hede] the cuer *added in outer margin in an Elizabethan hand*
15 lay] no*ta added in outer margin in a late hand*

Glasgow, GUL, Hunter MS 513, ff. 2r–37r *Basel, Ö.B.U., MS D.II.11, ff. 172r–177v*

    wolde shaue as barbours done w*ith* a Rasour | And yif thou doste thus thou shalte departe of þ*at* | pece of stone fro the tonicle / And yif that hole be | moche putte therin than vertu of god y yeue & | on the eyȝe lay cotun y wette in the white
20 of a | ney twies a·day / and onys a·nyght and he shall | be deliu*e*red in thre dayes / And yif suche be nought | y Cured And yif that pece abide there any while | on that tonicle of the eyȝe till the tonicle wexeþ | white and lesithe his lyght ·/· ||

Oxford, Bodleian Library, Ashmole MS 1468, pp. 1–6

Biblio.-Médiathèques de Metz, MS 176, ff. 1r–16r

    pa|ciens in tribus diebus. Et si
ta|les non sunt curati et illud
15 ferra|mentum per aliquod tempus
fuerit | et steterit super tunicam
oculi, tota tu|nica dealbabitur siue
dealbescet, | et sic paciens amittit
lumen de | oculo pacienti.

20 **70.** Adhuc dicimus | vobis de
predicta infirmitate a|liam similem
curam contra infirmi|tatem que
uenit et accidit ex a|ristis que
intrant oculos. Tempore | quo nos
25 eramus in Tuscia in ciui|tate que
vocatur Luca, homines | de terra
illa adduxerunt coram nobis |
quendam hominem qui habebat
in | oculo quandam aristam spice
fru|menti que intrauerat oculum
30 suum | cum ipse metebat. Et erat
illa aris|ta ex transuerso ita quod
capita a|riste non apparebant super
tuni|cam sed apparebant sicut

London, British Library, Sloane MS 661, ff. 32r–46r

Glasgow, GUL, Hunter MS 503, pp. 1–135

w*ith*oute | lay a plaster of flaxen
hurdys wyth | the whyte of an
egge. twyes on the | day. and   10
oonys of the nyght. And w*ith*|yn.
iij dayes he shall be hoole. and yf |
the fragment be long þ*er*on and be
not | cured on this seyd wyse. all
the tony|cle shall wex whyte. and
the pacyent | shall lese hys sy3te.
Moreou*er* here | wyll I teche yow   15
p*r*actysers a crafte to || take out   [116]
an hawe from the eye be en|sample
of a cure that I dyd oonys yn. |
Tuskayne. In a cite callyd. Luk, |
where was brou3t to me a man
þat | hade an hawe yn hys ey. of   5
the smy|tyng of a whete yere. ou*er*
thwart. but | the nethyr ende
appered outwarde on | the tonycle.
and yt appered as it doth. | when it

---

1 ensample] the hawe in | the eye.
*added in outer margin in an
Elizabethan hand* 3 Luk] no*ta
added in outer margin in a late hand*

Glasgow, GUL, Hunter MS 513, ff. 2r–37r

Basel, Ö.B.U., MS D.II.11, ff. 172r–177v

32v **Of aneyl ·i· awne or of a straw in the | ey3e and of the cure therof. |**

And yit we shull saye a·nother cure liche | to that of a·n eyl of strawe
5 entryng in to | the pacientes ey3en ¶ In the Cite that | men clepen Luca · ther was y browght afore vs a· | man that hade aneyl in his ey3e of a·whete ere | And that neyl was ouertward so that the poynte | of that neil that it appered
10 nought on the tonicle | But it

---

1 Of] 28 *added in outer margin*

Oxford, Bodleian Library, Ashmole MS 1468, pp. 1–6

[70] Of a neyl .i. awne or of a · strawe in þe ey3e | & of þe cure þerof ·/·
And yit we shull saye a · nother cure liche | to þat · of a · neyl of strawe entryng | into   5
þe pacientes ey3en ¶ In þe Cite | þat men clepen Luca · þer was y brou3t afore vs | a ·
man þat hade a neyl in his ey3e of a · whete | ere / and þat neyl was ouertward so þat
þe | poynte of þat neill þat it appered | nou3t on þe tonicle / But it appered as it | 10
appereth whan þe fyngers entren atwene þe | flesshe and þe nayl / But we kutte þe
tonicle | on þe neyl fro þat party where þat it entred | so   euyn and so softelich þat we   15
distourbled | nou3t þat tonicle ¶ And afterward we hadde | two nedyll in þe maner of a ·
peire twicches | y bounde and þo we putte hem in to þe ey3e | of on poynt vnder þe nayl
and þat ar aboue | fro þat side þat we kutte þe tonicle and after|ward   softely boþe nedils   20
in maner of a · peire | twycches turnyng and sumdel streynyng wiþ | oure fyngers we

---

10 þat¹] nedill *deleted*

Biblio.-Médiathèques de Metz, MS 176, ff. 1r–16r

      appa|rent cum intrant digitum
35   inter | carnem et ungulam. Et nos
      tunc | incidimus tunicam super
      aristam | ab illa parte ubi intra-
      uerat, tam | plane et suauiter quod
      non turba|uimus tunicam. Postea
40   habuimus | et cepimus duas acus
      ad modum | tenallie insimul
      ligatas, postea | immisimus vnam
      punctam vnius duarum | illarum
      acuum subtus uel subter aristam |
      ab illo latere ubi incidimus
45   tunicam | et aliam punctam acus
      posuimus | desuper. Postea
13vb suauiter strinximus || ambas acus
      tenallie, et stringendo et | tor-
      quendo cum digitis nostris, acus |
      illas extraximus illam supra-
      dictam | aristam de oculo illius
5   pacientis. | Ex alia parte postea
      habuimus de virtute | a Deo data et
      posuimus in illo oculo, | sicut
      habetis in incisura de tunicis |
      oculorum, bis in die donec tunica

London, British Library, Sloane MS 661, ff. 32r–46r

Glasgow, GUL, Hunter MS 503, pp. 1–135

is on a mannys fynger. betwe|ne   10
the fleshe and the nayle. and yn |
thys. I dyde thus in dede
proceden. | Fyrst y avysed me
wele and wysely | wher the hawe
entred. and þere sotylly | I kut
without any trouble of the tony|cle.   15
and þan hade I rede. ij. nedyls ||
myghtyly knytt to geder by the   [117]
eyon | yn maner of a twycch. Of
whych oon | I put the poynt vnder
the hawe on the | same syde wher
yt went yn. and be|twene the   5
tonycle and the poynt of | the
toþer nedyl. I put a boue the
hawe. | and after that sotylly I
streyned them | to gydder. and so
wyth softe wyndyng | of þat oon
honde. and sotyll rollyng | it wyth   10
the oþer honde. I drew oute | the
hawe. whych doon. a noon I put |
yn to the eye of the oynement
afore|sayd callyd. Virtus a deo
data. twyes | on the day tyl the

Glasgow, GUL, Hunter MS 513, ff. 2r–37r *Basel, Ö.B.U., MS D.II.11, ff. 172r–177v*

    apperethe as it appereth whan the
fyngers | entren atwene the flesshe
and the nayle ¶ But we kutte | the
tonicle on the neyl fro that party
where that | it entred so euyn and
so softeliche that we distour|blede
nought that tonicle ¶ And after-
15 ward we had | two nedill in the
maner of a peire twicches y
bounde | and tho we putte hem in
to the ey3e of on poynt | vndre the
nayle and that ar a·boue fro that
side | that we kutte the tonicle and
afterward softely | bothe nedils in
maner of a·peire twicches
20 turnyng | and sumdel streynyng
w*ith* oure fyngers we drewe | oute
the neyl and on that other side we
hadde of þe | vertue of god y
3euen and we diden that in the
ey3e | as it is said a·boue in the
kuttyng of the tonicle of | ey3en
twies a·day till the tonicle were all

Oxford, Bodleian Library, Ashmole MS 1468, pp. 1–6

drewe out þat neyl And | on þat oþer side we hadde of þe vertue of | god y 3euen and we
diden þat in þe ey3e | as it is said aboue in þe kuttyng of þe tonicle | of ey3en twies a   25
day till þe tonicle were | all consouded & þe ey3e lefte y clarified · wher|fore and 3e
doeth ri3t on þe same maner ·/· |

Biblio.-Médiathèques de Metz, MS 176, ff. 1r–16r

    fuit | consolidata et [oculus]
10 remansit securus | et clarus. Vnde
vos similiter faciatis, et semper |
de pauperibus misericordiam
habeatis ut Do|minus Ihesus
Christus melius adimpleat |
operaciones et curas uestras. |

    71. Inter omnes curas nostri libri
15 docere | volumus uos istam que
est glorio|sissima et sanctissima
cura inter alias | probatas a nobis
pro oculis. Et est | proprie contra
illos qui sunt morsi | de aliquo
mortifero animali in oculo, sicut |
20 est morsus vesparum, aranearum,
et ali|arum similium istis – simili-
ter et ex aliquo | alio aere corrupto
uel infecto, vnde | tota facies
inflatur tali modo quod | paciens
non potest aperire oculos – et |
25 multi de illis mirabiliter dolent

---

9 oculus] M colera, VP2 (f. 309v),
VR (f. 57v) oculus

London, British Library, Sloane MS 661, ff. 32r–46r

Glasgow, GUL, Hunter MS 503, pp. 1–135

tonycle was sow|dyd and the ey   15
hoole. And þus do || ȝe yn lyke   [118]
wyse yf ȝe wyll gett your |
worschyp and your pacyent helth. |

¶ It also happeneth sum tyme
folkys | by the styngyng of sum
venemous beste | yn the eye as by   5
waspys. or att*er*cop|pys. or ony
such oþ*er*. or w*ith* any infecte |
ayre. that men calle blastyng.
wher|thorugh the ey wexeth so
bolnyn*n*. that | the pacyent may
not opyn hus eye. | And the payne   10
growyth so greueo*us* | þat he may
haue no rest. wherfore | when ȝe
see any such. haue the recours | to

---

5 attercoppys] *stinging of wasps
added in outer margin in an Elizabethan hand* 7 wherthorugh] infect
ayere *added in outer margin in an
Elizabethan hand*

Glasgow, GUL, Hunter MS 513, ff. 2r–37r

33r   consouded || and the ey3e lefte y
clarified wherfor and ye dothe
right | on the same maner ·/·

Basel, Ö.B.U., MS D.II.11, ff. 172r–177v

**Of bityng of vene|mous best*es* a
boute þe ey3e as waspes spidrez |
& of the cure.** |

5   Also it appethe sumtyme that su*m*
ben y bite of | su*m*me venemous
beste and su*m*me in the ey3e be |
stongen or biten as w*ith* waspes or
of spi|dres or suche other or of
su*m*me aer y corrupt or in|fecte
where for all the face is for
10   swollen in soch | maner that the
pacient may nought open his |
ey3en and many of soche bityng*es*
wonderfulliche | sorwyn and for

---

24 consouded] and *added in lower
margin* 2 venemous] 29 *added in
outer margin*

Oxford, Bodleian Library, Ashmole MS 1468, pp. 1–6

[71] Of bytyng of venemous bestes aboute þe | ey3e as waspes spydres & of þe   30
cure ·/·
Also · it happeth su*m*tyme þat su*m*me ben | y bite of su*m*me venemous beste and |
su*m*me in þe ey3e be stongen or biten as | with waspes or of spidres or suche other or | of
su*m*me aer y corrupt or infecte · wherefor*e* | all þe face is forswollen in soche maner   35
þat | þe pacient may nou3t open his ey3en and | many of soche bityng*es* wonderfulliche
sorwyn | and for akþe mowe nat haue reste ¶ And 3e see | any suche ye shull hele hem
alwey w*ith* þe holy | herbe þat we clepen þe holy Thistell // And || Romayns clepen it   40 | 4a
Erispinal / and these ben þe | signes to knowe hem for he hath two lyknes | in her self
first for it hath litell leuys / and | 2ᵉ grete leuys and brode / and we sayne þat | all ben   5
of one complexion and of one sauour*e* & | hauen one vertue and it makeþ a citren flour*e* |
¶ Taketh hir and grynde of hir .M.j. and med|le in hem in þe maner of a · plastre on |
stupys or on cotun þe ey3e y shitte lay it aboue | and bynde it w*ith* a · bonde and leue it

Biblio.-Médiathèques de Metz, MS 176, ff. 1r–16r

et | non possunt requiescere. Vnde
cum vide|ritis talem pacientem
aliquem, sem|per concurratis ad
istam sanctissimam | herbam que
30 aput quosdam vocatur | cardus
benedictus, apud Romanos crispi‑
na, | et hec sunt signa cognoscendi
eam: ideo | quia habet duas
similitudines in se, primo | habet
folia minuta, secundo habet magis
lata. | Et dicimus quod omnes sunt
35 de vna complexione | et de vno
sapore et habent vnam et eandem |
virtutem et faciunt ambe florem
ci|trinum. Accipiatis eam et pistetis
de | ea ad quantitatem vnius
manipuli, et po|natis cum ea
40 medietatem albuminis | vnius oui
et misceatis hoc et ducatis | ad
modum emplastri. Et super stup‑
pam uel | bombacem extensum
super oculum clausum | ponatis et
cum fascia ligetis et di|mittatis
ipsum donec desiccetur super |

London, British Library, Sloane MS 661, ff. 32r–46r

Glasgow, GUL, Hunter MS 503, pp. 1–135

the gr*a*cy*o*us herbe callyd.
Cardus | b*e*nedictus. sowthystyl.
Take þ*er*of an*n* | handful and   15
stampe it. & temp*er* it || wyth   [119]
halfe the whyte of an egg. and |
þ*er*eof make a plaster wyth coton
or | flexe herdys. and the eye shitt.
ley it | theron. and bynd it þereto
w*ith* a lynne*n* | bend. so that it   5
remoue nat therfro. | And so let it
leye. tyl it be drye. and | aft*er* þat
it is drye. ley to a nother. | and so
tyl the bolnyng be hoole. | Thys
plast*er* ys callyd. Gracio*u*s. | for it   10
swagyth bolnyng. and yt | puttyth
a wey blode from the eye. | it
swagyth the peyne and dystroyth |
the venym. and yf it happen
sum|tyme sodeynly. that that the
eye | wex rede and sore bre*n*nyng.   15
so þat || the pacyent thenk þat hys   [120]

---

6 And] blode *added in outer margin in a late hand*

Glasgow, GUL, Hunter MS 513, ff. 2r–37r

 akthe mowe nat haue reste // And |
 ye see any suche ye shull hele hem
 alwey w*ith* the | holy herbe that
 we clepen the holy Thistell ¶ And |
15 Romanys clepen it Crispinal / and
 these ben the sig|nes to knowe hem
 for he hathe two lyknes in her |
 selfe / firste for it hathe litell leuys
 and the·2$^{e.}$ grete | leuys and brode
 / and we sayne that all ben of on |
 complexion and of one sauour &
20 hauen one vertue | and it makethe
 a·citren flour ¶ Takethe hir & |
 grynde of hir ·M·j· and medle in
 hem in the maner | of a plaster on
 stupis or on cotun the ey3e y
 shitte | lay it a·boue and bynde it
 w*ith* a·bounde and leue it | there
 till it be drye on the ey3e ¶ And
33v afterward || take the remen*a*nt of
 this emplastre and eftesones ley it
 on | the ey3e till the ey3e be

Basel, Ö.B.U., MS D.II.11, ff. 172r–177v

---

20 &] ℞ *added in outer margin*

Oxford, Bodleian Library, Ashmole MS 1468, pp. 1–6

þere till | it be drie on þe ey3e ¶ And afterward take þe | remen*a*nt of þis emplastre and 10
eftsones ley it | on þe ey3e till þe ey3e be a · swaged ¶ This | glorious emplastre abateth
swellyng of ey3en | and it casteth out blode and fornemyþ akþe | and distroyeth 15
venym // And whan þe ey3en | sodenly begynne to wexe rede and þe pacie*n*t | felith
grete brennyng and he wenyth þat he | hath his ey3en full of sande / he shall be
deliu*er*ed | wiþ þis glorious emplastre alsone as ye laye | it on þe ey3e / and we clepen 20
it glorious for | it hath many vertues gracious ·/· |

Biblio.-Médiathèques de Metz, MS 176, ff. 1r–16r

45 oculum. Postea habeatis de
14ra residuo pre||dicti emplastri, et
iterum ponatis donec ocu|lus
detumescat. Vultis uos au|dire
quanta bona facit istud glorio|sum
graciosum et sanctissimum
5 emplastrum in | oculo tumefacto?
Primo detumescit oculum | et
expellit sanguinem et alleuiat
do|lorem et venenum destruit, et
quan|do oculi subito rubescunt et
paciens | sentit magnum ardorem
10 et videtur ei | quod habeat
oculum plene arene, liberabitur |
ipse paciens cum isto emplastro
gracioso | glorioso et sanctissimo,
quam cicius posuistis | super
oculum suum. Et vocamus ipsum |
emplastrum gloriosum, graciosum,
15 et sanctissimum ideo | quia
multas virtutes habet, que sunt |
plene gracia, gloria, et sanctitate.
Operamini | ergo ipsum cum

Glasgow, GUL, Hunter MS 503, pp. 1–135

eye were | ful of grauel. w*ith* thys
g*ra*cious plast*er* | he shall ben
holpen assone as it is | leyd
þereon. And for thies causes & |
oþ*er*. thys playst*er* ys callyd. 5
Gracio*us*. | Thys þan tau3th by
thys autor, | Benemicius. the
specyall hurtys | of eyon boyth
Inwardly & outward|ly caused. and
the specyall cures of | the same. 10

London, British Library, Sloane MS 661, ff. 32r–46r

Glasgow, GUL, Hunter MS 513, ff. 2r–37r

    a·swaged ¶ This glorious em|plastre abatethe swellyng of ey3en and it castethe oute | blode and fornemythe akthe and
5 Distroyethe venym ¶ | And whan the ey3en sodenly begynne to wexe rede | and the pacient felithe grete brennyng and he we|nythe that he hathe his ey3en full of sande he | shall be deliu*e*red w*ith* this glorious emplastre alsone | as ye laye it on the ey3e and we clepen it
10 glorio|us for it hathe many vertues gracious ·/· |

Basel, Ö.B.U., MS D.II.11, ff. 172r–177v

Oxford, Bodleian Library, Ashmole MS 1468, pp. 1–6

Biblio.-Médiathèques de Metz, MS 176, ff. 1r–16r

salute et cum benedic|tione Dei et nostra.

72. Contra nebulam siue pannum.

| Hec est cura pro nebula de
20 qua di|cemus in nomine Christi: ℞ lapidem mar|garitarum, terantur et subtiliter pulueri|zentur – hic puluis positus super pupil|lam oculi ubi est nebula sparsa quasi | in aere claro, quam quidam vocant
25 pan|num, mirabiliter sanat ipsam. Item | ad eandem valet cristallus pulueriza|tus et superpositus. Item iaspis pul|uerizatus corrodit nebulam predictam | et sanguinem expellit si oculus est san|guinolen-
30 tus uel rubicundus. Item | corallus rubeus subtiliter pulueri-zatus | idem facit quod et iaspis et eciam ampli|ficat oculum. Item saphirus tria | facit in oculo:
35 corrodit nebulam, acu|it lumen, pupillam constringit – et | clarificat totum oculum et postquam |

London, British Library, Sloane MS 661, ff. 32r–46r

Glasgow, GUL, Hunter MS 503, pp. 1–135

¶ Now here yn the | laste ende of thys booke he techeth | gen*er*all medycyns. and fyrst he | techyth powders. and aft*er* colery*ous*. | & fynally he techyth a gen*er*al dya|torye for al man*er* of such   15
pacyentis || Fyrst as towchyng   [121]
powd*er*s. I ley | to yow. In the name of Ih*esu*. that | powd*er* mayde of the margaryte. | put yn the eye whych hath a clow|de lyke   5
a thynne clowde sprede a|brode yn the clere eyer. hit help*ith* | it. The same doth a Jasper pow|dryd. Also yf the eye be red or blo|dy. it

---

1 Fyrst] the laste p*ar*te of | this bocke *added in outer margin in an Elizabethan hand* as] poudre *added in upper margin in a late hand, followed by* for the Eyes *written in an Elizabethan hand* **4** put] clowde *added in outer margin in a late hand*

Glasgow, GUL, Hunter MS 513, ff. 2r–37r   Basel, Ö.B.U., MS D.II.11, ff. 172r–177v

Of þe cure of nebula þat is þe clowde in the eyȝe |
IN the name of Crist the cure of
nebula ·i· clowde ·℞· | take the
margerye stonys & poudre hem
ryght sotil|liche and this poudre y
15 do in to the eyȝe on the ap|pull of
the eyȝe where that the Clowde ys
abrode | that is in a·clere aer it
helith ¶ Also the same ys | Cristall
of the same valour y pulueriezd ·
Item Also | Jaspis y poudred
forfretithe away the forsaid
clowde | and castithe oute blode ¶
20 Also Rede Corall dothe the | same
¶ Also that Jaspis sotilliche y
poudred it ma|kethe the eyȝe more
¶ Also the zaphir dothe ·iij·
þinges | it fretethe the clowde it

---

11 Of] 30 *added in outer margin*
20 same] ℞ *added in outer margin*

Oxford, Bodleian Library, Ashmole MS 1468, pp. 1–6

[72] **Of þe cure of nebula þat is þe clowde | in þe eyȝe** ·/· |
In þe name of Crist þe Cure of nebula | .i. clowde .℞. take of margerye stonys | and   25
poudre hem riȝt sotillich and þis | poudre y do in to þe eyȝe on the appull of þe | eyȝe
where þat þe Clowde ys a brode þat is | in a · clere aer it helyþ ¶ Also for þe same ys |
Cristall of þe same valour y puluerized . Item // | Also Jaspis y poudred forfretyþ a way   30
þe for|said Clowde and casteth out blode ¶ Also rede | Corall dothe þe same ¶ Also þat
Jaspis sotillich | y poudred it makeþ þe eyȝe more ¶ Also þe ȝan|phyr dothe .iij. þinges it   35
freteþe þe clowde / it | clerith þe siȝt / it constreyneth þe appill of þe | eyȝe / and it
clereth all þe eyȝe ¶ And after þat | it is done in to þe eyȝe it may nouȝt apair | also longe
as þe pacient leuyth ¶ Also berell | y poudred it forfreteth þe Clowde and confor|teth þe   40
humours of þe eyȝe

---

24 In] C *added in outer margin*

Biblio.-Médiathèques de Metz, MS 176, ff. 1r–16r

    intrat oculum, oculus non potest
deteriorari | dum paciens viuat.
Item berillus | puluerizatus cor-
40 rodit nebulam et con|fortat
humores oculorum, scilicet
albugineum, | cristallinum, et
vitreum.

73. Docuimus vos | pulueres et
virtutes quorumdam lapi|dum
preciosorum. Sciatis quod cum
medi|caueritis aliquos nobiles
45 homines, debe|tis cum eis operari
14rb et dare laudem Deo || qui suas
virtutes misit in eis et mag|nificare
altitudinem Artis Nostre Pro|ba-
tissime Oculorum vt uos reci-
piatis | honorem. Sed tamen

London, British Library, Sloane MS 661, ff. 32r–46r

Glasgow, GUL, Hunter MS 503, pp. 1–135

puttyth it a wey. Also cri|stall   10
sotylly powderd. doth the sa|me
that the Jasper doth. and also |
largyth the eye. Also a saphire |
powderd dooth. iij. thyngys in
the | eye. It fretyth the webbe. It
shar|pyth the sy3te. and   15
constrenyth || the pupyll. and   [122]
clarifyeth all the eye. | And after
that it ys onys entryde | into the
eye. It may neuer be apeyred |
wythout grete hurte. Also powder |
of the berall fretyth a way yn the | 5
eye an comfortyth all the humers, |
But here it ys to be markyd. þat |
wyth all thies powders wyth eche |
of them must be medled powder
of | suger captyn to temper and to   10
res|treyne her my3ty vyolens. And
in | thys proporcyonn. ij. partys
ben of suger. | and oon of the oþer

---

9 of] the tempering of | pouders for |
the eyes. *added in outer margin in an
Elizabethan hand*

De Probatissima Arte Oculorum

Glasgow, GUL, Hunter MS 513, ff. 2r–37r *Basel, Ö.B.U., MS D.II.11, ff. 172r–177v*

    clerethe the sight it constrey|nethe
the appill of the ey3e and it
clerethe all the ey3e | ¶ And after
that it is done in to the ey3e it may
34r no||ught apaire as longe as the
pacient leuythe ¶ Also | berell y
poudred it fretethe the clowde and
confortethe þe | humours of the
ey3en

¶ These poudres ben for Rich |
men / Butt ye shull putte with hem
5 and medle of poudre | of zuccar
captiuo and temper hem to giders
for his vio|lens and oo partye shall
be of poudre and two parties | of
zucre captiuo and this poudre shall
be kepte in | a·boxe of golde or of
siluer and twies in the day ye |

Oxford, Bodleian Library, Ashmole MS 1468, pp. 1–6

[73] ¶ Thise poudres benn || for Ryche men / But 3e shull putte with | hem and medle   4b
of poudre of zuccre captiuo and | tempre hem to giders for his violens and oo | partye
shall be of poudre and two parties of | zucre captiuo / And þis poudre shall be kept in | 5
a · boxe of golde or of siluer and twyes in þe day | 3e shull do in to þe ey3e erly and at
eue . / . |

Biblio.-Médiathèques de Metz, MS 176, ff. 1r–16r

5 debetis cum ipsis | miscere de
puluere facto de zucaro cap|tiuo ut
temperetur sua malicia quia | sunt
uiolenti. Et sciatis quod debetis |
ponere duas partes de puluere
zucari et | vnam tantum de puluere
10 lapidis et miscere. | Facto puluere
reseruetis eum in vase | aureo uel
argenteo et pacientem | medicetis
bis in die, scilicet mane et sero. |
Et sciatis quod hec experimenta
probata | sunt a nobis, et innume-
15 rabiles homines | cum istis
preciosissimis pulueribus libe|ra-
uimus. Non nobis sed Domino Deo
nostro | gracias referamus – et uos
referatis | gracias et gloriam, qui
dedit nobis cog|nicionem de eis.
74. Contra Nebulam. | Hic
superius hucusque docuimus uos |
20 pulueres preciosos et bonos
contra | nebulam predictam.
Ammodo docebi|mus pro eadem
infirmitate quod cum | volueritis

Glasgow, GUL, Hunter MS 503, pp. 1–135

powd*er*. and thys | powd*er* must
be kept yn a boxe of gold | or of   15
syluer. and twyes in the day ||
morn and euyn put into the eye. | [123]

and not oonly of p*re*cyo*us* stonys.
but | also of go*m*mys and of oþ*er*
thyngys | may be made ful holsom
powd*er*s for | eyon. And as for   5

London, British Library, Sloane MS 661, ff. 32r–46r

Glasgow, GUL, Hunter MS 513, ff. 2r–37r
shull do in to the ey3e erly and at
eue ·/·

Basel, Ö.B.U., MS D.II.11, ff. 172r–177v

10   **Of | diuers medicynes for þe
forsaid nebula |**
For the same infirmite other
medycynes we | shull teche you as

---

9 Of] 31 *added in outer margin*

Oxford, Bodleian Library, Ashmole MS 1468, pp. 1–6
[74] Of diuerse medicynes for þe forsaide | nebula ·/· |
For þe same infirmite oþer medicynes | we shull teche you as whanne ye may | nou3t   10
fynde one medicyne / 3e shall take | a · nother / And first of gummes Take þe gumme
of | olyue treys and poudre it and do it in to þe | ey3e   it fretyþ þe webbe and clerith þe   15
si3t / Gumme | fenil dothe þe same and it quyckeþ þe spirit visi|ble / it sharpeþ þe si3t as
it is wonte and it | bringeth it into þe first helthe ¶ Also þe gumme | of þe bitter almounde
treys it fretyth þe clowde | and   it clerith þe ey3e // Also þe gumme doth of | soure   20
plumme treis þe whiche growen amonge | vyne treis /

Biblio.-Médiathèques de Metz, MS 176, ff. 1r–16r

    operari contra ipsam, et si uos non | poteritis inuenire vnam
25 istarum medici|narum, id est puluerum – concurratis ad aliam | sicut est ista: ℞ gummam oliuarum et pul|ueriza et mitte in oculum. Hoc corrodit | pannum et clarificat oculum. Item | gumma feniculi
30 corrodit pannum et | clarificat oculum, spiritum visibilem viui|ficat, acuit lumen et visum, sicut | consueuit ad pristinum statum et sa|nitatem. Item gumma amigdalarum | amarum corrodit nebulam
35 illam et cla|rificat visum et lumen oculorum. | Item gumma puarum acerbarum que inue|niuntur iuxta vineas idem facit. |

75. Scripsimus vobis uirtutes gummarum | que ualent contra
40 nebulam que | apparet in oculo

---

36 puarum acerbarum] VP2 (f.311r) priuorum acerborum, VR (f. 59r) prunarum acerbarum

London, British Library, Sloane MS 661, ff. 32r–46r

Glasgow, GUL, Hunter MS 503, pp. 1–135

    ge*m*mys. Take the | go*m*me of olyues and make þereof pow|der. and þat fretyth the webbe and | claryfyeth the eye. Gomme of fen|kyll doth the same. And also
10 quyke|nyth the visible spiritys. And sharp*ith* | the sy3th. Also gu*m*me of bitt*er* almond*is* | doth the same. And the bitt*er* plu*m*bes | gu*m*me. the same.

And wete 3e well | wheresoeu*er* the powd*er* of the seid gu*m*mes |
15 be put yn the eyon for the webbe

---

6 gomme] gom*m*a *added in outer margin in a late hand*

Glasgow, GUL, Hunter MS 513, ff. 2r–37r

    whanne ye may nought | fynde one
medicyne ye shall take a·nother | //
And first of gummes Take the
15 gumme of olyue treys | and
poudre it and do it in to the ey3e it
freteth the | webbe and clerethe the
sight ¶ Gumme feniculi dothe | the
same and it quickeþ the spirite
visible it sharpeþ | the sight as it is
wonte and it bringethe it in to | the
first helthe ¶ Also the gumme of
20 the bitter almo|unde treys it
fretethe the clowde and it clerethe
ey3e | ¶ Also the gumme dothe of
soure plumme treis the | whiche
growen amonge vyne treis

    ¶ And vnderstand | that the
poudres of the forsaid Gummes of
34v the forsaide || treys where euer
they be don in the ey3e For the

Basel, Ö.B.U., MS D.II.11, ff. 172r–177v

---

14 treys] ℞ *added in outer margin*

Oxford, Bodleian Library, Ashmole MS 1468, pp. 1–6

[75] and vnderstande þat þe poudres | of þe forsaid gummes of þe forsaid treys where |
euer þey be don in þe ey3e ffor þe forsaid pan|niclos þey helpen þey neuer offendenn | 25
ne trespassynn ¶ Also zuccre nabatis þat men | clepeth zucre candi wasshe hym well
and | wype hym on a fayre lynnen clothe till he | be drie from water and poudre hym · It
corro|dith and freteth þe webbe and clarifyeth þe | si3t and many merveyles it doth whan 30
it | is don in to þe ey3e ¶ Also thutye of Alisaundre | þat is sotill and grene y poudred and
medle hymm | with zuccre captiuo þey freten þe forsaid webbe | and   Clowdes and 35
clerith þe si3t and constrayneth | teres and it þenneth þe ey3e liddes forswollen | and it
distroyeth þe redenes and þe 3iche of þe | ey3e liddes / and it makeþ þe ey3e þe more ¶
Also | þe strenys of þe eyren with zuccre captiuo medle | hem ana .ʒ.ß. and medle hem 40
in a morter in þe | maner of Sauce and drie it at þe sunne in | glasyn vessell and poudre

---

25 þey²] clepen *deleted*

Biblio.-Médiathèques de Metz, MS 176, ff. 1r–16r

    sparsa sicut facit ne|bula que est in
aere claro, ut opera|mini ipsam
cum salute, quia cum | sanctissi-
mis istis gummis innumerabiles |
homines liberauimus et curauimus,
14va || adiuuante Domino Deo nostro
Ihesu Christo | qui est verus
medicus salutis. | Habeatis ipsos
pro probatissimis | pulueribus quia
5 uere ubicumque po|nuntur in
oculis pro illis dictis | panniculis,
iuuant et nunquam of|fendit et de
hoc experti sumus – ergo |
operamini ipsis cum salute. Item |
℞ zucarum nabetis quod candis
10 vo|catur et abluas ipsum bene
cum aqua, | et terge ipsum cum
panno lini | donec desiccetur ab
aqua, postea | puluerizetur. Hic
enim puluis cor|rodit panniculum
15 illum et clarifi|cat lumen ocu-
lorum et multa qui|dem mirabilia
facit cum intrat | oculum. Item ℞
tutyam alexan|drinam subtilem et

London, British Library, Sloane MS 661, ff. 32r–46r

Glasgow, GUL, Hunter MS 503, pp. 1–135

or || pannyclu*n*s. they shall helpe.   [124]
and no|thyng hurte. ¶ Also take
suger can|dy and washe it wele.
and wype it | wyth a ly*n*nen cloth
tyl it be drye. & | þan powd*er* it.   5
thys powd*er* fretyth the | webbe
and clarifyeth the syght. and |
doyth many oþ*er* woond*er*ful
thyngys. | when it is entred into
the eye. ¶ | Also take tutie of
alexandre sotyl | and grene. and   10
powd*er* it and medyl | it wyth
suger captyn even q*ua*ntitees. |
Thys powd*er* restrenyth teres.
and | fretyth the webbe. puttyth a
weye | bolnyng of the eye ledys.
and dys|troyth the ycche þereof.   15
and the blode || of the eyon. ¶   [125]
Also take the strenys | of egg. and

---

9 sotyl] totij *added in outer margin in a late hand* **2** egg] *The drawing of the brevigraph for* er *at the end of this word appears to have stopped midway*

Glasgow, GUL, Hunter MS 513, ff. 2r–37r

for|said paniclos they helpen and
neu*er* offenden ne tres|passyn ¶
Also zucc*re* nabat*is* that men
clepethe zuc*re* | candi wasshe hym
well and wype hym on a fay*re* |
5 lynnen clothe till he be drie from
water and poudre | hym · It
corrodithe and fretethe the webbe
and cla|rifithe the sight and many
merveyles it dothe wha*n* | it is don
in to the ey3e ¶ Also thutye of
Alisaund*re* | that is sotill and grene
10 y poudred and medle hym | w*ith*
zuc*re* captiuo they freten the
forsaide webbe and | clowdes and
clerithe the sight and constraynethe
teres | and it thennethe the ey3e
liddes for swllen and it |
distroyethe the redenes and the
3iche of the ey3e |liddes and it
makethe the ey3e the more ¶ Also
15 the | strenys of eyren w*ith* zuccre

---

15 strenys] ℞ *added in outer margin*

Oxford, Bodleian Library, Ashmole MS 1468, pp. 1–6

and lay it on*n* þe ey3e | and it shall frete þe Clowde w*ith*oute penaunce | or violence and
clereth þe ly3t of þe ey3e // ‖ Also þe rote drage se*r*pentine make it clene | from his 5a
barke and stampe it and clense it & | wiþ þe Colature medle poudre y made of au3oron
.i. | sarcocolla .ʒ.ß. and of þe Juce .ʒ.j. and | do hem to gidres in a · vessell and drie 5
hem | at þe sonne and poudre hem asonys and it is | good ayenst þe Clowde / and to hem
þat suffre*n* | narabin and in*n* many stedes it is cleped mobi|lion / And in Cesile and in
Calabre and in poile | pustile me fyndeþ many suche / And 3e shull | hele þese pacientes
first whiles þey ben new | and fresshe erly and at euen / and these medecy|nes þat 3e 10
fynden good and y proued · 3e | shull haue hem afore honde /

---

1 Also] No*t*a ben*e added on top margin in a different hand; some letters, apparently by the same hand and then deleted, follow*

Biblio.-Médiathèques de Metz, MS 176, ff. 1r–16r

20 viridem, et pulueriza | et misce
cum puluere pre|dicto facto de
zucaro captiuo, et | pone tantum
de vno quantum de alio – hic |
puluis corodit nebulam pre|dictam,
lucem seu lumen clari|ficat, lacri-
25 mas constringit, palpe|bras
tumefactas subtiliat, ru|bedinem
palpebrarum et pruritum | destruit,
et totum oculum ampliat. | Item ℞
germina ouorum et cum zuc|caro
captiuo, misce ana et ducantur |
30 simul in mortario, et pistentur |
ad modum salse. Postea desic-
cen|tur ad solem in vase vitreo et |
iterum puluerizentur et de hoc
puluere | valde subtili facto
35 ponatur in | oculum. Corrodit
enim hic puluis | predictam
nebulam sine dolore et | violencia
et multum clarificat | lumen. Item
℞ radicem drage | id est serpentine
40 et mundetur a cor|tice, postea
pistetur et coletur | ut exeat sucus,

London, British Library, Sloane MS 661, ff. 32r–46r

Glasgow, GUL, Hunter MS 503, pp. 1–135

medyll them wyth suger | captyn
and bray them to gheder In | a
brasyn morter yn the maner of a |
sawce. and it yn a wesyll of glas | 5
and dry it all at the son. and þan |
powder it. & þerof put yn þine
eye. | in whych ys a webbe. and it
shall | frete it wythoute peyn or
vyolence. | an claryfie the sy3te. ¶ 10
Also take | the dragons roote. and.
scrape a|wey clene the berke. and
stampe | it. and wryng out the Jus.
and | medyl it wyth powder of
sarcocolle | yn thys maner 15
proporcion. That ys || ii. ʒ. of the [126]
Jows and halfe ann vncer of | the
powder. and drye yt at the son.
and | powder it. and thys ys goode
for the webe | In the eye. Also ann
vncer of spyce cal|lyd. Lignum 5
aloes. And brenn it betwe|ne. ij.

---

5 sawce] nota *added in outer margin in a late hand* wesyll] g *deleted*

Glasgow, GUL, Hunter MS 513, ff. 2r–37r

captiuo medle hem ana | ·ʒ·ß· and medle hem in a·morter in the maner of | Sauce and drie it at the sunne in glasyn vessell and | poudre and lay it on te eyʒe and it shall frete the | clowde w*ith* oute penaunce or violence and clerethe
20   þe | lyght of the eyʒe ¶ Also the rote drage s*er*pentine ma|ke it clene from his barke and stampe it and clense | it & w*ith* the Colature medle poudre y made of anzoron | ·i· sarcocola ·ʒ·ß and of the Juce ·ʒ·j· and do hem to |gideres in a· vessell and drie hem at the sonne
25   and | poudre hem a·sonys and it
35r   is good a yenst the clowde || and to hem that suffren narabin and in many stedis it is | cleped mobilion and in Cesile and in calabre and in poi|le pustile me fyndeth many suche and ye shull hele þese |

Basel, Ö.B.U., MS D.II.11, ff. 172r–177v

---
20 make] ℞ *added in outer margin*

Oxford, Bodleian Library, Ashmole MS 1468, pp. 1–6

Biblio.-Médiathèques de Metz, MS 176, ff. 1r–16r

  colaretur et ad|misceatur de pul-
  uere facto de an|zarut, id est
  sarcocolla, et sicut ʒ ij | de suco
45 illius radicis et ʒ ß zucari | predicti
  et admisceantur insimul. | Postea
14vb desiccentur ad solem et || desiccatis
  iterum puluerizentur. Valet hic |
  puluis contra nebulam et ad illos |
  qui paciuntur naralum et in
  multis | locis dicuntur morbiliom,
5 in Cicilia uero | in Calabria et in
  Pullia uocantur et | dicuntur
  pustule. Vere dico uobis karissi-
  mi | si a principio cum sunt
  recentes, is|tam infirmitatem
  pacientes sunt | curati cum isto
10 puluere, continuato | mane et
  sero et operamini ipso cum sa|lute.

Glasgow, GUL, Hunter MS 503, pp. 1–135

bassyns so that the smoke goo |
not out. whych doone. that take. j
ʒ. | of suger captyn and stampe it
i*n* the | ouer bassyn*n* wyth the
smoke & ma|ke apowder of them 10
both. After thys | stampe the
brend. lignu*m* aloes. In | the same
basyn þat it was brend | yn. and
medyll þe*r*ewyth a drame of |
goode muske. and iiij. dramys of |
amber wele smellyng. Than put || 15
both powde*r*s yn on basyn. and [127]
make | of all oon sotyl powde*r*.
This powder | fretyth the forseyd
clowde and clari|fyeth the syʒte
and comforteth the | vysible spirit. 5
and restrenyth teres | causyd of
colde hume*r*s. and comforteth | the
brayn lyftyng vp the eyledys. | and
dystroyth the peyn of the
my|greym. ¶ Also the gall of a

---

10 thys] loke her *added* *in* *outer*
margin in a late hand

London, British Library, Sloane MS 661, ff. 32r–46r

Glasgow, GUL, Hunter MS 513, ff. 2r–37r   *Basel, Ö.B.U., MS D.II.11, ff. 172r–177v*

    pacientis first whiles they ben
5 newe and fresshe erly | and   at
euen / and these medicynes that ye
fynde good | and y proued ye shull
haue hem afore honde /

Oxford, Bodleian Library, Ashmole MS 1468, pp. 1–6

Biblio.-Médiathèques de Metz, MS 176, ff. 1r–16r   *Glasgow, GUL, Hunter MS 503, pp. 1–135*

beste cal|lyd. Castor. medled w*ith*   10
the Juys of | an herbe. clepyd.
Morsus galline. | Of whych herbe
be. ij. spyces. oon*n*. | beryth a rede
floure. the oþ*er* a violet | floure.
that whych beryth the rede | floure   15
ys callyd. Domina. the oþ*er*. ||
Ancilla. and not wyth stondyng | [128]
this diu*er*sytee of floures. þei ben*n*
both | of oon complexion*n*. And
of oon sa|uor. and of oon*n*
similitude. saue þat | floure. ¶   5
Take the Jous of thys | herbe and
put yn the thyrde p*ro*por*c*ion. | and
medyl it to ghed*er*. and so myche |
of the powd*er* of sarcacolle. that
yt | be as sade as past. þan dry it at
the | son. Than powd*er* it ageyn.   10
and me|dyll it wyth suger captyn.
for it is | vyolet.

76. Tamen recordor uobis illud
quod | hoc quod uobis uidebitur
bonum | et probatum, habeatis pre
manibus | uestris, quia omne

London, British Library, Sloane MS 661, ff. 32r–46r

Glasgow, GUL, Hunter MS 513, ff. 2r–37r　　　　*Basel, Ö.B.U., MS D.II.11, ff. 172r–177v*

Also sponge | marina y clensed
from sonde and y brent in a newe
potte | and make poudre and it
shall freten the clowde and |

Oxford, Bodleian Library, Ashmole MS 1468, pp. 1–6

[76] Also sponge | marina y clensed from sonde and y brente in | a · newe potte and
make poudre and it shall | fretenn þe Clowde and blacketh þe tonicle & | it clereth þe 15
siȝt ¶ Also ligni aloes y brente | a twene two basyns So þat no smoke passe | out / whan
þis is y do · haue ȝe zuccre cap|tif .ℨ.j. and grynde it in þe ouer bacynn with | þe forsaid 20
fumo and make poudre to gidres | and after grynde þe brente tre in þe bacynn | byneþe
þere þat it lay and with hym medle | ℨ.ß of gode muske and .ℨ.iiij. of fyn ambre | oriental
moste swetest in sauour / and after|ward medle alle þoo poudres to gidres and | make 25
riȝt a sotill poudre · this poudre fretith | away þe Clowde and it clarifyeth þe siȝt | and it
conforteth þe visible spirit and it con|strayneth teres .s. yif þey come by cause | of 30
colde / and it conforteth þe • braynn. Item | it lyfteth vp þe eyȝe liddes and it distroyeth |
penaunce and akþe ¶ But wyselich doth | þat noo asshes falle in to þe bacynn noþer |
coles and all shalt þou poudry and kepe it | in a boiste of siluer // Also for þe forsaid 35
Cloude | take þe galle of þat best þat is y cleped a · | Brocke and with it medle þe Juse of

Biblio.-Médiathèques de Metz, MS 176, ff. 1r–16r   *Glasgow, GUL, Hunter MS 503, pp. 1–135*

15 certum et probatum | reddit
    hominem artificem. Item spon|gia
    marina mundata ab arena et | in
    olla noua combusta postea pul-
    ue|rizata et superposita corrodit
    nebulam | predictam, nigrescit
20 tunicam et cla|rificat lumen
    oculorum. Item accipite lignum |
    aloes ʒ 1 comburatur inter duos |
    baciles ita quod fumus non exeat,
    hoc | facto habeatis sucarum
    captiuum et de | ipso accipiatis ʒ 1
25 illius zucari in su|periori bacile
    cum predicto fumo ut fiat | inde
    puluis insimul. Postea pistetis |
    lignum combustum in bacile
    inferori, | in quo iam est, ut
    reuertatur in pul|uerem, et cum eo
30 misceatis ʒ ß boni | musci et ʒ 4
    bone ambre vnde odori|fere. Postea
    misceatis omnes pulueres | in vno
    bacile insimul et ducantur |
    adinuicem ut fiat puluis subti-
    lissimus. | Corrodit enim puluis

London, British Library, Sloane MS 661, ff. 32r–46r

De Probatissima Arte Oculorum

Glasgow, GUL, Hunter MS 513, ff. 2r–37r   *Basel, Ö.B.U., MS D.II.11, ff. 172r–177v*

  blackethe the tonicle and it
10 clerethe the sight ¶ Also | ligni
  aloes y brente atwene two basyns
  So that no | smoke passe out /
  whan this is y do haue ye zuccre |
  captif ·ʒ·j· and grynde it in the ouer
  bacyn w*ith* the | forsaid fumo and
  make poudre to gedres and after |
  grynde the brent tre in the basyn
15 byneth there þ*at* | it lay and w*ith*
  hem medle ʒ·ß of gode muske
  and·ʒ·iiij· | of fyn ambre oriental
  moste swettest in sauour & |
  afterwarde medle alle thoo poudres
  to gidres and | make right a sotill
  poudre this poudre fretith a· | way
  the clowde and it clarifyethe the
20 syght and | it confortethe the
  visible spirit and it constrayne þe |
  teres ·s· yif they come by cause of
  colde / and it confor|tethe the
  brayn Item liftethe vp the eyʒe
  liddes | and it distroyethe
  penaunce of akthe ¶ But

Oxford, Bodleian Library, Ashmole MS 1468, pp. 1–6

an | herbe þat is cleped morsus galline .i. an*glice* | pymp*er*nell and þ*er*of is two maners
one þat | haþe rede floures / and a noþer þat hath ‖ vyolet floures / but take it þat hath 40 | 5b
rede | floures and þat is þe lady y saide / but þat | other ys y cleped þe s*eru*ant but
neu*er*þelesse | þey bene of one complexion and hauen one | vertue and one sauour*e* ¶ 5
Drawe oute þe | iuse and putte þe thridde party with þe | forsaid galle and bringe hem to
gidres w*ith* | þe poudre y made of auʒoron or of sarcocolle | and there shall be only
somoche of þe poudre | þat it be as it were a paste and drie it at þe | sonne and poudre it 10
ayen and do it on þe | Clowde / and it forfreteth and it shall clarifie | þe sight and medle
w*ith* hit zuccr*e* captiuo for | it is violent

Biblio.-Médiathèques de Metz, MS 176, ff. 1r–16r

35   iste predictam | nebulam, lumen oculorum clarificat, | et confortat spiritum visibilem, lacrimas | constringit si sint de humore frigido, | et confortat cerebrum et supercilia, dolo|rem emigraneum
40   reprimendo destruit, | alleuiat, et auffert. Tamen discrete faci|atis ne cadant in bacilibus cineres | uel carbones, et sciatis quod debetis omnes | res predictas puluerizare quamlibet per | se. Facto sic
45   puluere de omnibus predictis | et de qualibet per se, reseruetis eum ||
15ra   primo bene mixtum in pixide de vitro. | Item ad predictam nebulam: Recipe fel de | illo animali quod vocatur casu, et cum | eo misceatis de succo illius herbe
5   que | dicitur morsus galline in libris | medicinalibus – Arabes vocant ipsam | uilcande, Greci uero que-curat-dolorem, | ac si diceretur in Latina lingua domina |

London, British Library, Sloane MS 661, ff. 32r–46r

Glasgow, GUL, Hunter MS 513, ff. 2r–37r

35v
    wyse|lyche dothe that noo asshes
    falle in to the bacyn noþer ‖ coles
    and all shalt thou poudry and kepe
    it in a boiste of | siluer ¶ Also for
    the forsaide clowde take the galle
    of | that best that is y cleped
    a·brocke and w*ith* it medle | the
    Iuse of an herbe that is cleped
5   morsus galline | ·i· an*glice*·
    pymp*er*nell and ther of is two
    maners on that | hathe rede floures
    / and a·nother that hathe vyolet |
    floures and that is the lady y saide /
    but that other | ys y cleped the
    s*eru*ant but neue*r*thelesse they ben
    of one | complexion and hauen
10   one vertue / and one sauour | ¶
    Drawe oute the yuse and putte the
    thridde party | w*ith* the forsaid
    galle and bringe hem to gidres
    w*ith* | the poudre y made of
    anzoron or of sarcocolle and | ther

Basel, Ö.B.U., MS D.II.11, ff. 172r–177v

---

2 siluer] ℞ *added in outer margin*

Oxford, Bodleian Library, Ashmole MS 1468, pp. 1–6

Biblio.-Médiathèques de Metz, MS 176, ff. 1r–16r *Glasgow, GUL, Hunter MS 503, pp. 1–135*

et ancilla. Et dicemus uobis qua
10   de | causa   dicitur domina et
ancilla, ideo quia | facit duos
flores, scilicet vnum rubeum | et
alterum uiollaceum, vnde illa que |
habet florem rubeum dicitur
domina | alia uero ancilla, scilicet
15   que habet florem | violaceum.
Tamen sunt de vna com|plexione et
habent eandem uirtutem, et | vnum
saporem et vnam similitudinem. |
Extrahatis ex ea sucum et ponatis |
terciam partem cum dicto felle, et
20   du|cantur   simul cum alio supra-
dicto pul|uere facto de anzareto, id
est de sarco|colla. Et sit tantum de
puluere quod sit quantum | pasta,
et desiccetur ad solem et iterum |
puluerizetur, et de isto puluere
25   super ne|bulam   ponatis. Iste
puluis corrodit | eam et lucem
clarificat, tamen miscea|tis cum eo
de puluere facto de zucaro |

London, British Library, Sloane MS 661, ff. 32r–46r

Glasgow, GUL, Hunter MS 513, ff. 2r–37r

    shall be only somoche of the poudre that it be | as it were a paste and drie it at the sonne and |
15 poudre it ayen and do it on the clode/ and it forfreteþe | and it shall clarifye the sight and medill with hit | zuccre captiuo for it is violent

Basel, Ö.B.U., MS D.II.11, ff. 172r–177v

Oxford, Bodleian Library, Ashmole MS 1468, pp. 1–6

Biblio.-Médiathèques de Metz, MS 176, ff. 1r–16r

    optimo quia mollis est aliquan-
tulum. |
    77. Item ad predictam nebulam: ℞
30   fel ur|sinum et misceatis cum
puluere facto | de margaritis et
incorporatur, ad so|lem siccetur, et
iterum puluerizetur sub|tiliter. Hic
puluis potenter corrodit ne|bulam
35   illam et clarificat lumen ocu|lorum,
et sint due partes de felle et vna |
de lapidibus. Item fel aquile cum |
puluere iaspidis lapidis et incorpo-
retur | ad modum paste, postea
desiccetur ad | solem et iterum
40   puluerizetur, et cum pul|uere
captiuo misceantur. Et sint due |
partes ipsius zucari et vna illius
pulueris | facti de felle et iaspide.
Corrodit | enim iste puluis nebu-
lam, et sanguinem | expellit, et
45   grauedinem palpebrarum | alleuiat.
15rb Item oleum oliue uetus posi||tum
in oculis mirabiliter corrodit |
nebulam et clarificat lumen. Sed |

London, British Library, Sloane MS 661, ff. 32r–46r

Glasgow, GUL, Hunter MS 503, pp. 1–135

¶ Also take the galle of | of a bere.
and medyll it wyth the | powder of
margarytys. and drye | them at the   15
soon. Than powder it || a geyn.   [129]
and loke þer be. ij. partys of
galle | and oon of powder. ¶ Also
take the | galle of an Eglee. and
yncorperate þer|wyth the powder
of iaspe. and drye | it yn the son.   5
than mdyl it wyth | the powder of
suger captyn. so that. | ij. partys be
suger. and oon of galle | and of the
Jaspe. ¶ Also the oyle | of Olyfe
put yn to the ey meruelusly |
fretyth the webbe. or clowde. but   10
it | ys ry3te vyolent. wherfore at
euyn | when 3e put the oyle yn the
eye. | ley a boue the plaster þat is
callyd. | Emplastrum laudabile. to
temper the | vyolens of the oyle.   15

De Probatissima Arte Oculorum 487

Glasgow, GUL, Hunter MS 513, ff. 2r–37r   Basel, Ö.B.U., MS D.II.11, ff. 172r–177v

```
        ¶ Also to the same | take Beres
        galle and medle therwithe poudre
        of mar|gerie stones and drye it at
   20   the sonne and eftesones | poudre
        it · For myghtiliche it fretethe the
        cloude and | it clarifithe the sight
        and ther shall be two partyes | of
        the galle and one partie of the
        Margerye stones | ¶ Also the galle
        of anegle with the poudre of
        Jaspis | encorpore hem to gidres in
   25   maner of paste and drie | it at the
        sonne and with the poudre of
  36r   zuccre captin || medle it / and of it
        shall be two parties / and of the
        galle | and of the Jaspe be o partie
        / it shall frete the clowde and |
        causte oute blode and it shall
        allight and swagen the gre|uance
        of the ey3e liddes // Also olde oyle
```

---

18 take] ℞ *added in outer margin*

Oxford, Bodleian Library, Ashmole MS 1468, pp. 1–6

[77] ¶ Also to þe same take beres galle | and   medle therwith poudre of margerie sto|nes   5
and drie it at þe sonne and eftesones | poudre it · ffor my3tiliche it freteþ þe cloude | and
it clarifieþ þe sight and þer shall be two | parties of þe galle / and one partie of þe |
margerye   stones ¶ Also þe galle of anegle with | þe poudre of Jaspis encorpore hemm to   10
gidres | in maner of paste *and* drie it at þe sonne & | wiþ þe poudre of zuccre captiuo
medle it / and | of it shall be two parties / and of þe galle and of | þe Jaspe shall be o
partie / it shall frete | þe Clowde and causte out blode / and it shall | allighte and   15
swagen þe greuance of þe ey3e | liddes ¶ Also olde oyle of olyue y putte into | þe ey3e
meruelously it freteþ þe Clowde | and clarifieþe þe ly3t / but neuerþelesse it is moche |

Biblio.-Médiathèques de Metz, MS 176, ff. 1r–16r

    tamen quia uiolens est in sero, semper cum | medicacueritis
5 ipsum ponatis super oculum | de emplastro laudabili nostro ad [sedandam] | illam uiolenciam.

    78. Item succus | uue acerbe, antequam incipiat per xx di|es maturare, cum puluere alexan|drino
10 misceatur ad modum paste | et ad solem siccetur. Et iterum pulueri-zetur | confectio hec et sit vna pars de ipso pul|uere et due partes de puluere zuccari cap|tiui, et hos duos misce insimul. Iste enim | puluis intus positus corrodit
15 pan|num predictum rubedinem

---

5 sedandam] M suadendum, VP2 (f. 311v) sedandum, VR (f. 61r) sedandam

London, British Library, Sloane MS 661, ff. 32r–46r

Glasgow, GUL, Hunter MS 503, pp. 1–135

¶ Also Jow*us* || of a sowre crape. [130]
Take xx^{ti} crapes | ere they be rype. confecte them wyth | oure powd*er* callyd. Alexander. yn | the man*er* of a past. and drye it i*n* the | sone.   5
and powd*er* it aȝen. and medle | it wyth the powd*er* of suger captyn. | dowble to the oþ*er* powd*er*. Thys fre|tyth myghtely the sayd clowde. and | dystroyeth the rednes of the eye ledys | and claryfyeth the   10
syȝte, |

---

15 Jowus] of a sowre. *added in lower margin*

Glasgow, GUL, Hunter MS 513, ff. 2r–37r *Basel, Ö.B.U., MS D.II.11, ff. 172r–177v*

5 of olyue y putte | in to the ey3e meruelously it fretethe the clowde and cla|rifieth the lyght but neuerthelesse it is moche violent | but euermore at euen whan ye do your medicyne to þe | pacient lay ye on the ey3e of the gloryous plastre that | is y wrete afore gracious

10 ¶ Also the Juse of soure grape | a twenty dayes er that it begynne to ripe neme it and | medle wi*th* hym wi*th* poudre of Alisaunder and make hem | in maner of paste and drie hem at the sonne and ther shall | be oo p*ar*tie of the Juse and two of the poudre whan it | is drie poudre it eftesones · This poudre

15 fretethe the | forsaide Clowde and it distroythe the Reddenes of the | ey3e liddes and it clarifiethe the light ·/·

Oxford, Bodleian Library, Ashmole MS 1468, pp. 1–6

violent / but euermore at euen whan ye do | your medicyne to þe pacient lay ye on þe | 20
ey3e of þe gloryous plastre þat is y write | gracious
[70] ¶ Also þe Juse of soure grape | a twenty daies er þat it begynne to ripe | neme it 25
and medle wi*th* hym wi*th* poudre of | Alisaunder and make hem in maner of paste | and
drie hem at þe sonne / and þere shall be | oo p*ar*tie of þe Juse / and two of þe poudre |
whan it is drie poudre it eftesones · This | poudre freteth þe forsaid Clowde and it | 30
distroyeth þe redenes of þe ey3e liddes and | it clarifyeth þe light .;. ||

---

23 gracious] *the preceding word, apparently* afore, *has been rubbed out. Such action has also damaged slightly the words over (*ey3e*) and under it (*a twenty*).*

Biblio.-Médiathèques de Metz, MS 176, ff. 1r–16r

palpe|brarum destruit et lumen oculorum | clarificat. |

79. Expleuimus uobis tractatum | de diuersis pulueribus et docui|mus vos varia et diuersa genera, | et quomodo debetis illos pulueres compo|nere pro illa nebula que apparet | in oculo quasi nebula sparsa in aere | claro, vt quando vos inuenietis pacien|tes cum talibus panniculis seu ne|bulis in oculis, debetis vnumquemque | medicare secundum possibilitatem suam | et magnificare Deum et dare honorem | nobis et [Arti Nostre Probatissime] Oculorum. | Et quando non poteritis vnum puluerem | illorum habere seu inuenire, recur|ratis ad alium, quia omnes sunt | probati a nobis pro illa infirmi|tate. Et multos de ista

29 Arti...Probatissime] M Arte Nostra Probatissima, VP2 (f.312v) Arti Nostre Probatissime

London, British Library, Sloane MS 661, ff. 32r–46r

Glasgow, GUL, Hunter MS 503, pp. 1–135

*Now fynally drawyng | to the ende of thys booke. | Bennemic*ius*. spekyth | to hys dysciplis concludyng thus. | O ȝe my dyscyples whych wyll | be p*ra*ctysers yn cures off sore eyon. | lyke os ȝe haue herde me teche. || herde me teche so werke. and pray | god wyth laude and thankyng þat | he wyll wytsayff of hys specyall | grace. to p*er*forme your cures to hys | worshype and your pacyentys helth. | And alwey haue a warenes i*n* your | cures to mesurable dyet. of your | pacyentys. and to kepe them from | cont*ra*ryo*us* metys. tyll þei recoue*re* per|fyȝte helth. That ys to wyt. froo | beef. gootys flech

[135,9]

15

[136]

5

10

9 Now] *This paragraph (§79) appears in the MS after §81*

Glasgow, GUL, Hunter MS 513, ff. 2r–37r   Basel, Ö.B.U., MS D.II.11, ff. 172r–177v

Of | gouuernaunce & dietyng of pacientz |
KEpethe well your paciens from contrarie metes | and drinkes also longe as ye shull haue hem in |
20   your Cure that is from thinges trespassyng | that men vsen moste / as from oxe flesshe / Cowe flessh | gotes flesshe and from olde olde kyddes flesshe and | fro Salades from muscherons from Elys counger sa|mon from swyvyng from stuphes and from
25   Saucis | from trauayle from werynes of body from lekys ||
36v from oynons fram garlik they shull nought fasten neiþer | wake moche and that they gone nought out of her | hous for the clerenes

---
16 Of] 32 *added in outer margin*
18 Kepethe] K *over deletion*

Oxford, Bodleian Library, Ashmole MS 1468, pp. 1–6

[79] Of gouernaunce and dietyng of pacientz | þat hauen infirmitez in þe ey3en ·/· | 6a
Kekepeth well your pacientes from | contrarie metes and drinkes also | longe as ye shull haue hem in youre | Cure þat is from þinges trespassyng þat men | vsen moste / as from   5
oxe flesshe / cowe flesshe | gotes flesshe / and from olde kyddes flesshe and | fro Salades from muscherons from Elys coun|ger Samon from swyuyng from stuphes & | from Saucis from trauayle from werynes | of body from lekys from oynons fram garlik | 10
þey shull nou3t fasten neiþer wake moche and | þat þey gone nou3t out of her hous for þe clere|nes of þe sunne ne by nyght lete hem se | none li3t neyþer lanterne neyþer fire ne   15
none | white shynyng thinge yonge folke shulde drinke | water olde men wyne watred and 3eue hem | rere eyren and sumtyme flesshe of weder yonge | kydes and lambrem rosted oþer y sodde / And | 3if þe Cure shall be longe in doyng with broþis | with spices   20
of Clowes of comyn and of saffron |

492

Biblio.-Médiathèques de Metz, MS 176, ff. 1r–16r

35   infirmi|tate cum alijs accidentijs
supradictis | curauimus et libera-
uimus semper gracia | Dei
mediante. Sed debetis custodire |
omnes infirmos vestros ab omnibus
eis | contrarijs dum medicatis
40   ipsos, do|nec reducantur ad
pristinam sani|tatem. Custodiant se
ab accumini|bus, a carne bouina,
yrcina, vac|cina, caprina, salitina, a
fungis, ab | anguillis, a coitu, a
45   stuphis, a | salsamentis, labore, et
fatigacione | corporis – et ab alijs
15va   hijs similibus. || Et cum medicatis
eos, non permittatis eos ieiunare,
nec multum vigilare, nec exire de
domo ubi manent propter clarita-
5   tem solis et | aeris, nec debet
paciens respicere | in lumen
lucerne quia multum | offenderet
eos, donec peruenerint ad | pris-
tinam sanitatem. Et semper | fac
10   ipsos stare in obscuris locis | ad
plus quam possint, et comedant |

London, British Library, Sloane MS 661, ff. 32r–46r

Glasgow, GUL, Hunter MS 503, pp. 1–135

salted. from stoke | fysshe. from
elys. from onyons. | from garlyk.
from co*mm*eny*n*g of | women.
from bathes. from sawcys. | from   15
grete werynes. from grete || labour.   [137]
from ou*er* myche wacche and |
fastyng. lete hym not goo a
broode | yn the wynde. nor yn the
soon. nor | loke yn no lant*er*ne
ly3te. tyll they | be recou*er*ed. lete   5
them ete rere egg*is* | wyth breed
yff þei be yong. lete | them drynk
water. And yff they | be olde. lete
them drynk wyne. w*ith* | water.
And yff the cure tarye. þat | nature   10
helpe not. yeve them fleshe | of
yong gootys gelded soden. and |
not rooste tyll they be re-
cou*er*ede. |

Glasgow, GUL, Hunter MS 513, ff. 2r–37r   **Basel, Ö.B.U., MS D.II.11, ff. 172r–177v**

    of the sonne ne by nyght lete he*m* |
    se none light neyther lanterne
5 neyther fire ne none whi|te
    shynyng thinge yonge folke shulde
    drinke water olde | men wyne
    watred and yeue hem rere eyren
    and su*m* |tyme flesshe of weder
    yonge kydes and lambrem rosted |
    or y sodde ¶ And yif the Cure shall
    be longe in doyng | w*ith* brothis
    w*ith* spices of Clowes of Comyn &
    of saffroun |

Oxford, Bodleian Library, Ashmole MS 1468, pp. 1–6

Biblio.-Médiathèques de Metz, MS 176, ff. 1r–16r

    oua sorbilia assata cum pane. | Et
si sint iuuenes bibant aquam, | et si
sint senes bibant vinum bene |
limphatum. Sed si cura pro-
15 lon|gatur ita quod natura non
adiuuet | eos cito, detis eis
aliquando de carnibus | castratiuis
et edulinis, elixatis, | cum pane si
habent cursum lacrimarum. | Vel si
oculi non lacrimantur, et semper |
20 habeant paratum brodium cum |
speciebus gariofilorum cimini, et
croci, et | paulatim elongetis eis
dietam | donec eant de bono in
melius. |
    80. Ammodo ueniamus ad
25 colliria | pro alijs diuersis infir-
mitatibus | qui accidunt in palpe-
bris oculorum, | et prohibent
lumen, et deuastant | tunicas
oculorum, et non dimittunt |
pacientem habere requiem die ac |
30 nocte. Dicimus ergo de primo
de | rubedine et grauedine pal-

Glasgow, GUL, Hunter MS 503, pp. 1–135

Now after the doctryne of | [130,11]
powders. the autor techith |
dyuers. Colories. for diuers |
sekenes that fallyth yn the eye
ledys | and letten the sy3te. and   15
wasten the || tonycle. and lette the   [131]
pacyent to ha|ue hys rest. ¶ And
fyrst ayen red|nes of the eye
lyddys. take totye of | alexandre.

London, British Library, Sloane MS 661, ff. 32r–46r

Glasgow, GUL, Hunter MS 513, ff. 2r–37r   Basel, Ö.B.U., MS D.II.11, ff. 172r–177v

10   **Of coliries of diuerse infirmitez in the ey3en** |
Go we nowe to coleries for diuerse infirmitees | whiche that fallen in to the ey3eliddes that | otherwhile defenden lyght and wasten the | tonicles and they suffren nought

---

10 Of] 33 *added in outer margin*

Oxford, Bodleian Library, Ashmole MS 1468, pp. 1–6

[80] Of Coliries for diuers infirmitez in þe ey3enn ·/· |
Go we nowe to coleries for diuerse infir|mitez whiche þat fallen into þe | ey3eliddis · þat other while defen|den ly3t and wasten þe tonicles and þey | suffren nou3t þe pacient to   25
haue reste // Ayenst | þe Redenes of ey3en and þe greuaunce of þe | ey3e liddes of what maner þat euer it be of | ¶ Take gode tuthie of Alisaundre þe Adaman|dston Sang dragon   30
rede corall gode aloes ana | ℥.ß. Sarcocoll Spykenard ana ℨ.j. candi | ℥.j. camphor mirre olibani masticis ana ℨ.ß rotes | of fenell rotis of persili wormode ana .M.j. | of white wyne gode and fyn ℔.iij. after þat | þe rotes ben y clensed and grounde with þe   35
wor|mode well y grounde all and ri3t small sethe | hem well in þat white wyne till þat wyne | be halvendele y wasted and þan clansed · þan | medle all þe forsaid þerwith and sethe hem | efte and clense it eftesonys and kepe þat licoure || in glasse and kepe it for   40 | 6b
thyne store / And erlich | and late at euyn doþ it in þe sore ey3en till þe | pacient be heled ¶ Also to þe forsaid greuance of | ey3en and for þe redenes of þe ey3e liddes /

Biblio.-Médiathèques de Metz, MS 176, ff. 1r–16r

pe|brarum de quocumque modo fit
causa: ℞ | tutye alexandrini,
lapidis ematitis, sanguinis |
draconis, coralli rubei, boni aloe
35 epatice | ana ʒ ß, sarcocolle,
spice nardi, | croci ana ʒ 1, candi
alexandrini ʒ 1, | camphore, mirre,
olibani, masticis ana | ʒ ß. ℞
petrocilii, feniculi, absinthij ana |
manipulum 1. Hec omnia terantur
40 in | mortario et in vno mundo
va|sile ponantur, et distempe-
rentur | cum tribus libre boni vini
albi, | et super ignem bulliant
donec | vinum reuertatur et
45 consumatur | ad medietatem, et
tollatur ab | igne et coletur per
15vb pannum || lineum, et in vase
uitreo reseruetur. | Et de hoc
collirio pro predicta infirmi|tate in
oculis mittatis mane et sero |
donec paciens curetur et liberetur |
5 ad plenum. Item ad predictam
gra|uedinem palpebrarum et

London, British Library, Sloane MS 661, ff. 32r–46r

Glasgow, GUL, Hunter MS 503, pp. 1–135

and of amatist stone. | sandragon. 5
reed corall. good aloes. | epatik
euyn porc*i*onn. of eche halfe | an
vnc*er*. sarcacolle. spykenard.
sa|ffron. of eche a drame. suger
candy | an*n* vnc*er*. Camphir.
Mir*r*a. olibani. | mastyk. of eche 10
halfe a dra*m*me. the | rootys of
p*er*cely. fenel. and wormo|de of
eche halfe an*n* hanful. Breke | all
thyes thyngys to gydd*er* yn a
mor|ter. And aft*er* put them yn a
feyr | basyn. and temp*er* þem 15
wyth. iij. || pyntyns of good whyte [132]
wyne. and | after put yt yn an*n*
erthen pott. boylle | it to ghed*er*
wyth a softe fyre. tyll the | wyne
be halfe wasted. Then clense | it 5
thorught a ly*n*nen cloth. and kepe |
it yn glasse. and put þ*er*of yn the
pa|cyentys eye. mor*n*n and eve. tyll
it be | hoole. Also aȝen the seyd
sekenes of | the ey ledys and the
rednes therof. | ¶ Take totye of 10

Glasgow, GUL, Hunter MS 513, ff. 2r–37r

15 the pacient to | haue reste ¶
Ayenst the redenes of ey3en and
the | greu*a*nce of the ey3elyddes
of what maner that eu*er* | it be of ¶
Take gode tuthie of alisaundre the
Ada|mandston Sang dragon rede
corall gode Aloes an*a* | ᴈ ß
Sarcocoll Spykenard an*a* ᴈ·ß rotis
20 of fenell | rotis of p*er*sili
wormode an*a* M j of white wyne
gode | and fyn ℔·iij· after that the
rotes ben y clensed and | grounde
w*ith* þe wormode well y grounde
all and | right small sethe hem well
in that white wyne | till that the
vyne be halvendele y wasted and ||
37r than clensed than medle all the
forsaid therw*ith* and seþ*e* | hem
ofte and clense it eftesonys and
kepe that licour | in glasse and
kepe it for thyne store / and erliche
and | late at euyn dothe it in the

Basel, Ö.B.U., MS D.II.11, ff. 172r–177v

---

17 it] ℞ *added in outer margin*

Oxford, Bodleian Library, Ashmole MS 1468, pp. 1–6

Take | tuthie of Alisaundre .ᴈ.ß autidi eres vsti ana | ᴈ.j. & ᴈucc*re* capt*iu*o ᴈ j. ros*arum*   5
rub*rarum* siccar*um* ᴈ i & ß | of alle þese make poudre saue þe roses and in thre | pounde
of white wyne lete hem sethen till þe | halfnendele oþ*er* more þan streyne it and do | it   10
vp ¶ Also anoþ*er* for þe same / Take tuthie | of Alisaundre ᴈ.j. fourty branches of a
spanne | lengþe of þe rede bremble and grynde hem ri3t | small as þou shuldist make
Sauce wiþ þe | poudre of tuthie and sethe hem in two pounde | of white wyne into þe   15
myddildele be y soden | away and doo þerwith as it is said abouen |

Biblio.-Médiathèques de Metz, MS 176, ff. 1r–16r

oculorum et | ad palpebras rubeas:
℞ tucie alexandrini | ℥ ß, anti-
monij, eris usti ana ℥ 1, zuc|cari
captiui ℥ 1, rosarum siccarum semi
10   ℥ 1 | et ß. Hec omnia pulueri-
zentur preter | rosas et in olla noua
cum tribus | libris boni vini
bulliant donec vinum | consumatur
usque ad medietatem. Postea |
coletur et colatura illa in vase
15 vi|treo reseruetur, et de colatura
seu | collirio mane et sero in oculis
pona|tis donec paciens sanetur.
Item ad | supradictum infirmi-
tatem: ℞ tucye | alexandrini ℥ 1 et
20 xl tallos rubi qui pis|tentur bene
ad modum salse, et cum pre|dicto
puluere tucye in olla noua po|natis
cum duabus ℔ boni vini al|bi, et
tantum bulliat quod vinum
consumatur | et reuertatur usque
25 ad medietatem. | Postea coletur
per pannum lineum, et | illud
collirium in vase vitreo re|seruetur

London, British Library, Sloane MS 661, ff. 32r–46r

Glasgow, GUL, Hunter MS 503, pp. 1–135

alexander halfe | an vnc*er* of
antemonie. erys vsti. | suger
captyn. of eche an*n* vnc*er* and
an*n* | halfe. and roses dryes.
asmuche. | all thyes thyngys saue
roses pon|derd. put yn a Erthen   15
pote wythe ‖ iij pyntys of whyte   [133]
wyne boyllyng | wyth soft fyre tyll
halfe be wastede. | and vse thys as
the oþer beforn. ¶ | Also anoþer
colerie for the same. Ta|ke an*n*   5
vnc*er* of totye alexandre. and | xl.
Croppys of bremel. and stampe |
them to ghedyr as it were sawce |
wyth iij. pyntys of whyte wyne |
yn a new erthen potte boyle it
to|gheder to the halfe. and vse it as   10
the | toþer.

---

14 ponderd] *The drawing of the brevigraph for* er *at the end of this word appears to have stopped midway*

De Probatissima Arte Oculorum

Glasgow, GUL, Hunter MS 513, ff. 2r–37r *Basel, Ö.B.U., MS D.II.11, ff. 172r–177v*

5   sore ey3en till the | pacient be helyd ¶ Also to the forsaid greu*a*nce of | ey3en and for the redenes of the ey3e liddes ¶ Take | tuthie of Alysaundre ·ʒ j ros*arum* rub*earum* sicc*arum* ·ʒ i & ß of all | these make pouder saue the roses and in thre pound | of white wyne
10 lete hem sethen till the halfuen|dele other more than streyne it and do it vp ¶ Also | a nother for the same ¶ Take tuthie of Alysaundre | ·ʒ·j fourty braunches of a·spanne lengthe of rede | bremble and grynde hem right small as thou shul|diste make Sauce w*ith* the
15 poudre of tuthie and | sethe hem in two pounde of white wyne into the | myddildele be y soden a way and doo therwith as | it is said abouen

---

11 Alysaundre] ℞ *added in outer margin*

Oxford, Bodleian Library, Ashmole MS 1468, pp. 1–6

Biblio.-Médiathèques de Metz, MS 176, ff. 1r–16r

et utatur sicut alijs tantum | et donec paciens plenarie sit curatus. |

81. Scripsimus vobis colliria
30 probatis|sima contra palpebras rubeas | et grauedinem oculorum, quia nos | cum istis collirijs innumerabiles homines | curauimus et liberauimus, habentes | predictam infirmitatem, non
35 nobis | sed altissimo Deo nostro Ihesu Christo re|ferentes gloriam. Sed ista colliria | que sunt a nobis composita non va|lent contra pannum – immo nocent, | ideo quia vinum est constrictiuum et
40 con|firmatiuum. Et ideo si posueritis in oculis | colliria facta cum vino super pannum | oculorum, nunquam pacientes | postea ad conualescenciam reuerterentur.

London, British Library, Sloane MS 661, ff. 32r–46r

Glasgow, GUL, Hunter MS 503, pp. 1–135

Thies forseyd coleryes byth | moyst preuyd for the seyd sekenes | of the eye ledys. but þei arnn not | good for the webbe yn the eye. but | raþer neyous. for 15
wyne ys constriktyfe || and [134]
confyrmatyffe. And þerfore yf | colerie be made wyth wyne and be | put yn the eye that hath a webbe. | the pacyent shall neuer be hoole. nor | holpyn þere wyth. 5
but rather and | appayred.

¶ Also take totye and | sarcacolle of eche halfe ann vncer. ro|ses sedys. ij. vncer camphyr. ij. dram|mys. pouder thyes to gheder. and bo|yll them in a quarte of 10
whyte wy|ne to the thyrd parte. And put. ij. | dropys yn the sore eye. and it wyll | put a wey rednes of the eyon. & | restreyne teres. ¶

Glasgow, GUL, Hunter MS 513, ff. 2r–37r   *Basel, Ö.B.U., MS D.II.11, ff. 172r–177v*

¶ These ben colleries moste y |proued ayenst the forsaid infirmitees but the avayle | nought ayent the webbe but it noyeþ it /
20   For one | is constraynyng and confirmyng and therfore yiff þer | be y putte a collerie y made w*ith* wyne on a webbe | of the ey3e the pacient shall neuer haue his sight |

Oxford, Bodleian Library, Ashmole MS 1468, pp. 1–6

[81] ¶ Thise ben coliries moste y proued ayenst þe | forsaid infirmitees but þey avayle nou3t ayenst | þe webbe but it noyeþ it / ffor one is constray|nyng and confirmyng and   20
therefore 3if þer be | y putte a collerie y made with wyne on a | webbe of þe ey3e þe pacient shall neuer haue | his si3t

Biblio.-Médiathèques de Metz, MS 176, ff. 1r–16r

Glasgow, GUL, Hunter MS 503, pp. 1–135

Also a ʒen wa|trye eyon. yff the
pacyent drynk || erely fastyng.
Auream alexandri|nam, wyth wyne.
streyneth teres | meruelously. ¶
Also medyll sarca|coller wyth
womans mylke. and | dry it at the
son. and eftsones do | the same.
and than powder it. and | put it yn
the eye whych is dusty | or mysty
it cleryth well the syʒth. |

15
[135]

5

82. Vnde | audiuistis contraria
contra pannum | et conua-
lescenciam contra palpebras
ru||beas et ipsarum grauedinem et
similiter | oculorum. Operamini
ergo ipsa cum sa|lute et cum
benedictione mea, et red|datis
graciam et gloriam Deo nostro
Ihesu | Christo, qui nobis dedit
cognicionem | de eis et ea co-
gnoscendi. Et oretis | eum ut ipse
dignetur consummare et | ad

45

16ra

5

8 syʒth] *§79 follows in the MS*

London, British Library, Sloane MS 661, ff. 32r–46r

De Probatissima Arte Oculorum 503

Glasgow, GUL, Hunter MS 513, ff. 2r–37r *Basel, Ö.B.U., MS D.II.11, ff. 172r–177v*

¶ And therfore ye haue y herde my
worching & | w*ith* hele ȝilde
thonkyng to almyghti god be-
seching | and praying hym that
he wolde vouchesauf to | ende
your Cures

25
5

Oxford, Bodleian Library, Ashmole MS 1468, pp. 1–6

[82] ¶ And therfore ye haue y herde my wor|ching wiþ hele ȝilde þonkyng to almyȝti god | beseching and praying hym þat he wolde | vouchesauf to ende your*e* Cures .   25
Amen .;. |

Biblio.-Médiathèques de Metz, MS 176, ff. 1r–16r	Glasgow, GUL, Hunter MS 503, pp. 1–135	
effectum tradere et ducere curas | vestras. |		
10 Explicit Ars probatissima | de cura oculorum composita | a magistro Beneuenuto Grapheo | de Iherusalem.	Deo gracias.	[137,13]

---

9 vestras] amen *expunged*

London, British Library, Sloane MS 661, ff. 32r–46r

Glasgow, GUL, Hunter MS 513, ff. 2r–37r

Amen.

Basel, Ö.B.U., MS D.II.11, ff. 172r–177v

Oxford, Bodleian Library, Ashmole MS 1468, pp. 1–6

Explicit Benevenut*us* de Jerusalitanens*is* .;.

Of tonicle of the eyzen and the humours and cataractus

Oculus anglice an eyze is harde holowe rounde full of water and y set in the myddewarde of the fronte of the hened that it mynystre and yeue lyght to the body thorowe helpyng of the visible spirit and the outward lyght ¶ And the eyze is said of the senwe optico that is said holowe wherfore opticus is twelue and hit is said holowe in latyn and Johannici saith that ther ben seuene tonicles of the eyzen ¶ The first he clepeth retentiua ¶ The secund sedina ¶ The 3. sclros ¶ the firthe aranea ¶ the 4. vnea ¶ the 6. cornea ¶ the 7. coniunctiua ¶ These bene seuene tonicles of the eyze and yif the first happeth to be broke or thorowe any thinge ys forate and for that hole may not holde the humors of the eyzen ware pozibe it semeth that all the substance of the eyzen is wasted and the eyze with his humors ys consumed ¶ The tonicle of the eyze ys that clere sercle the which to many it apperethe blak to other appereth pari mixe and by the myddell of the eyze ther is an hole the which hole is said pupilla an the appell of the eyze in the whiche the visible spirite comyth by the holwe nerffe hathe his oute goyng and taketh lyght of a

Glasgow, Glasgow University Library, Hunter MS 513 (V.8.16), f. 2r

References

Agrimi, Jole 1976. *Tecnica e scienza nella cultura medievale: inventario dei manoscritti relativi alla scienza ed alla tecnica medievale (secc. XI-XV): biblioteche di Lombardia*. Firenze: La Nuova Italia.

Albertotti, Giuseppe 1896. L'opera oftalmojatrica di Benvenuto nei codici, negli incunabuli e nelle edizione moderne. *Memorie della Regia Accademia di Scienze, Lettere ed Arti di Modena* (sezione di lettere), ser. 2, vol. 12, parte 1a, 27–101. [Separately published 1897.]

Albertotti, Giuseppe 1897. Benvenuti Grassi Hierosolimitani doctoris celeberrimi ac expertissimi de ocvlis eorvmque egritvdinibvs et cvris. Incunabulo ferrarese dell'anno MCCCCLXXIIII con notizie bibliografiche. *Annali di ottalmologia* 26, 1–60.

Albertotti, Giuseppe 1898. I codici Riccardiano Parigino ed Ashburnhamiano dell'opera oftalmojatrica di Benvenuto. *Memorie della Regia Accademia di Scienze, Lettere ed Arti di Modena* (sezione di lettere), ser. 3, vol. 1, 3–88.

Albertotti, Giuseppe 1902. I codici napoletano, vaticani e Boncompagni ora Albertotti dell'opera oftalmojatrica di Benvenuto. *Memorie della Regia Accademia di Scienze, Lettere ed Arti di Modena* (sezione di lettere) ser. 3, vol. 4, iii–xiv, 1–166. [Pp. 10–147 (texts of the four MSS only) published separately (1901) with the same title; pp. iii–xiv, 1–9, 148–66 (all material except the texts of the four MSS) published separately (1903) under the title *I codici di Napoli e del Vaticano e il codice Boncompagni ora Albertotti reguardanti la opera oftalmojatrica di Benvenuto con alcune considerazioni e proposte intorno all'abbassamento della catarata*.]

Albertotti, Giuseppe 1906. Il libro delle affezioni oculari di Jacopo Palmerio da Cingoli ed altri scritti di oculistica, tratti da un codice del secolo XV di Marco Sinzanogio da Sarnano. *Memorie della*

Regia Accademia di Scienze, Lettere ed Arti di Modena (sezione di lettere), ser. 3, vol. 6, 3–60, 61–80. [Separately published 1904.]

Alcock, Thomas / Wilmot, John [1687] 1961. *The Famous Pathologist; or, The Noble Montebank.* (Edited by de Sola Pinto, Vivian). Nottingham: Sisson and Parker.

Alonso Almeida, Francisco Jesús 2002. Punctuation Practice in a Late Medieval English Medical Remedybook. *Folia Linguistica Historica* 21.1–2, 207–232.

Anderson, Frank Joseph 1977. *An Illustrated History of the Herbals.* New York: Columbia University Press.

Austin, Thomas [1888] 1964. *Two Fifteenth-Century Cookery-Books: Harleian MS. 279 (ab.1430), & Harl. MS. 4016 (ab.1450), with Extracts from Ashmole MS. 1429 Laud MS. 553, & Douce MS. 55.* London: Oxford University Press. Available at <http://name.umdl.umich.edu/CookBk>.

Avicenna 1556. *Liber Canonis, De medicinis cordialibus, et Cantica.* Basle: Joannes Heruagios.

Baayen, R. Harald / van Halteren, Hans / Tweedie, Fiona J. 1996. Outside the Cave of Shadows: Using Syntactic Annotation to Enhance Authorship Attribution. *Literary and Linguistic Computing* 11.3, 121–132.

Ball, Catherine N. 1996. A Diachronic Study of Relative Markers in Spoken and Written English. *Language Variation and Change* 8.2, 227–258.

Beaujouan, Guy 1972. Manuscrits médicaux du moyen âge conservés en Espagne. *Mélanges de la Casa de Velázquez* 8, 161–221.

Berger, Albrecht Maria / Auracher, T. M. 1884–1886. *Des Benvenutus Grapheus "Practica oculorum." Beitrag zur Geschichte der Augenheilkunde.* 2 vols. München: J. Lindauer / C. Fritsch.

Biblioteca Nacional de España 1953–2002. *Inventario general de manuscritos de la Biblioteca Nacional.* 15 vols. Madrid: Ministerio de Educación Nacional / Dirección General de Archivos y Bibliotecas.

Black, William Henry 1845. *A Descriptive, Analytical, and Critical Catalogue of the Manuscripts Bequeathed unto the University of Oxford by Elias Ashmole.* Oxford: Oxford University Press.

Brinegar, Claude Stout 1963. Mark Twain and the Quintus Curtius Snodgrass Letters: A Statistical Test of Authorship. *Journal of the American Statistical Association* 58.301, 85–96.

British Museum [1837–1840]. *Catalogus librorum manuscriptorum bibliothecæ Sloanianæ.* [n. p.: n. n.]

Burchfield, Robert 1994. Line-End Hyphens in the *Ormulum* Manuscript (MS Junius I). In Godden, Malcolm / Gray, Douglas / Hoad, Terry F. (eds.) *From Anglo-Saxon to Early Middle English. Studies Presented to E. G. Stanley.* Oxford: Clarendon Press, 182–187.

Burrow, John Anthony / Turville-Petre, Thorlac [1992] ²1996. *A Book of Middle English.* Oxford: Blackwell.

Burrows, John F. 2002. 'Delta': a Measure of Stylistic Difference and a Guide to Likely Authorship. *Literary and Linguistic Computing* 17.3, 267–287.

Burrows, John F. 2007. All the Way Through: Testing for Authorship in Different Frequency Strata. *Literary and Linguistic Computing* 22.1, 27–47.

Cabello de la Torre, Pedro 1990. *Macer Floridus.* León: Universidad de León.

Calle Martín, Javier 2004. Punctuation Practice in a 15th-century Arithmetical Treatise (MS Bodley 790). *Neuphilologische Mitteilungen* 105, 407–422.

Calle Martín, Javier 2009. Line-final Word Division in Late Middle English *Fachprosa*: the Case of GUL MS Hunter 497 (V.7.24). In Díaz Vera, Javier Enrique / Caballero, Rosario (eds.) *Textual Healing: Studies in Medieval English Medical, Scientific and Technical Texts.* Bern: Peter Lang, 35–53.

Calle Martín, Javier forthcoming. Line-final Word Division in Early English Handwriting. In Thaisen, Jacob / Rutkowska, Hanna (eds.) *Scribes, Printers, and the Accidentals of Their Texts.* Frankfurt am Main: Peter Lang.

Calle Martín, Javier / Miranda García, Antonio 2005. Editing Middle English Punctuation. The Case of MS Egerton 2622 (ff. 136–152). *International Journal of English Studies* 5.2, 27–44.

Campbell, Alistair 1959. *Old English Grammar*. Oxford: Clarendon Press.

Cappelli, Adriano [1912] ⁶1990. *Lexicon abbreviaturarum*. Milano: Ulrico Hoepli.

Castan, Auguste Ferréol François Joseph 1897. *Catalogue général des manuscrits des bibliothèques publiques de France. Départements. Tome XXXII-XXXIII. Besançon.* 2 vols. Paris: Plon.

Clemens, Raymond / Graham, Timothy 2007. *Introduction to Manuscript Studies*. Ithaca / London: Cornell University Press. Available at <http://www.loc.gov/catdir/toc/ecip0714/2007010667.html>.

Collins, Minta 2000. *Medieval Herbals: the Illustrative Traditions*. London: British Library / University of Toronto.

Couderc, Camille Jean / Lavalley, Gaston / Albanès, Joseph Mathias Hyacinthe 1890. *Catalogue général des manuscrits des bibliothèques publiques de France. Départements. Tome XIV, Clermont-Ferrand, Caen, Toulon, Draguignan, Fréjus, Grasse, Nice, Tarascon*. Paris: Plon.

Cox, David Roxbee / Brandwood, Leonard 1959. On a Discriminatory Problem Connected with the Works of Plato. *Journal of the Royal Statistical Society. Series B (Methodological)* 21.1, 195–200.

Crellin, John K. / Scott, J. R. 1969. Pharmaceutical History and Its Sources in the Wellcome Collections. II. Drug Weighing in Britain, c. 1700–1900. *Medical History* 13.1, 51–67.

Cross, Rowin A. 2004. *A Handlist of Manuscripts Containing English in the Hunterian Collection Glasgow University Library*. Glasgow: Glasgow University Library.

Cummings, Michael 2005. The Role of Theme and Rheme in Contrasting Methods of Organization of Texts. In Butler, Christopher / Gómez-González, María de los Ángeles / Doval Suárez, Susana María (eds.) *The Dynamics of Language Use: Functional and Contrastive Perspectives*. Amsterdam: John Benjamins, 129–154.

Curme, George O. 1912. A History of the English Relative Constructions. *Journal of English and Germanic Philology* 11, 355–380.

Choulant, Ludwig (ed.) 1832. *De viribus herbarum: una cum Walafridi Strabonis, Othonis Cremonensis et Joannis Folez carminibus similis argumenti, quae recensuit et adnotatione critica instruxit Ludovicus Choulant; accedit anonymi carmen Graecum de herbis quod edidit Julius Sillig*. Lipsiae: sumptibus Leopoldi Vossii.

Daly, Walter J. / Yee, Robert D. 2001. The Eye Book of Master Peter of Spain – a Glimpse of Diagnosis and Treatment of Eye Disease in the Middle Ages. *Documenta Ophthalmologica* 103.2, 119–153.

De Laey, Jean Jacques 2008. The Eye in Vesalius' Works. *Sartoniana* 21, 115–127.

Dekeyser, Xavier 1984. Relativizers in Early Modern English: a Dynamic Quantitative Study. In Fisiak, Jacek (ed.) *Historical Syntax*. Berlin / New York / Amsterdam: Mouton, 61–87.

Denholm-Young, Noël [1954] ²1964. *Handwriting in England and Wales*. Cardiff: University of Wales Press.

Derolez, Albert 2003. *The Palaeography of Gothic Manuscript Books: from the Twelfth to the Early Sixteenth Century*. Cambridge: Cambridge University Press.

Eggins, Suzanne [1994] ²2004. *An Introduction to Systemic Functional Linguistics*. London: Continuum.

Eldredge, Laurence M. 1993. The Textual Tradition of Benvenutus Grassus' «De arte probatissima oculorum». *Studi medievali* (3rd series) 34.1, 95–138.

Eldredge, Laurence M. 1998. A Thirteenth-Century Ophthalmologist, Benvenutus Grassus: his Treatise and its Survival. *Journal of the Royal Society of Medicine* 91.1, 47–52.

Eldredge, Laurence M. 1999. The English Vernacular Afterlife of Benvenutus Grassus, Ophthalmologist. *Early Science and Medicine* 4, 149–163.

Eldredge, Laurence M. 2002. Did Benvenutus Grassus Lecture at Montpellier? In Iyeiri, Yoko / Connolly, Margaret (eds.) *And Gladly Wolde he Lerne and Gladly Teche: Essays on Medieval English Presented to Professor Matsuji Tajima on his Sixtieth Birthday*. Tokyo: Kaibunsha, 155–167.

Eldredge, Laurence M. 2004. A Newly Identified Manuscript of Benvenutus Grassus' Treatise on the Eye. *Studi medievali* (3rd series) 45.2, 947–951.

Eldredge, Laurence M. 2007. A Locator List of Some Medieval Ophthalmological Texts. *Canadian Bulletin of Medical History / Bulletin canadien d'histoire de la médecine* 24, 467–477.

Eldredge, Laurence M. (ed.) 1996. *Benvenutus Grassus. The Wonderful Art of the Eye. A Critical Edition of the Middle English Translation of His De probatissima arte oculorum.* East Lansing (MI): Michigan State University Press.

Ellegård, Alvar 1962. *A Statistical Method for Determining Authorship: the Junius letters, 1769–1772.* Göteborg: Acta Universitatis Gothoburgensis.

Esteban Segura, María Laura 2009. Punctuation Practice in MS GUL Hunter 509. In Díaz Vera, Javier Enrique / Caballero, Rosario (eds.) *Textual Healing: Studies in Medieval English Medical, Scientific and Technical Texts.* Bern: Peter Lang, 93–107.

Esteve Ramos, María José 2008. 'Thys Manner of Infirmyte the Grete Lechys of Salerne Clepyd Obtalmyam': A Study of Medical Terms in Benvenutus Grassus. *Miscelánea* 37, 39–51.

Finneran, Richard J. (ed.) 1996. *The Literary Text in the Digital Age.* Ann Arbor: University of Michigan Press.

Finzi, Angelo Attilio 1899. *Il codice Amploniano dell'opera oftalmojatrica di Benvenuto ed il Collirium Jerosolimitanum nella pratica oculare.* Modena: Clinica oculistica, Reale Università di Modena.

Fischer, Olga 1992. Syntax. In Blake, Norman F. (ed.) *The Cambridge History of the English Language. Vol. II: 1066–1476.* Cambridge: Cambridge University Press, 207–408.

Fischer, Olga / van der Wurff, Wim 2006. Syntax. In Hogg, Richard M. / Denison, David (eds.) *A History of the English Language.* Cambridge: Cambridge University Press, 109–198.

Fischer, Olga / van Kemenade, Ans / Koopman, Willem / van der Wurff, Wim 2000. *The Syntax of Early English.* Cambridge: Cambridge University Press.

Foys, Martin K. 2008. The Reality of Media in Anglo-Saxon Studies. *The Heroic Age, a Journal of Early Medieval Northwestern Europe*. Available at <http://www.mun.ca/mst/heroicage/issues/11/forumc.php>.

Fries, Peter Howard 1995. Patterns of Information in Initial Position in English. In Fries, Peter Howard / Gregory, Michael (eds.) *Discourse in Society: Systemic Functional Perspectives*. Norwood (N.J.): Ablex, 1–19.

Fries, Peter Howard 2002. The Flow of Information in a Written English Text. In Fries, Peter Howard / Cummings, Michael / Lockwood, David / Spruiell, William (eds.) *Relations and Functions within and around Language*. London / New York: Continuum, 117–155.

Frisch, Stefan 1997. The Change in Negation in Middle English: a NEGP Licensing Account. *Lingua* 101, 21–64.

Frischer, Bernard D. / Guthrie, Donald / Tse, Emily / Tweedie, Fiona J. 1996. Sentence Length and Word-Type at 'Sentence' Beginning and End: Reliable Authorship Discriminators for Latin Prose? New Studies on the Authorship of the *Historia Augusta*. *Research on the Humanities Computing* 5, 110–142.

Frisk, Gösta (ed.) 1949. *A Middle English Translation of Macer Floridus De Viribus Herbarum*. Uppsala: Almqvist & Wiksells Boktryckeri AB.

Hale, William Gardner / Buck, Carl Darling 1966. *A Latin Grammar*. University, Alabama: University of Alabama Press.

Halm, Carl Felix / Laubmann, Georg / Meyer, Wilhelm / Schmeller, Johann Andreas ²1873–1894. *Catalogus codicum Latinorum bibliothecae regiae Monacensis*. 7 vols. Monachii: Sumptibus Bibliothecae Regiae.

Halliday, Michael Alexander Kirkwood 1967. Notes on Transitivity and Theme in English, Part II. *Journal of Linguistics* 3, 177–274.

Halliday, Michael Alexander Kirkwood / Matthiessen, Christian M. I. M. [1985] ³2004. *An Introduction to Functional Grammar*. London: Edward Arnold.

Härtel, Helmar / Ekowski, Felix 1982–1989. *Handschriften der niedersächsischen Landesbibliothek Hannover*. 2 vols. Wiesbaden: Harrassowitz.

Hector, Leonard Charles 1958. *The Handwriting of English Documents*. London: Edward Arnold.

Hickes, George 1705. *Linguarum vetterum septentrionalium thesaurus grammatico-criticus et archæologicus*. 2 vols. Oxoniæ: e Theatro Sheldoniano.

Hilton, Michael L. / Holmes, David I. 1993. An Assessment of Cumulative Sum Charts for Authorship Attribution. *Literary and Linguistic Computing* 8.2, 73–80.

Hladký, Josef 1985a. Notes on the History of Word Division in English. *Brno Studies in English* 16, 73–83.

Hladký, Josef 1985b. Word Division in Caxton and Dryden. *Philologica Pragensia* 28, 135–141.

Holmes, David I. 1994. Authorship Attribution. *Computers and the Humanities* 28.2, 87–106.

Holmes, David I. 1998. The Evolution of Stylometry in Humanities Scholarship. *Literary and Linguistic Computing* 13.3, 111–117.

Holmes, David I. / Forsyth, Richard S. 1995. *The Federalist* Revisited: New Directions in Authorship Attribution. *Literary and Linguistic Computing* 10.2, 111–127.

Hoover, David L. 2001. Statistical Stylistics and Authorship Attribution: an Empirical Investigation. *Literary and Linguistic Computing* 16.4, 421–444.

Hoover, David L. 2003. Another Perspective in Vocabulary Richness. *Computers and the Humanities* 37, 151–178.

Hoover, David L. 2004a. Delta Prime? *Literary and Linguistic Computing* 19.4, 477–495.

Hoover, David L. 2004b. Testing Burrows's Delta. *Literary and Linguistic Computing* 19.4, 453–475.

Houseman, Alfred Edward 1921. The Application of Thought to Textual Criticism. *Proceedings of the Classical Association* 18, 67–84.

Ingham, Richard 2006. Negative Concord and the Loss of the Negative Particle *ne* in Late Middle English. *Studia Anglica Posnaniensia* 42, 77–97.

Iyeiri, Yoko 2001. *Negative Constructions in Middle English*. Fukuoka: Kyushu University Press.

Iyeiri, Yoko (ed.) 2005. *Aspects of English Negation*. Amsterdam: John Benjamins.

Jenkinson, Hilary 1926. Notes on the Study of English Punctuation of the Sixteenth Century. *Review of English Studies* 2.6, 152–158.

Jordan, Richard 1974. *Handbook of Middle English Grammar: Phonology*. The Hague / Paris: Mouton.

Jourdan, Antoine Jacques Louis ²1840. *Pharmacopée universelle*. 2 vols. Paris: J.-B. Baillière.

Katritzky, M. A. 2006. *The Art of Commedia: a Study in the Commedia dell'Arte 1560–1620 with Special Reference to the Visual Records*. Amsterdam: Rodopi.

Keller, Karl Heinz / Schmolinsky, Sabine 1994–2001. *Katalog der lateinischen Handschriften der Staatlichen Bibliothek (Schlossbibliothek) Ansbach*. 2 vols. Wiesbaden: Harrassowitz.

MED = Kurath, Hans / Kuhn, M. / Reidy, John / Lewis, R. E. (eds.) 1954–2001. *Middle English Dictionary*. Ann Arbor: University of Michigan Press.

Labbé, Dominique 2007. Experiments on Authorship Attribution by Intertextual Distance in English. *Journal of Quantitative Linguistics* 14.1, 33–80.

Laborde, Charles 1901. *Un oculiste du XIIe siècle. Bienvenu de Jérusalem. Le manuscript de la Bibliothèque de Metz*. M.D. Thesis, Université de Montpellier.

Laborde, Charles / Pansier, Pierre / Teulié, Henri (eds.) 1901. *Le Compendil pour la douleur et maladie des yeulx qui a esté ordonné par Bienvenu Graffe maistre et docteur en Médecine*. Paris: A. Maloine.

Laurans, M. 1903. *Bienvenu de Jérusalem, le manuscrit de Besançon*. M.D. thesis, Université de Montpellier.

Lee, Stuart D. *Ælfric's Homilies on Judith, Esther, and the Maccabees.* <http://users.ox.ac.uk/~stuart/kings/main.htm>.

Lezcano, Emma 1996. The Choice of Relativizers in Early Modern English: Evidence from the Helsinki Corpus. *Sederi* 7, 61–71.

Liddell, Henry George / Scott, Robert / Jones, Henry Stuart / McKenzie, Roderick (eds.) ⁹1996. *A Greek-English Lexicon. With a Revised Supplement.* Oxford / New York: Clarendon Press.

Lindberg, David C. 1975. *A Catalogue of Medieval and Renaissance Optical Manuscripts.* Toronto: Pontifical Institute of Mediaeval Studies.

Lindberg, David C. 1976. *Theories of Vision from Al-Kindi to Kepler.* Chicago / London: University of Chicago Press.

Love, Harold 2002. *Attributing Authorship: an Introduction.* Cambridge: Cambridge University Press.

Lucas, Peter J. 1971. Sense-units and the Use of Punctuation-markers in John Capgrave's *Chronicle. Archivum Linguisticum* 2, 3–24.

Lutz, Angelika 1986. The Syllabic Basis of Word Division in Old English Manuscripts. *English Studies* 67.3, 193–210.

Madan, Falconer F. / Hunt, Richard William / Craster, H. H. Edmund / Denholm-Young, N. 1895–1953. *A Summary Catalogue of Western Manuscripts in the Bodleian Library at Oxford Which Have not Hitherto Been Catalogued in the Quarto Series.* 7 vols. Oxford: Clarendon Press.

Marqués Aguado, Teresa 2009a. The Dialectal Provenance of G.U.L. MS Hunter 513 (ff. 1r–37r). In Díaz Vera, Javier Enrique / Caballero, Rosario (eds.) *Textual Healing: Studies in Medieval English Medical, Scientific and Technical Texts.* Bern: Peter Lang, 109–121.

Marqués Aguado, Teresa 2009b. Punctuation Practice in the Antidotary in GUL MS Hunter 513 (ff. 37v–96v). *Miscelánea* 39, 55–72.

Marqués, Teresa / Miranda, Antonio / González, Santiago 2008. *The Use of the Eyes: A Middle English Ophthalmic Treatise in GUL MS Hunter 513 (ff.1r–37r). An Annotated Edition and Study.* Málaga: Servicio de Publicaciones de la Universidad de Málaga.

Martin, James Robert 1992. *English Text: System and Structure*. Amsterdam: John Benjamins.
Martin, James Robert / Rose, David 2003. *Working with Discourse: Meaning beyond the Clause*. London: Continuum.
LALME = McIntosh, Angus / Samuels, Michael L. / Benskin, Michael 1986. *A Linguistic Atlas of Late Mediaeval English*. 4 vols. Aberdeen: Aberdeen University Press.
Mendenhall, Thomas Corwin 1887. The Characteristic Curves of Composition. *Science* 9.214, 237–246.
Merriam, Thomas 1994. Letter frequency as a Discriminator of Authors. *Notes and Queries* 239, 467–469.
Michaelson, S. / Morton, A. Q. / Wake, W. C. 1978. Sentence Length Distributions in Greek Hexameters and Homer. *Association for Literary and Linguistic Computing Bulletin* 6.3, 254–267.
Miguel Alonso, Aurora. *La imprenta renacentista y el nacimiento de la ciencia botánica*. <http://www.ucm.es/BUCM/foa/exposiciones/11JardinesPapel/la_imprenta_renacentista.htm>.
Milroy, James 1992. Middle English Dialectology. In Blake, Norman F. (ed.) *The Cambridge History of the English Language. Vol. II: 1066–1476*. Cambridge: Cambridge University Press, 156–206.
Milwright, Marcus 2003. The Balsam of Maṭariyya: An Exploration of a Medieval Panacea. *Bulletin of the School of Oriental and African Studies* 66.2, 193–209.
Miranda García, Antonio / Calle Martín, Javier 2005. The Validity of Lemma-Based Lexical Richness in Authorship Attribution: a Proposal for the Old English Gospels. *ICAME Journal* 29, 115–130.
Miranda García, Antonio / Calle Martín, Javier 2007. Function Words in Authorship Attribution Studies. *Literary and Linguistic Computing* 22.1, 49–66.
Miranda García, Antonio / Garrido Garrido, Joaquín forthcoming. *TexSEn*. Málaga: SPICUM.
Mitchell, Bruce 1980. The Dangers of Disguise: Old English Texts in Modern Punctuation. *Review of English Studies, New Series* 31 (124), 385–413.

Mitchell, Bruce 1985. *Old English Syntax. Volume II: Subordination, Independent Elements, and Element Order*. Oxford: Clarendon Press.

Moreno Olalla, David 2006. *Yn dyuerse parties of the worlde*. Dialectal Blend in G.U.L. Hunter 503. Paper read at the 18th International SELIM Conference, Málaga.

Moreno Olalla, David / Miranda García, Antonio 2009. An Annotated Corpus of Middle English Scientific Prose: Aims and Features. In Díaz Vera, Javier Enrique / Caballero, Rosario (eds.) *Textual Healing: Studies in Medieval English Medical, Scientific and Technical Texts*. Bern: Peter Lang, 123–140.

Mossé, Fernand 1952. *A Handbook of Middle English*. Baltimore: The Johns Hopkins University Press.

Mosteller, Frederick / Wallace, David L. 1963. Inference in an Authorship Problem. *Journal of the American Statistical Association* 58.302, 275–309.

Mosteller, Frederick / Wallace, David L. 1964. *Inference and Disputed Authorship: the Federalist*. Reading (MA): Addison-Wesley.

Mustanoja, Tauno F. 1960. *A Middle English Syntax. Part I: Parts of Speech*. Helsinki: Société Néophilologique.

Nicoud, Marilyn 2004. La médecine à Milan à la fin du Moyen Age: les composantes d'un milieu professionnel. In Collard, Franck / Samama, Evelyne (eds.) *Mires, physiciens, barbiers et charlatans: les marges de la medicine de l'Antiquité au XVIe siècle*. Langres: Dominique Gueniot, 101–131.

Noreen, Adolf [2]1892. *Altisländische und altnorwegische Grammatik, unter Berücksichtigung des Urnordischen*. Halle: Max Niemeyer.

Obegi Gallardo, Nadia 2006. Punctuation in a Fifteenth-century Scientific Treatise (MS Cambridge L1.4.14.). *Linguistica e Filologia* 22, 99–114.

Paoli, Cesare / Rostagno, Enrico / Lodi, Teresa 1887. *I codici Ashburnhamiani della R. Biblioteca Mediceo-Laurenziana di Firenze*. Roma: La Libreria dello Stato.

Parkes, Malcolm Beckwith 1978. Punctuation, or Pause and Effect. In Murphy, J. J. (ed.) *Medieval Eloquence. Studies in the Theory and Practice of Medieval Rhetoric*. Berkeley / Los Angeles / London: University of California Press, 127–142.

Parkes, Malcolm Beckwith [1969] ²1979. *English Cursive Book Hands: 1250–1500*. London: Scolar Press.

Pearson, David 2003. Illustrations from the Wellcome Library. Joseph Fenton and His Books. *Medical History* 47.2, 239–248.

Petti, Anthony Gaetano 1977. *English Literary Hands from Chaucer to Dryden*. London: Edward Arnold.

Pormann, Peter 2005. The Physician and the Other: Images of the Charlatan in Medieval Islam. *Bulletin of the History of Medicine* 79, 189–227.

Porter, Roy 2001. *Quacks, Fakers and Charlatans in English Medicine*. Stroud: Tempus.

Powell, Marcy S. 1984. Word Division. *English Studies* 65.5, 452–458.

Quicherat, Jules Étienne Joseph / Michelant, Henri Victor / Raynaud, Gaston Charles 1879. *Catalogue général des manuscrits des bibliothèques publiques de des départements. Tome V (Metz, Verdun, Charleville)* Paris: Imprimerie Nationale.

Quirk, Randolph / Greenbaum, Sidney / Leech, Geoffrey / Svartvik, Jan 1985. *A Comprehensive Grammar of the English Language*. London: Longman.

Reuter, Ole 1937. Some Notes on the Origin of the Relative Combination 'the which'. *Neuphilologische Mitteilungen* 38, 146–188.

Roberts, Jane 2005. *Guide to Scripts Used in English Writings up to 1500*. London: The British Library.

Robinson, Peter 2005. Current Issues in Making Digital Editions of Medieval Texts – or, Do Electronic Scholarly Editions Have a Future? *Digital Medievalist* 1.1. Available at <http://www.digitalmedievalist.org/journal/1.1/robinson>.

Schuba, Ludwig 1981. *Die medizinischen Handschriften der Codices Palatini Latini in der vatikanischen Bibliothek*. Wiesbaden: Ludwig Reichert.

Schum, Wilhelm 1887. *Beschreibendes Verzeichniss der Amplonianischen Handschriften-Sammlung zu Erfurt, im Auftrage und auf Kosten des königlich preussischen Unterrichts-Ministeriums bearbeitet und herausgegeben, mit einem Vorworte über Amplonius und die Geschichte seiner Sammlung*. Berlin: Weidmann.

OED = Simpson, John Andrew / Weiner, Edmund S. C. (eds.) ²1994. *The Oxford English Dictionary*. Oxford: Oxford University Press.

Squires, Ann / Timbrell, Nicola 1994. *The Dream of the Rood*. Oxford: ITTI Products.

Stehle, Raymond Louis 1942. Weights and Measures in Medicine. *Canadian Medical Association Journal* 46.5, 463–465.

Steinschneider, Moritz 1893. *Die hebräischen Übersetzungen des Mittelalters und die Juden als Dolmetscher. Ein Beitrag zur Literaturgeschichte des Mittelalters, meist nach handschriftlichen Quellen*. Berlin: Kommissionsverlag des Bibliographischen Bureaus.

Taavitsainen, Irma 2001. Language History and the Scientific Register. In Diller, Hans-Jürgen / Görlach, Manfred (eds.) *Towards a History of English as a History of Genres*. Heidelberg: Universitätsverlag Carl Winter, 185–202.

Taavitsainen, Irma / Pahta, Päivi. *Corpus of Early English Medical Writing*. <http://www.helsinki.fi/varieng/CoRD/corpora/CEEM/STSteam.html>.

Taavitsainen, Irma / Pahta, Päivi 1997. The Corpus of Early English Medical Writing. In Nevalainen, Terttu / Kahlas-Tarkka, Leena (eds.) *To Explain the Present: Studies in the Changing English Language in Honour of Matti Rissanen*. Helsinki: Société Néophilologique, 209–295.

Taavitsainen, Irma / Pahta, Päivi (eds.) 2004. *Medical and Scientific Writing in Late Medieval English*. Cambridge: Cambridge University Press.

Tabanelli, Mario 1973. *Tecniche e strumenti chirurgici del XIII e XIV secolo*. Firenze: Olschki.

Tallentire, David R. 1973. Towards an Archive of Lexical Norms: a Proposal. In Aitken, Adam Jack / Bailey, Richard Weld / Hamilton-Smith, N. (eds.) *The Computer and Literary Studies*. Edinburgh: Edinburgh University Press.

Tannenbaum, Samuel Aaron 1930. *The Handwriting of the Renaissance*. New York: Columbia University Press.

Tieken-Boon van Ostade, Ingrid / Tottie, Gunnel / van der Wurff, Wim (eds.) 1999. *Negation in the History of English*. Berlin: Mouton de Gruyter.

Toth, Margaret K. 1959. Early Herbals. *University of Rochester Library Bulletin* 15.1. Available at <http://www.lib.rochester.edu/index.cfm?PAGE=3360>.

Tweedie, Fiona J. / Baayen, R. Harald 1998. How Variable a Constant Be? Measures on Lexical Richness in Perspective. *Computer and the Humanities* 32, 323–352.

[Udina y Martorell, Federico / Casas Homs, José María] (eds.) 1967. *Las curas de las enfermetats del uelhs faitas per Benvengut de Salern = Las curas de las enfermedades de los ojos hechas por Bienvenido de Salerno*. Masnou: Instituto Cusí-Laboratorios del Norte de España.

van Kemenade, Ans 1999. Sentential Negation and Clause Structure in Old English. In Tieken-Boon van Ostade, Ingrid / Tottie, Gunnel / van der Wurff, Wim (eds.) *Negation in the History of English*. Berlin: Mouton de Gruyter, 147–166.

van Kemenade, Ans 2000. Jespersen's Cycle Revisited: Formal Properties of Grammaticalization. In Pintzuk, Susan / Tsoulas, George / Warner, Anthony (eds.) *Diachronic Syntax: Models and Mechanisms*. Oxford: Oxford University Press, 51–74.

Voigts, Linda Erhsam / Kurtz, Patricia Deery 2000. *Scientific and Medical Writings in Old and Middle English: An Electronic Reference* (ver. 1.0). Ann Arbor: University of Michigan Press.

von Heinemann, Otto 1898. *Die Handschriften der herzoglichen Bibliothek zu Wolfenbüttel*. Wolfenbüttel: J. Zwissler.

Wilmart, André 1937–1945. *Codices reginenses latini*. 2 vols. Città del Vaticano: Bibliotheca vaticana.

Wood, Casey Albert 1929. *De oculis eorumque egritudinibus et curis. Translated with Notes and Illustrations from the First Printed Edition, Ferrara, 1474, A. D.* Stanford: Stanford University Press.

Wright, Thomas / Halliwell-Phillipps, James Orchard [1841–1843] ²1845. *Reliquiæ Antiquæ: Scraps from Ancient Manuscripts, Illustrating Chiefly Early English Literature and the English Language*. 2 vols. London: J. R. Smith.

Young, John / Aitken, Patrick Henderson 1908. *A Catalogue of the Manuscripts in the Library of the Hunterian Museum in the University of Glasgow*. 2 vols. Glasgow: James MacLehose & Son.

Yule, George Udny 1939. On Sentence-Length as a Statistical Characteristic of Style in Prose: With Application to Two Cases of Disputed Authorship. *Biometrika* 30.3/4, 363–390.

Yule, George Udny 1944. *The Statistical Study of Literary Vocabulary*. Cambridge: Cambridge University Press.

Zeeman, Elizabeth 1956. Punctuation in an Early Manuscript of Love's Mirror. *Review of English Studies* 7, 11–18.

Notes on Contributors

ALEJANDRO ALCARAZ-SINTES is Lecturer at the University of Jaén (Spain) where he teaches English Language and Linguistics at undergraduate, master and doctoral levels. He has worked on the complementation of Old English adjectives, resulting in a number of papers presented at national and international Conferences, and book chapters. He has also published on the application of new technologies in teaching practice in the *International Journal of English Studies*.

JAVIER CALLE-MARTÍN is Senior Lecturer in the Department of English at the University of Málaga (Spain). His research interests range from Historical Linguistics to Manuscript Studies, focusing on the use of punctuation in early English documents. He has published in *Neuphilologische Mitteilungen* (2004), *Folia Linguistica Historica* (2005) or *The Review of English Studies* (2008). Recently, he has also developed an interest in stylometric approaches to authorship attribution, publishing in journals like *Language Resources and Evaluation* (2005), *Literary and Linguistic Computing* (2007) and *Ecdotica* (2008).

LAURENCE ELDREDGE, a retired English Professor from the University of Ottawa in Canada, now lives and works in England. Medieval ophthalmology is his immediate focus, on which he has published extensively.

LAURA ESTEBAN-SEGURA is Lecturer at the Department of English Philology of the University of Murcia (Spain). Her main research interests lie in the History of the English Language, Textual Criticism, Palaeography/Codicology, Manuscript Studies and Translation. The more specialist aspects of her research focus on the study of unedited medical manuscripts in Middle English. Dr Esteban-Segura has published in specialised journals such as *Linguistica e Filologia* (2005), *SELIM* (2007), *English Studies* (2010) or *Neuphilologische Mitteilungen* (2011).

TERESA MARQUÉS-AGUADO is Lecturer in the Department of English at the University of Murcia (Spain), where she teaches English Language at various levels and some undergraduate courses on English Historical Linguistics. Her research interests include Palaeography, Codicology, Manuscript Studies and English Historical Linguistics. She is currently involved in the electronic edition of unedited late Middle English texts, and has published in *English Studies* and other specialised journals, as well as in Peter Lang or Wiley-Blackwell.

DAVID MORENO OLALLA is Lecturer in the Department of English at the University of Málaga (Spain). A linguist by training, he has a strong interest in Historical Phonology and Morphology, and Comparative Linguistics. Most of his work deals with the dialectological aspects of Middle English scientific *Fachprosa*, Historical Corpus Linguistics, Textual Criticism and History of the Book, but he has occasionally dabbled in other areas such as English Language Teaching, exploring the possibilities of Diachronic Linguistics in the teaching of Present-Day English, or the analysis of Translation techniques in Anglo-Saxon England.